BASIC PATHOLOGY

SECOND EDITION

AN INTRODUCTION TO THE MECHANISMS OF DISEASE

Sunil R. Lakhani
BSc, MBBS, MD, MRCPath
Department of Histopathology
University College London Medical School,
London

Susan A. Dilly
BSc, MBBS, FRCPath
Department of Histopathology
St George's Hospital Medical School, London

Caroline J. Finlayson
MBBS, FRCPath
Department of Histopathology
St George's Hospital Medical School, London

A member of the Hodder Headline Group
LONDON • NEW YORK • NEW DELHI

First edition published in Great Britain 1993
Second edition published in 1998
This impression reprinted in 2002 by
Arnold, a member of the Hodder Headline Group,
338 Euston Road, London NW1 3BH
http://www.arnoldpublishers.com

Distributed in the United States of America by
Oxford University Press, Inc.,
198 Madison Avenue, New York, NY 10016
Oxford is a registered trademark of Oxford University Press

British Library Cataloguing-in-Publication Data
A catalogue record for this book is available from the British Library

Library of Congress Cataloging-in-Publication Data
A catalog record for this book is available from the Library of Congress

ISBN 0 340 67787 2

3 4 5 6 7 8 9 10

Publisher: Fiona Goodgame
Production Editor: Julie Delf
Production Controller: Helen Whitehorn
Illustrator: Peter Lamb
Text designer: Julie Martin
Cover design: T. Griffiths

Typeset in 9.5/13 pt Sabon by Scribe Design
Printed and bound in India by Replika Press Pvt Ltd. 100% EOU,
Delhi-110 040

CONTENTS

PREFACE

'What is the use of a book', thought Alice, 'without pictures or conversations'

Lewis Carroll

Any artist will tell you that in drawing objects, you cannot ignore the spaces in between. The picture ceases to exist when only one aspect is viewed in isolation. Musical pieces composed entirely of notes and without pauses would be nothing more than noise and an irritation. Yet when it comes to teaching, we ignore this fact and fail to put our own speciality into the context of the whole curriculum.

Recently there has been a trend towards a more integrated approach to medical education. We are delighted that such an approach, which we have used in our teaching for the last 7 years, is now adopted widely in the UK and abroad.

Our aim has been to create a tutorial on the mechanisms of disease over a background of history, science and clinical relevance. The goal is to give the students a sense of belonging to a movement – the movement from past to present and from laboratory to the patient.

The book has been written in the hope that students will read the text fully and at leisure. This not only contains details about the disease processes but also historical anecdotes and clinical scenarios. Since examinations and assessments are an inevitable part of student life, questions and lists are also included to aid revision. The cartoons are intended to amuse as well as illustrate the importance of certain topics and we sincerely hope that the dull, dreary image of histopathology that all students seem to be born with will be shed after

reading the book. Pathology is one of the most fascinating and fun subjects a student is likely to encounter during their undergraduate training.

Many of the tables and lists have logos attached to them and the key is provided below:

Oral Examiner:
Short questions appropriate for MCQs, oral exams and ward round 'quiz'

Written exam:
Subjects likely to appear in the written paper of the examination

Small print:
Details which will amaze and worry your friends (they may not be your friends afterwards!)

Definitions:
Saves you having to put down this book and look for a dictionary

Although the book is primarily intended for under-graduate medical students, we hope that it will also be amusing and useful to students of dentistry, human biology and some paramedical specialities. Postgraduate students studying for Pathology or Surgical examinations may also wish to consult the book.

SRL, SAD, CJF
London, February 1998

ACKNOWLEDGEMENTS

It is 5 years since the publication of the first edition and considerable progress has been made in the understanding of disease processes. Updating a book sounds a much simpler task than writing one from scratch, however, this has been far from the truth.

In keeping with our desire for an integrated approach to teaching, we have added in new chapters on microbiology and haematology as they apply to the understanding of inflammation and cardiovascular disease. The work to bring this book into 1998 has been aided considerably by the help and efforts of many of our clinical and scientific colleagues including Prof. MJ Davies, Prof. A Dalgleish and Dr M Patton. We would particularly like to thank Dr Philip Butcher at St George's Hospital for his contribution to the chapter on microbiology, Dr Grant Robinson also at St George's Hospital for help with the haematology in Section 2, Dr Rosemary Scott at University College London for help and comments for Section 5 on Genes and Disease, Prof. Richard Carter for help with the section on chemical carcinogens and Mr Chi Wah Lok, Medical Technical Officer at UCLMS for photographic assistance.

We would like to acknowledge Macmillan London Ltd., The Publication Division (copyrights) HMSO, HarperCollins Publishers, Oxford University Press, Cordon Art B.V., Holland, Gryphon Editions Ltd., Oriel Press Ltd., The Journal of Clinical Pathology (BMJ) the Office for National Statistics and The Wellcome Institute for the History of Medicine for the photographs and quotations used in the book.

Fiona Goodgame, Julie Delf, Peter Lamb, Georgina Bentliff and all the staff at Arnold have given us a great deal of help and their patience and support throughout the planning and production of this edition is greatly appreciated.

Finally we would like to thank our families who have made enormous sacrifices and continue to support us in our, sometimes, selfish endeavours.

PART *1*

INFLAMMATION, HEALING AND REPAIR

CHAPTER 1

ACUTE INFLAMMATION

- What is inflammation?
- Acute inflammation
- Systemic effects of inflammation

> No natural phenomenon can be adequately studied in itself alone, but to be understood must be considered as it stands connected with all nature.
>
> Sir Francis Bacon

WHAT IS INFLAMMATION?

Inflammation is a mechanism by which the body deals with an injury or insult. When living tissue is attacked, for example by physical, chemical or microbial agents, a series of local processes are initiated in order to contain the offensive agent, neutralise its effect, limit its spread and hopefully eradicate it. As part and parcel of this process, there is initiation of healing and repair of the injured tissue. Inflammation, healing and repair are like the black and white stripes of the zebra: in order truly to understand the zebra, one cannot study the stripes in isolation. In the same way, the processes of healing and repair have to be addressed in their relationship to the process of inflammation.

The circulatory system is of fundamental importance in the inflammatory response. In general terms, the offending agent, whatever it may be, causes a change in the microvasculature of the injured area, leading to a massive outpouring of cells and fluid. This collection of cells and fluid is known as the **inflammatory exudate**, and within this exudate we find ingredients that are needed to combat the offending agent and to begin the process of healing and repair. However, this is only half the story. It is romantic to imagine an army being sent to deal with an invading force and to restore the peace and tranquillity to the area. Life is not quite so simple; there is a price to be paid for war. The ugly side of it ranges from cosmetic problems, such as keloid scars, to life-threatening illnesses, such as autoimmune diseases.

John Hunter, surgeon to St George's Hospital from 1768 to 1793, was interested in inflammation and repair. He was an incredible man whose aim was the total understanding of mankind. Hunter was born in Scotland on 14 February 1728, the last of 10 children. He spent the first 20 years there and his childhood has been described as 'wasted and idle'. This is because he 'wanted to know all about the clouds and the grasses, and why the leaves changed colour in the autumn'. Hunter's inquisitiveness and fascination with nature stood him in good stead when he began to unravel the mysteries of the human body. His book, *A treatise on the blood, inflammation, and gunshot wounds*, is a monument to his thoroughness and powers of observation in delineating the processes of disease. Hunter was one of the first to observe that inflammation was not a disease but

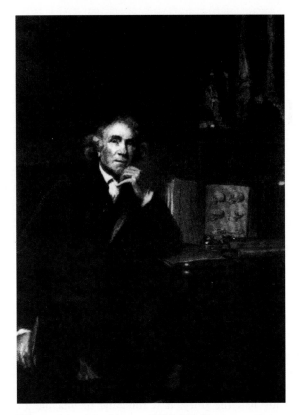

Figure 1.1 John Hunter (1728–93) (Courtesy of the Wellcome Institute for the History of Medicine)

a response to tissue injury whose attempts at repair were sometimes more harmful than the original disease.

Many of Hunter's experiments are absolutely fascinating as well as crazy and amusing, but more of that later, so keep reading.

> 'inflammation in itself is not to be considered as a disease, but as a salutary operation, consequent either to some violence or to some disease. But this same operation can and does go vary; it is often carried further even in sound parts ...
>
> Where it can alter the diseased mode of action, it likewise leads to a cure; but where it cannot accomplish that salutary purpose, as in cancer, scrofula, venereal disease, etc. it does mischief.'
>
> John Hunter

Anyone who has had a boil or any other skin infection will be familiar with the four cardinal signs of inflammation: **rubor (redness)**, **calor (heat)**, **tumour (swelling)** and **dolor (pain)**. These were first described by a Roman physician, Cornelius Celsus in the first century AD. To this a fifth sign was later added – **functio laesa (loss of function)**; however, this is not a necessary accompaniment of the inflammatory process.

So what is the pathophysiology behind these clinical signs?

MICROVASCULATURE

As previously mentioned, the microvasculature plays a central role in inflammation and the *redness* is caused by **vasodilatation**. This is important for increasing the flow of blood to the affected area and hence delivering cells and plasma-derived substances needed for combat. Vasodilatation also produces the *heat*. The *swelling* results from **increased permeability** of the vessel walls, leading to the outpouring of fluid and cells: the inflammatory exudate. In some circumstances, the swelling may cushion the affected part and lead to immobilisation (*loss of function*). The sign that is the most difficult to explain is *pain*. This probably arises from the combination of stretching of tissue by exudate and the action of some of the **chemical mediators** involved in inflammation.

We are indebted to Julius Conheim (1839–84) for investigating the pathophysiology of inflammation. He was a German pathologist, a pupil and later assistant to the father of cellular pathology, Rudolf Virchow. He delineated the vascular changes of inflammation using living preparations of thin membranes, such as the mesentery, and demonstrated the vasodilatation and the subsequent exudation of fluid. But what are the underlying mechanisms of this process? In broad terms, there are two aspects to consider:
- the cells of inflammation
- the chemical mediators.

CELLULAR MEDIATORS

The principal **cells of inflammation** are the lymphocytes, plasma cells, macrophages and

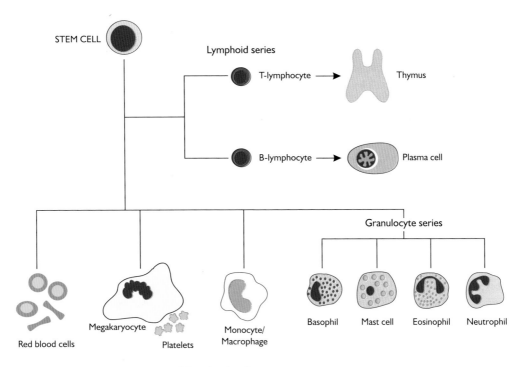

Figure 1.2 Origins of haemopoietic and lymphoid cells

polymorphonuclear leucocytes or granulocytes, which include neutrophils, eosinophils and basophils. A Russian microbiologist, Elias Metchnikoff, working at the Pasteur Institute in Paris in 1884, demonstrated that leucocytes **phagocytose** bacteria and concluded that the purpose of the inflammatory response was to bring phagocytic cells to the area to kill the organisms. Inflammatory cells descend on a focus of tissue damage in 'waves'; the first cell type recruited is the neutrophil polymorph (an 'acute' inflammatory cell), which is followed by macrophages, lymphocytes and plasma cells ('chronic' inflammatory cells). Later, the tissue generates new blood vessels and fibrous scar tissue as reparative work begins.

Phagocytosis: the process of engulfing foreign or damaged material. Macrophages and neutrophils are phagocytic cells

CHEMICAL MEDIATORS

In 1927 Sir Thomas Lewis identified **histamine**, present in tissue mast cells, as a mediator of acute inflammation. Since then, a vast array of mediators has been identified, but not all have a proven role *in vivo*. They may be derived from the plasma, the participating inflammatory cells or the damaged tissue itself.

The **cell-derived products** include:
- vasoactive amines
- cytokines and growth factors
- arachidonic acid derivatives (eicosanoids)
- platelet activating factor
- lysosomal enzymes
- oxygen-derived free radicals
- nitric oxide.

The **plasma-derived mediators** include:
- the kinin system
- the coagulation and fibrinolytic system
- the complement system.

Some are important in the amplification of the inflammatory response, others play their role in the elimination of the offending agent. The media-

Table 1.1 Cells involved in inflammation

Cell category	Cell type	Origin	% white cells	Major function
Circulating cells				
Granulocytes (polymorphonuclear leucocytes)	Neutrophils	Bone marrow	75	Acute inflammatory cell involved in bacterial killing and phagocytosis. Granule contents for increasing vascular permeability, chemotaxis, killing organisms and digesting extracellular matrix
	Eosinophils	Bone marrow	1	Acute inflammatory cell particularly common in allergic and parasitic conditions. Granules include major basic protein.
	Basophils	Bone marrow	<1	Circulating cells that give rise to **mast cells**. Granules include histamine
Lymphocytes	T cells	Lymphoid organs and thymus	20	Various subtypes involved in antigen recognition and presentation, cell killing and regulation of immune responses (e.g. helper, suppressor and natural killer cells)
	B cells	Lymphoid organs and bone marrow	20	On antigen stimulation, proliferate and give rise to specific **plasma cells**, which synthesise specific immunoglobulins
Macrophage system	Monocytes	Bone marrow	4	Migrate into tissues to be macrophages capable of phagocytosis, cytokine production and antigen processing and presentation
Non-circulating cells				
Kupffer cells (liver sinusoids) Macrophages (bone marrow, spleen and lymph nodes)				Fixed phagocytic cells lining sinusoids and filtering large molecules/particles from blood or lymph
Megakaryocytes in bone marrow				Produce platelets, which contain serotonin, platelet-derived growth factor, etc. Also important in haemostasis
Hepatocytes				Produce proteins important in: • clotting and fibrinolytic system • complement system • kinin system • acute phase proteins

tors and their role in inflammation will be discussed in more detail later.

CAUSES OF INFLAMMATION

We have considered the reaction to tissue injury, but what are the causes? Because infections are so common, there is a tendency to think that infection and inflammation are synonymous, and it is easy to overlook other important causes. Causes of inflammation include :

• mechanical injuries
• bacteria, viruses, fungi and parasites
• ischaemia

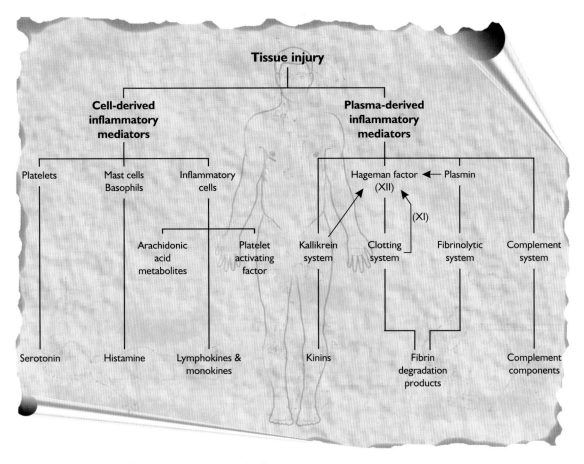

Figure 1.3   Origins of important mediators of inflammation

- chemical injuries
- extremes of temperature
- radiation (e.g. ultraviolet light)
- immune mechanisms (e.g. autoimmune disease).

The common feature is that the agent first damages the patient's cells, initiating the fascinatingly complex process of inflammation. The patient with the boil on the bum will, however, be less impressed than we are with the inflammatory processes taking place. He may regard the fact that the injury has caused microvascular changes via mediators, leading to cellular and humoral factors accumulating at the site of injury, as being of less importance than the burning question, 'What will happen next?'

There are a number of possibilities. The process may restore the tissue to its normal state, with nothing to suggest that anything has been amiss. Healing may take place but leave a scar. The injury and the inflammation may grumble on for a long time, or the injury may completely overwhelm the body and lead to death. This last outcome is especially likely where inflammatory defences are deficient, such as in those with AIDS, in cancer patients treated with cytotoxic drugs or in patients receiving immunosuppressive drugs for autoimmune diseases or following organ transplantation. The final outcome depends on the interactions between the various processes involved in inflammation. Just as the zebra is neither black with white stripes nor white with black stripes, so it is the combination of the various inflammatory components that determines the texture of the whole.

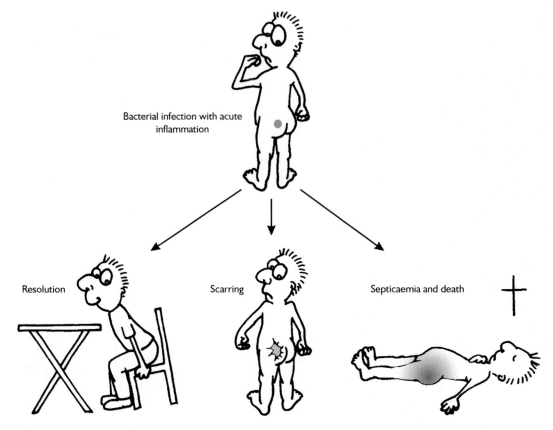

Figure 1.4 Possible outcomes of acute inflammation

Acute inflammation

Inflammation is divided into acute and chronic forms based on the duration and the predominant inflammatory cell type. **Acute inflammation** is generally of short duration, lasting from a few minutes to a few days, and the cellular exudate is rich in neutrophil polymorphonuclear leucocytes, with some macrophages arriving after the initial insult. **Chronic inflammation** tends to be more variable and may last for months or years, the chief cells involved being lymphocytes, plasma cells and macrophages. The inflammatory process, whether acute or chronic, may be modified by a whole host of factors, such as the cause of the damage, nutritional status, the competence of the immune system and intervention with antibiotics, 'anti-inflammatory drugs' or surgery.

LOBAR PNEUMONIA

A disease exemplifying acute inflammation is lobar pneumonia, named because the lung parenchyma is involved in continuity so that a whole lobe or lobes are affected by the process. *Streptococcus pneumoniae*, a Gram-positive diplococcus bacterium, is the most common cause of lobar pneumonia. This invades the lung, leading to changes in the microvasculature and a massive outpouring of fluid into the alveolar spaces, resulting in **congestion** (Fig. 1.5(a)). This fluid is rich in fibrin.

Soon afterwards, neutrophils follow, and the fibrin-rich fluid and cells spread from alveolus to alveolus via the pores of Kohn. The neutrophils attack the organisms and phagocytose them, leading to the death of both organisms and many neutrophils. Not surprisingly, the alveoli are airless, and the lung is now firm and red with the

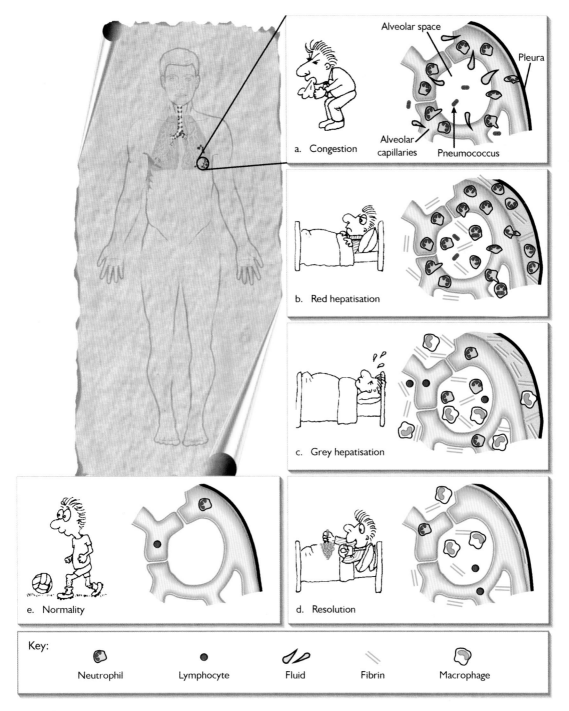

Figure 1.5 Lobar pneumonia

texture of liver. This stage is termed 'red hepati-sation' (b).

As this process progresses, the macrophage is recruited not only to phagocytose dead neutrophils

and bacteria but also to digest the fibrin mesh. The lung is still firm, but the large inflammatory cell infiltrate and reduction in vasodilatation give it a grey colour, hence the term 'grey hepatisation' (c).

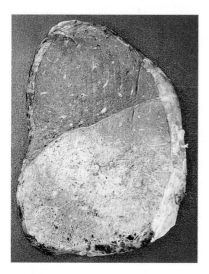

Figure 1.6 Left lung with consolidation (grey hepatisation) of the lower lobe

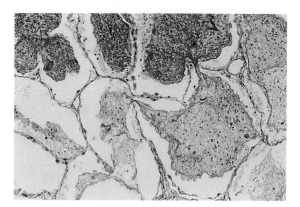

Figure 1.7 Photomicrograph of lung alveoli filled with inflammatory exudate and fibrin passing through the pores of Kohn

The final outcome will depend on the competence of this system and whether the basic framework of the lung tissue is intact. Ideally, the alveoli will be cleared and re-aerated, and **resolution** (d) will take place. If the alveolar framework has been destroyed or the exudate has not been cleared, **organisation** will occur, leading to scar formation. The infection may persist in destroying lung tissue but become localised so that an **abscess** is formed. This is a collection of pus walled off by fibrous tissue. Alternatively, the infection may spread to the rest of the lung, involve the pleura, cause an empyema, disseminate via the blood stream to other areas of the body or even lead to death.

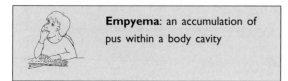

Empyema: an accumulation of pus within a body cavity

ACUTE APPENDICITIS

Another good example of acute inflammation is acute appendicitis. The classical symptoms of appendicitis are pain (first in the periumbilical region and then localising to the right iliac fossa), nausea, vomiting and fever. The point of maximum tenderness in the right iliac fossa is known as McBurney's point after the American surgeon Charles McBurney (1845–1913). His description appears in the *New York Medical Times* in 1889 and states that the pain is to 'be determined by pressure of one finger, and the point lies 1 1/2 in. from the anterior superior iliac spine on a straight line drawn from that process to the umbilicus'. McBurney also described the muscle-splitting or grid-iron incision used for appendicectomy.

The initiating event of appendicitis is not always clear, but it may be obstruction of the lumen by a faecolith (hardened calcified faecal material) or collections of pinworms. The build-up of pressure from the obstruction may affect the blood supply and lead to ischaemic injury of the appendiceal wall, which is then invaded by bacteria normally present within the gut. This triggers the process of inflammation. Neutrophils migrate out of the damaged vessels and into the appendix wall, together with large amounts of fibrin, which are deposited on the serosal surface. The inflammation may settle down but more usually does not. If there is a delay in surgical intervention, destruction of the appendiceal wall may produce a perforation, resulting in inflammatory and necrotic debris spilling into the peritoneal cavity. Here it sets up a widely disseminated inflammatory response over the entire peritoneal membrane (peritonitis). At this stage, the inflammatory response causes severe shock and is life-threatening.

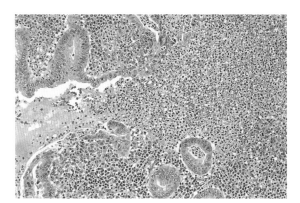

Figure 1.8 Photomicrograph of an appendix showing ulceration and acute inflammatory exudate between damaged glands

What is the predominant cell of acute inflammation?
Neutrophil polymorph

What are the predominant cells of chronic inflammation?
Lymphocytes
Macrophages/monocytes
Plasma cells
N.B. These cells are sometimes called **mononuclear** cells, in contrast to polymorphonuclear leucocytes

What are the cardinal features of inflammation?
Redness
Swelling
Pain
Heat
Loss of function

Summarise the events in inflammation
Changes in microvasculature
Exudate formation
  Fluid
  Cells
Various possible outcomes
  Resolution
  Scarring
  Chronic inflammation/abscess
    formation
  Spread
  Death

Now that we have the overall concept of inflammation and its clinical relevance, we must look more closely at the complex cellular and molecular events of this process. We shall first examine the changes in the microvasculature.

VASCULAR CHANGES

Many of the vascular events that follow injury were delineated by Julius Conheim, mentioned above. His experiments with frog mesentery beautifully demonstrated that injury produced vasodilatation, resulting in more blood entering the tissue but sometimes a slower flow of blood in capillaries. This allows white cells (leucocytes) to attach to the vessel wall (**margination**) and then move across the wall to the extravascular compartment (**diapedesis** or **emigration**).

Before we consider the causes of altered vascular permeability, it is worth revising the normal physiological factors that control the movement of fluid across a small vessel wall (Figure 1.8). Fluid flows away from areas of high hydrostatic pressure and towards areas of high osmotic pressure. Thus fluid leaves from the arterial end of the capillary network and is reabsorbed at the venous end (a), any excess being removed via lymphatics. A rise in hydrostatic pressure within the vessel without changes in permeability will increase leakage of fluid out of the vessel, but it

will have no protein in it (b). However, if the permeability of the vessel wall increases, fluid can move more readily, and protein molecules may also leak across. Movement of protein molecules will alter the osmotic pressure gradient, such that less fluid is reabsorbed into the blood at the venous end of the capillaries and tissue fluid will increase (c). In areas of inflammation, there is usually a rise in hydrostatic pressure and an increase in vascular permeability (d).

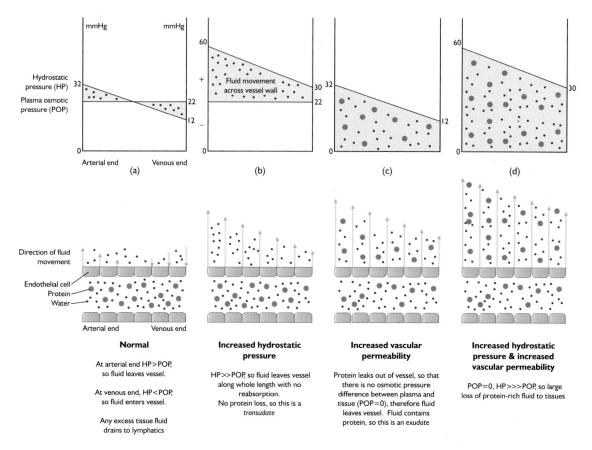

Figure 1.9   Factors affecting the movement of fluid across vessels

This is an appropriate time to introduce a number of new words. An **exudate** is the fluid within the extravascular spaces, which is rich in protein and hence has a specific gravity of greater than 1.020. On the other hand, a **transudate** has a low protein content and a specific gravity of less than 1.020. **Oedema** simply refers to the presence of excess fluid within the extravascular space and body cavities, and may be an exudate or transudate. **Pus** can be thought of as a special kind of

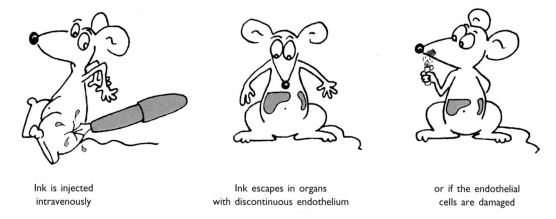

Ink is injected
intravenously

Ink escapes in organs
with discontinuous endothelium

or if the endothelial
cells are damaged

Figure 1.10

What is oedema?

It is excess fluid within extravascular space or body cavities

What is the difference between a transudate and an exudate?

A transudate is fluid of low protein content and specific gravity of <1.02, hence being an ultrafiltrate of blood. An exudate has a high protein content with a specific gravity of >1.02. It also contains fibrinogen and will clot spontaneously

Describe the different types of exudates?

- Fibrinous – cloudy white, with strands of fibrin to form adhesions
- Serous – watery. Occurs with bacteria (e.g. some Streptococci) that produce fibrinolysins to digest fibrin
- Purulent – discoloured by the presence of inflammatory cells and pyogenic organisms (e.g. Staphylococci)
- Fibrinopurulent – mixture of pus and fibrin
- Haemorrhagic – blood-stained owing to vessel damage

If we examine the fluid that forms during an inflammatory reaction, we find that it is an exudate. This means that large protein molecules have leaked out of the microvasculature. What is the mechanism of the increased permeability? Most vessels are lined by endothelium that is termed 'continuous'. In endocrine organs, intestines and renal glomeruli, the endothelium is normally more permeable because it contains 'windows', hence the name **fenestrated endothelium**, while in the spleen, liver and bone marrow the endothelium is **discontinuous**.

What happens following injury has been elegantly demonstrated using simple experiments involving the intravenous injection of Indian ink (Fig. 1.10). The ink will remain within the vascular compartment, except in the liver and spleen, where the discontinuous endothelium allows ink to escape. If a mild injury is produced (e.g. by using heat), the damaged area will turn black. Microscopical examination will reveal that the ink particles have crossed the endothelial layer and are trapped at the basement membrane. Injection of the vasoactive substance histamine will cause the endothelial cells of the small venules to contract, creating gaps through which the ink molecules can pass. In reality, the situation is more complicated as the vascular changes will depend on the severity of the insult.

Three types of vascular response have been demonstrated, although in real situations they generally overlap:
- the immediate-transient response
- the immediate-persistent response
- the delayed-persistent response.

exudate, a **purulent exudate**. Besides the protein-rich fluid, it contains dead or dying bacteria and neutrophils. The consistency of pus depends on the amount of digestion by neutrophil enzymes, and the colour depends on the type of organism and the presence of neutrophil-derived myeloperoxidase, which imparts a yellowish-green colour. Exudates generally contain fibrinogen, which is converted to fibrin through the action of tissue thromboplastin. The fibrin forms a mesh for cells to migrate on and later a scaffold for healing and repair.

Immediate-transient response

This occurs immediately following injury, reaches a peak after 5–10 minutes and ceases after 15–30 minutes. This response can be produced by histamine and other chemical mediators and is blocked by the prior administration of antihistamines. The leakage occurs exclusively from small venules that develop gaps between the endothelial cells as endothelial cells contract. This occurs following nettle stings or insect bites.

Immediate-transient response

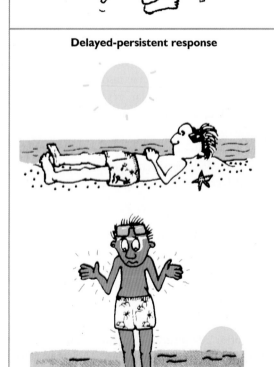

Immediate-persistent response

Delayed-persistent response

Figure 1.11 Types of vascular response

Immediate-persistent response

This results from severe injury such as burns, where there is direct damage to endothelial cells. The leak starts immediately and reaches a peak within an hour. As the endothelial cells are damaged and may even slough off, the leak will continue until the vessel has been blocked with thrombus or the vessel is repaired. Unlike the previous example, it can affect any type of vessel.

Delayed-persistent response

This is a very interesting type of response, familiar to anyone who has overindulged in a tropical holiday after a period under the clouds of England. There is an interval of up to 24 hours before the leak starts from both capillaries and venules. Small aggregates of platelets and endothelial cells are seen in some capillaries, and it seems that the endothelial cells are damaged directly.

We shall look next at the cellular component of the inflammatory response.

CELLULAR EVENTS

The principal cells of the acute inflammatory response are the neutrophils and macrophages. Following injury, the neutrophils migrate out of the vessels, the number recruited depending on the type of injury. For example, infections with bacteria attract more inflammatory cells than do purely physical injuries. After the neutrophils, there is a second wave of cells – the macrophages. The movement of neutrophils out of the vessels and their role in combat can be divided into discrete steps:

- margination
- adhesion
- emigration
- chemotaxis
- phagocytosis and degranulation.

Margination and adhesion

When haemodynamic changes take place in the vasculature during inflammation, white cells fall

Table 1.2 Adhesion molecules

Family	Some family members	Principally expressed on	Main function
Integrins	β1 family, e.g. VLA-4 β2 family, e.g. LFA-1	Lymphocytes and monocytes	Mediates immune and inflammatory responses including binding immunoglobulin superfamily molecules on endothelial cells to provide firm adhesion to vessel wall prior to migration
Immunoglobulin super family	ICAM 1, 2 and 3 VCAM-1	Endothelial cells, lymphocytes and monocytes	As above by binding to integrins
Selectins	E-selectin L-selectin P-selectin	Endothelium Lymphocytes, polymorphs and monocytes Platelets and endothelial cells	Initial phase of leucocyte adhesion to vessel wall
Cadherins	B, E, M, N, P, R, T	Range of tissues	Homophilic calcium-dependent cell–cell adhesion, e.g. at sites of desmosomes and adherens junctions. Not specifically involved in inflammation

ICAM-1 = intercellular adhesion molecule-1; LFA-1 = leucocyte function associated antigen-1; VCAM-1 = vascular cell adhesion molecule-1; VLA-4 = very late antigen 4.

out of the central axial flow and line themselves up along the wall (a little reminiscent of the school disco!). The cells then adhere to the endothelium, although precisely how this occurs is still a mystery. It appears that there are specific complementary 'adhesion molecules', which stick leucocytes to endothelial cells, the number of these molecules on the cell surfaces being increased by inflammatory mediators. One pair of such molecules is ICAM-1 (intercellular adhesion molecule-1) on endothelial cells and LFA-1 on leucocytes, which bind together like 'lock and key'. Resting cells express very few adhesion molecules, but some inflammatory mediators (e.g. complement fragments (C5a) and leukotrienes (LTB4)) increase the expression of LFA-1 , while other mediators (e.g. interleukin-1 and bacterial endotoxin) enhance ICAM-1 expression. This adhesion is of great importance, and people with a genetic deficiency of these

adhesion molecules suffer from repeated bacterial infections.

Our knowledge of adhesion molecules is rapidly expanding. Broadly speaking, there are four families, three of which are involved in inflammation: the **integrins**, the **immunoglobulin gene superfamily** and the **selectins**. Some (but not all) of their family members are listed in Table 1.2. Their expression changes during inflammation so that different types of cells adhere at different stages. Some of these molecules have been termed **addressins** because they act as address labels to allow cells to leave the circulation in a specific tissue. This is particularly important in the recirculation and 'homing' of lymphocytes, which is discussed on page 25.

Emigration and chemotaxis

Once the cells have adhered to the endothelium, they form foot-like processes termed **pseudopodia**

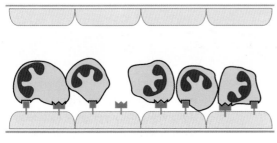

Neutrophils attach to endothelial cells lining vessels by binding through adhesion molecules

(a)

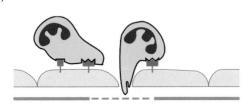

Basement membrane dissolved by proteases

(b)

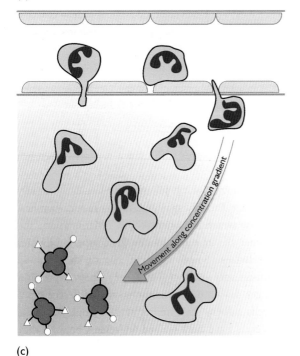

Movement along concentration gradient

(c)

Figure 1.12   (a) Margination. (b) Emigration. (c) Chemotaxis

that push their way between the endothelial cells. Eventually, the leucocyte lies between the endothelial cell and the basement membrane where it

releases a protease to digest the basement membrane, which allows it to reach the extravascular space. Neutrophils, basophils, eosinophils, macrophages and lymphocytes all use this route. Red blood cells may also pass through the gaps but only as passive passengers.

The cells are able to move towards a chemical signal, this specific movement being termed **chemotaxis**. (Note that this is different from **chemokinesis**, which is an increased and accelerated *random* movement.) The Boyden chamber is a popular system for demonstrating chemotaxis. It consists of two chambers separated by a micropore filter. The cells go into one chamber, and the putative chemical mediator is placed in the other. If cells move from the first to the second chamber, chemotaxis is demonstrated. The compounds that have been suggested as chemotactic agents include bacterial products, fragments of the complement system (e.g. C5a) and products of arachadonic acid metabolism (e.g. prostaglandins and leukotrienes).

How does this process work? Like so many cellular stimuli, the first stage depends on the chemotactic agents binding to specific receptors on the leucocyte cell membrane. This leads to an increase in ionised calcium level within the cytoplasm, which promotes construction of the contractile elements **actin** and **myosin**, responsible for movement. However, precisely how these interact to produce directional movement of the cell is not known.

Phagocytosis

Once the neutrophils and macrophages have arrived at the site of injury, they ingest the debris and bacteria, a process termed phagocytosis. This requires a number of distinct steps: the material has to be recognised as foreign or dead, it has to be engulfed and ingested, and finally it has to be killed or degraded.

Not all of the processes by which neutrophils and macrophages differentiate between normal tissue and foreign or dead tissue are known, but it is clear that bacteria coated with certain substances

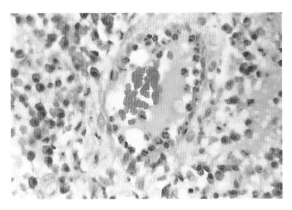

Figure 1.13 Photomicrograph illustrating margination and emigration

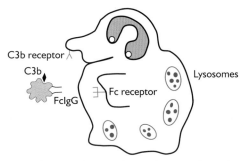

Pseudopodia extend toward opsonised particle

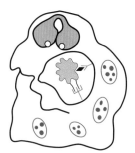

Phagosome forms

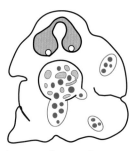

Lysosome fuses to phagosome to form a phagolysosome

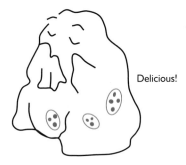

Delicious!

Figure 1.14 Phagocytosis

are ingested more readily. The factors that coat bacteria are called opsonins, and the process is termed **opsonisation**. This is derived from the Greek word *opson* meaning 'relish', i.e. getting ready for eating. There are two major opsonins:

• immunoglobulin (IgG)
• C3b component of complement.

In order for the neutrophils and macrophages to recognise these opsonins, there must be receptors on the cell surface. There are two such receptors, one for the Fc fragment of IgG (see Fig. 2.7) and the other for C3b (see p. 23). After the opsonised fragment attaches to the receptor, the cell puts out a pseudopodium. This extension of cell cytoplasm encircles the particle so that it becomes wrapped in what was originally cell surface membrane. This new intracytoplasmic membrane-bound sac is termed a **phagosome**. Another such sac, normally present in the cell and packed with destructive enzymes, is the **lysosome**. A lysosome fuses with the phagosome, producing a **phagolysosome**. This allows the enzymes to have access to the engulfed particle, and it is within this vesicle that the killing takes place. If some proteolytic enzymes leak out of the phagolysosome, as may occur if the lysosome fuses with the phagosome while the phagosome is still open to the cell surface, they may damage adjacent tissue, a phenomenon described, rather poetically, as 'regurgitation during feeding'. Fusion of a lysosome with the cell membrane, and hence the local release of toxic metabolites, is important for attacking large

organisms, such as worms, that are too large to ingest.

Mechanisms for bacterial killing

There are essentially two mechanisms for bacterial killing: oxygen-dependent and oxygen-independent.

The **oxygen-dependent system** involves toxic oxygen radicals that have an unpaired electron (indicated by a dot). These include superoxide ($O_2^{-\cdot}$), singlet oxygen ($O^{\cdot\cdot}$) and the hydroxyl radical ($OH^{-\cdot}$). These molecules are produced by the **respiratory burst** that occurs during the process of phagocytosis. Oxygen is reduced to superoxide ion, which is then converted to hydrogen peroxide (H_2O_2). This is not, however, the most powerful bactericidal chemical. Neutrophils contain the enzyme myeloperoxidase, which converts H_2O_2 to $HOCl^{\cdot}$ (hypochlorous acid) in the presence of halide ions (e.g. chloride), and nitric oxide, produced by macrophages, reacts with the superoxide anion to form the strong oxidant, nitrogen dioxide. These are powerful oxidants active against bacteria, fungi, viruses, protozoa and helminths. This system is of clinical importance as its absence produces 'chronic granulomatous disease of childhood', an inherited disease in which the neutrophils are able to ingest bacteria but unable to kill them. This is because the child lacks the enzyme NADPH oxidase, which leads to a failure of production of superoxide anion ($O_2^{-\cdot}$) and hydrogen peroxide.

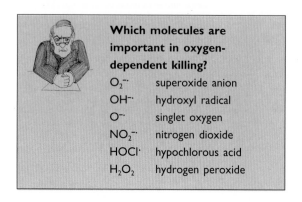

Which molecules are important in oxygen-dependent killing?

$O_2^{-\cdot}$	superoxide anion
$OH^{-\cdot}$	hydroxyl radical
$O^{\cdot\cdot}$	singlet oxygen
$NO_2^{-\cdot}$	nitrogen dioxide
$HOCl^{\cdot}$	hypochlorous acid
H_2O_2	hydrogen peroxide

There are a number of **oxygen-independent** mechanisms that are useful in microbial killing. These include:

- **lysozyme**, an enzyme that attacks the cell wall of some bacteria (especially Gram-positive cocci)
- **lactoferrin**, an iron-binding protein that inhibits the growth of bacteria
- **major basic protein** (MBP), which is a cationic protein found in eosinophils and is active principally against parasites
- **bactericidal permeability increasing protein** (BPI), which, as the name implies, causes changes in the permeability of the membranes of the microorganisms.

Also, the **low pH** found in the phagolysosomes, besides being bactericidal itself, enhances the conversion of hydrogen peroxide to superoxide. Unfortunately, the leucocyte is not successful in killing all organisms, and some bacteria, such as the mycobacterium that causes tuberculosis, can survive inside phagocytes, happily protected from antibacterial drugs and host defence mechanisms.

We shall now go on to consider the chemical mediators involved in inflammation.

CHEMICAL MEDIATORS

Since Sir Thomas Lewis demonstrated the role of histamine, an enormous number of possible mediators have been put forward, some remaining putative rather than having an established role.

Cell-derived mediators

Arachidonic acid derivatives
These are the **prostaglandins** and the **leukotrienes**. Just like the clotting and fibrinolytic system, they play a part in thrombosis as well as inflammation. They are best thought of as local hormones. They have a short range of action, are produced rapidly and degenerate spontaneously or are degraded by enzymes. Arachidonic acid, the parent molecule, is a 20-carbon polyunsaturated fatty acid that is derived either from the diet or from essential fatty acids. It is not found in a free state but is present esterified in the cell membrane phospholipid. The two pathways of arachidonic acid metabolism and

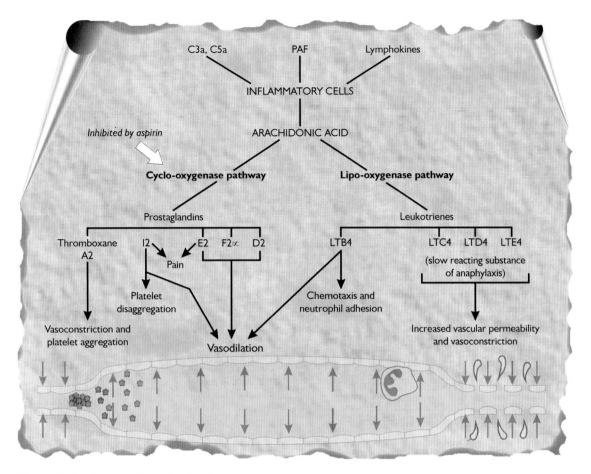

Figure 1.15 Arachidonic acid derivatives

its products are shown in Figure 1.14, which also depicts some of the roles of the products in inflammation. Drugs such as corticosteroids, aspirin and indomethacin act to reduce inflammation by inhibiting the production of prostaglandins.

Cytokines, lymphokines and monokines
A large array of polypeptides are being identified, and these act principally to regulate immune and haemopoietic cell proliferation and activity. In addition, they have effects in the inflammatory response. They are produced by many different cells in the body; those produced by lymphocytes are called **lymphokines,** and those from macrophages are termed **monokines.** Two of the most important are **interleukin-1** (IL-1) and **tumour necrosis factor** (TNF). They have a variety of important effects, as shown in Figure 1.15.

They can be grouped broadly as:
- interleukins
- colony stimulating factors
- interferons
- chemokines
- growth factors.

Growth factors have a role in chemotaxis as well as inducing healing and repair of the tissues and playing a part in the development of malignant tumours. The principal growth factors are:
- epidermal growth factor (EGF)
- platelet-derived growth factor (PDGF)
- fibroblast growth factor (FGF)
- transforming growth factor (TGF).

Most of these can be produced by macrophages, which are numerous in areas of chronic inflammation.

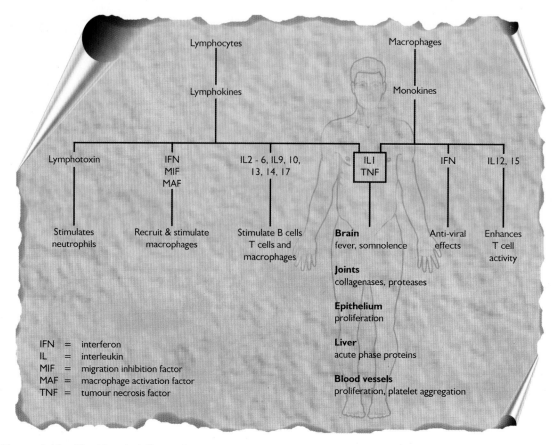

Figure 1.16   Cytokines in inflammation

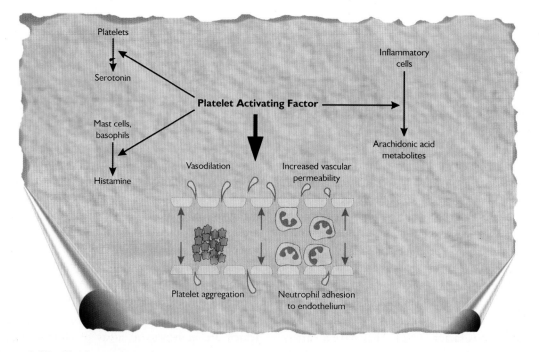

Figure 1.17   Platelet activating factor

Platelet activating factor (PAF)

This is derived from antigen-stimulated, IgE-sensitized basophils as well as neutrophils, macrophages and endothelial cells. In addition to activating platelets, it can cause vasodilatation, permeability changes, leucocyte adhesion and chemotaxis, and stimulate the production of other mediators, in particular the arachidonic acid metabolites.

Vasoactive amines

Histamine and serotonin (5-hydroxytryptamine) are stored in and released from mast cells, basophils and platelets. Their release causes vasodilatation and increases the permeability of venules. The action of histamine on vessels is mediated via H_1 receptors, while some of its other actions (e.g. bronchoconstriction) are effected via H_2 receptors.

Many factors can lead to release of these substances, including physical trauma, immunological reactions leading to the formation of C3a and C5a, releasing factors produced by neutrophils, monocytes and platelets, and interleukin-1. The role of these amines is thought to be in the early phase of inflammation as it has been shown that antihistamines blocking H_1 receptors have no effect on the permeability that is present after 60 minutes.

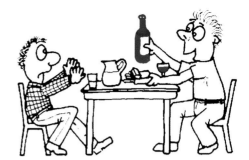

Figure 1.18 An individual with α-1-antitrypsin deficiency must avoid agents that damage the lungs or liver

them damaging their own cell. There are two types of granules: the smaller *specific* and the larger *azurophilic*. These contain substances that increase vascular permeability and are chemotactic. The enzymes destroy many extracellular components, including collagen, fibrin, elastin, cartilage and basement membrane, as well as producing intracellular killing in the phagolysosome, as already described. If these processes were unopposed, there would be massive tissue destruction, so there are antiproteases within the serum and tissue fluids to neutralise these enzymes and therefore regulate the extent of tissue damage. Does this seem a far-fetched idea, distant from clinical practice? Not at all.

A deficiency of one such antiprotease, **alpha-1-antitrypsin**, leads to the unopposed action of elastase and hence the destruction of elastic tissue, especially in the lungs and liver. Clinically, a patient

Lysosomal contents
Specific granules contain:
    Lactoferrin
    Lysozyme
    Alkaline phosphatase
    Collagenase
    Leucocyte adhesion molecule
Azurophilic granules contain:
    Myeloperoxidase
    Lysozyme
    Cationic proteins
    Acid hydrolases
    Neutral proteases (elastase)

Lysosomal contents

Lysosomal enzymes and accessory substances are present in neutrophils and monocytes, packaged in membrane bound vesicles ('granules') to prevent

Emphysema: abnormal permanent enlargement of the air spaces due to destruction of alveolar walls
Cirrhosis: Derived from the Greek meaning 'of yellow colour' because the patient (and internal organs) is jaundiced as a result of increased bilirubin. Cirrhosis is the end stage of chronic diffuse liver damage, leading to scarring and abnormal nodular architecture

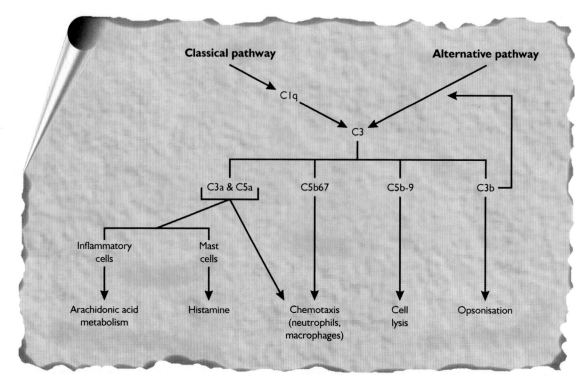

Figure 1.19 Complement system

with alpha-1-antitrypsin deficiency may suffer from emphysema of the lungs and liver cirrhosis.

Nitric oxide

Nitric oxide is produced by endothelial cells, macrophages and specific neurons in the brain and has roles in smooth muscle relaxation, reducing platelet aggregation and adhesion, and acting as a toxic radical to certain microbes and tumour cells. Macrophage nitric oxide production only occurs when induced by cytokines, such as gamma interferon, whereas endothelial and neural nitrous oxide is produced constitutively. Uncontrolled production by macrophages can lead to massive peripheral vasodilatation and shock (see p. 116).

Plasma-derived mediators

Kinin system

Bradykinin is the major active product of this system. It is a polypeptide that is one of the most

powerful vasodilators known to man, increases vascular permeability and also induces pain when injected into the skin. The kinin cascade is activated by Hageman factor, and its relationship to the coagulation system is shown in the figure. As with other cascades, this contains an amplification step because kallikrein itself acts to stimulate the production of Hageman factor.

Clotting and fibrinolytic system

This system is not only important in inflammation but is also central to blood clotting, which is discussed in Chapter 6 (see Figure 6.6, page 97). It is the fibrinopeptides that act as chemical mediators in inflammation. These increase vascular permeability and are chemotactic for neutrophils. As in the kinin system, the cascade is activated by Hageman factor and includes an amplification loop so that plasmin stimulates Hageman factor. Plasmin is a multifunctional protease that also lyses fibrin clots to produce fibrin degradation products, which themselves induce permeability changes and also trigger the complement system by cleaving C3.

Complement system

The system comprises a large number of proteins that are involved in increasing vascular permeability, chemotaxis, opsonisation and the direct lysis of organisms. The most important components concerned with the inflammatory reaction are:

- **C3a** and **C5a** increasing vascular permeability and chemotaxis
- **C3b** and **C3bi** opsonins
- **C5b–9** membrane attack complex, involved in cell lysis.

Activation of this system occurs rapidly through the **classical pathway** initiated by antigen-antibody complexes, or more slowly through the **alternative pathway**.

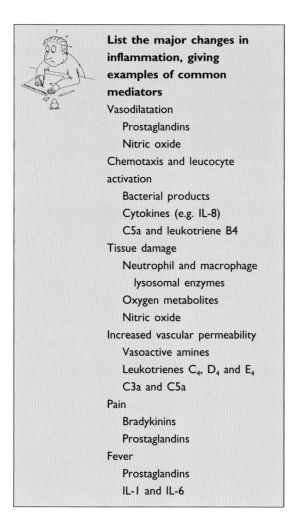

List the major changes in inflammation, giving examples of common mediators

Vasodilatation
    Prostaglandins
    Nitric oxide
Chemotaxis and leucocyte activation
    Bacterial products
    Cytokines (e.g. IL-8)
    C5a and leukotriene B4
Tissue damage
    Neutrophil and macrophage lysosomal enzymes
    Oxygen metabolites
    Nitric oxide
Increased vascular permeability
    Vasoactive amines
    Leukotrienes C_4, D_4 and E_4
    C3a and C5a
Pain
    Bradykinins
    Prostaglandins
Fever
    Prostaglandins
    IL-1 and IL-6

SYSTEMIC EFFECTS OF INFLAMMATION

Having considered lobar pneumonia, we have an idea of the *local* effects of inflammation. We have alluded to the fact that, at the same time, there are many *systemic* effects that may take place, such as fever, rigors, tachycardia, a drop in blood pressure, a loss of appetite, vomiting, skeletal weakness and aching. These are collectively known as **acute phase reactions**.

Fever is a regular accompaniment of inflammatory responses and occurs as a result of the 'resetting' of the thermoregulatory centre in the anterior hypothalamus. This probably produces a rise in temperature by constricting vessels in the skin, thus reducing blood flow and limiting heat loss, and by promoting heat production in the muscles by shivering. Biological substances that induce fever are called **pyrogens**. Many bacteria and viruses produce molecules that act as pyrogens, and these are called **exogenous pyrogens**. **Endogenous pyrogens** are produced by the body and are listed below. It is thought that exogenous pyrogens stimulate leucocytes to release the endogenous pyrogen IL-1, which acts on the hypothalamus by raising local prostaglandin E2 (PGE2) levels. Aspirin is useful for lowering the temperature because it interferes with PGE2 production.

Endogenous pyrogens
Tumour necrosis factor
Interleukin-1
Noradrenaline
α-interferon
Prostaglandin E1
Prostaglandin E2

Localised inflammatory responses lead to changes in plasma proteins owing to alterations in liver metabolism. These proteins are called **acute phase proteins**, and this change is thought to be mediated by IL-1, IL-6 and TNF. There is an

Acute phase protein response in disease

Major response in:

Bacterial infection

Rheumatoid arthritis

Systemic vasculitis

Trauma

Malignancy

Crohn's disease

Minor response in:

Viral infection

Connective tissue diseases, e.g. systemic lupus erythematosus

Ulcerative colitis

increased production of clotting factors and complement, which is of importance because these are consumed during the inflammatory process. Transport proteins, such as haptoglobins, may be important in regulating the amount of amines and oxygen free radicals. Many other acute phase proteins, such as C-reactive protein and serum amyloid A, are produced, but their role is not entirely clear. The acute phase reaction varies depending on the cause of inflammation. Viral infection is a poor inducer of acute phase proteins, whereas bacterial infections produce a major response, probably by bacterial endotoxins acting indirectly through raised TNF-α levels.

When investigating a patient, C-reactive protein is the most useful acute phase reactant to measure. If symptoms are equivocal, it may help to establish that there is organic disease rather than psychosomatic disease. In those patients with chronic diseases, a rise in the level may be an indication of an acute exacerbation or of intercurrent infection.

The number of leucocytes in the peripheral blood increases in many forms of inflammation so that they are available to fight infection. It is assumed that cytokines act through colony stimulating factors to increase the production and release of cells from the marrow. Again, there are differences depending on the type of infection, and this may be helpful in making a diagnosis. Bacterial infection provokes an increase in neutrophils, viral infections cause a rise in lymphocyte numbers and allergic reactions or parasitic infections result in more eosinophils.

Trauma or stress of any kind also affects the hypothalamus-pituitary-adrenal axis, resulting in the production of growth hormone, prolactin, antidiuretic hormone (ADH), adrenocorticotrophic hormone (ACTH) and adrenaline. These hormones are responsible for the breakdown of glycogen, changes in fatty acid metabolism and sodium-potassium transport. It is these metabolic changes that are responsible for the malaise, weakness, loss of appetite and other varied systemic effects observed during injury.

CHAPTER 2

THE IMMUNE SYSTEM

- The lymphatic system in inflammation
- Generation of diversity in the immune system
- What does immunoglobulin do?
- Tolerance and autoimmune disease
- Hypersensitivity

THE LYMPHATIC SYSTEM IN INFLAMMATION

Before we go on to discuss the other types of inflammatory response, we must consider the role of the lymphatic system in inflammation.

The lymphatic system comprises all the collections of lymphoid tissue that are present throughout the body. Lymphocytes are produced and mature in the bone marrow and thymus. They migrate in the blood to populate and proliferate in the lymph nodes, the spleen and the lining of the gut and respiratory tract, the so-called mucosa-associated lymphoid tissue or MALT.

The lymphatic system has a one-way circulation linked to, but separate from, the blood circulatory system. Generally, more fluid moves out of tissue capillaries than is returned, as we discussed when considering fluid flow across the vessel walls in inflammation. This excess fluid is termed lymph and drains into the lymphatic channels that are present in all tissues. In addition to the fluid, lymph also contains a variety of inflammatory cells, particularly lymphocytes and macrophages; the actual number of cells is very variable and increases if the tissue is inflamed. The lymphatic fluid filters through a chain of lymph nodes, most ultimately entering the blood via the thoracic duct at its junction with the left subclavian and internal jugular veins. Once immune cells are back in the blood, the cycle is repeated. This recirculation of lymphoid cells is important as it allows information about invading organisms to be shared with other areas of lymphoid cell production. A lymphocyte that has come from a specific area, such as the gut, recognises particular surface molecules on the endothelial cells of that area (**addressins**) that allow it to 'home' back to the same tissue.

Let us consider how this works in practice. Imagine that you have a severe sore throat, making it painful to swallow. Fairly soon, you will notice the lymph nodes on either side of the sternomastoid muscle enlarging and even becoming painful.

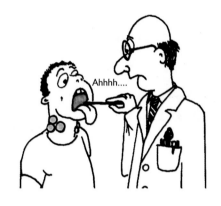

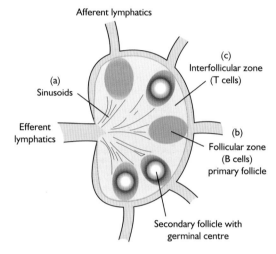

Afferent lymphatics

(c)
Interfollicular zone
(T cells)

(a)
Sinusoids

Efferent
lymphatics

(b)
Follicular zone
(B cells)
primary follicle

Secondary follicle with
germinal centre

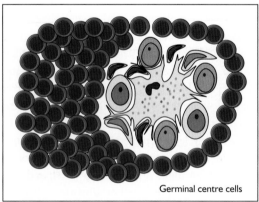

Germinal centre cells

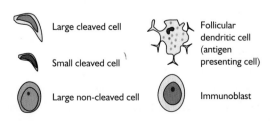

Large cleaved cell

Small cleaved cell

Large non-cleaved cell

Follicular
dendritic cell
(antigen
presenting cell)

Immunoblast

Figure 2.1   Basic architecture of the lymph nodes

If one of the nodes were to be excised for microscopical examination, it would show a number of changes.

First the sinusoids (a) would appear more prominent (**sinus histiocytosis**) because their lining cells, the macrophages, have an important job. The macrophages trap the organisms causing the sore throat (e.g. Streptococci) to prevent dissemination into the blood. The macrophages have another vital role, that of initiating a specific immune response to the offending agent. This requires cooperation between B lymphocytes, T lymphocytes, macrophages and other antigen-presenting cells in the node.

B lymphocytes are concentrated in the follicles (b) of the node and can develop into plasma cells that produce antibodies against the invading organisms. This is particularly important in bacterial infections, and the enlargement of the B cell areas is called **follicular hyperplasia**. If the sore throat is caused by a virus, which is more common, the T cells are most important. These reside outside the follicles in the interfollicular zone (c), which will enlarge.

The local lymph nodes trap the antigens in special cells that phagocytose antigens, process them and then display them on their cell surfaces. These are called **antigen-presenting cells** and include **follicular dendritic cells** in the follicles, **dendritic reticulum cells** in the interfollicular zones and **macrophages** in a variety of areas. This method of antigen presentation activates specific lymphocytes and promotes the immune response. Hopefully, this will contain the infection, but if it fails, the infection may reach the blood. Infection of the blood (septicaemia) may also occur by tissue organisms directly entering blood vessels. The septicaemic patient is gravely ill with fevers, shivering attacks (rigors) and dangerous lowering of the blood pressure ('shock'). Now it is the turn of the spleen to trap organisms and promote immune cell proliferation. Its structure and functions are analogous to those of the lymph node, with macrophages lining sinusoids and specific B and T cell areas, but the fluid percolating through is blood rather than lymph.

Some of the body's defences, such as the protective layers of skin or mucus lining the gut, are

Table 2.1 T lymphocyte subsets

	CD4+			CD8+	
	Suppressor/inducer	Helper/inducer		Suppressor cells	Cytotoxic cells
		Th1	Th2		
Genetic restriction (MHC)	II	II	II	I	I
Suppressor activity	++ (provide help)	–	–	++	–
Cytotoxic activity	–	+	–	–	++
Help for immunoglobulin	–	+	+++	–	–

MHC = major histocompatibility complex.

T cells are important against infections, in graft rejection, in graft-versus-host disease, in some hypersensitivity reactions and in tumour immunity. Th1 cells assist macrophages in stimulating cell-mediated immunity. Th2 cells assist B cells by stimulating immunoglobulin production and regulating immunoglobulin class.

innate, while the immune system provides a method for **acquiring** defences against the specific antigens that the individual encounters in life.

The immune response can be regarded as **humoral immunity** and **cell-mediated immunity**. Humoral immunity results from B cells transforming to plasma cells, which produce immunoglobulin (antibodies). Cell-mediated immunity occurs through T cells capable of direct attack and lymphokine production. T cells also act to regulate the immune response through subsets called helper T cells and suppressor T cells.

We know that, on the first encounter with an antigen, there is a proliferation of immunologically identical B cells, called a **clone**, together with memory cells. The clone will produce the antibody appropriate to the antigen. Initially, the antibody is of type IgM, and the clone later switches to producing IgG. If the antigen is encountered again, the memory cells will stimulate clonal proliferation of the appropriate antibody-producing cells.

T cells differ in their biological roles, some acting as **helper** cells, some as **cytotoxic** cells, some as **killer** cells and some as **suppressor** cells. They secrete a wide variety of cytokines (lymphokines) that act on other inflammatory cells (e.g. many interleukins, interferon-γ, TNF-α and TGF-β). T cells help B cells by direct cell contact through

CD (cluster designation) numbers indicate that a particular cell has a surface antigen that can be detected with a specific antibody. This has proved very useful for identifying leucocytes

Some CD antigens useful in leucocyte identification

Antigen	Principally expressed on
3	Mature T cells
4	Helper/inducer T cells
8	Suppressor/cytotoxic T cells
15	Monocytes and granulocytes
16 and 56	Natural killer (NK) cells
20	Most B cells
68	Monocytes/ macrophages

CD40 and B7 molecules on the B cell and CD28 antigen on the T cell, followed by lymphokine secretion promoting B cell growth and develop-

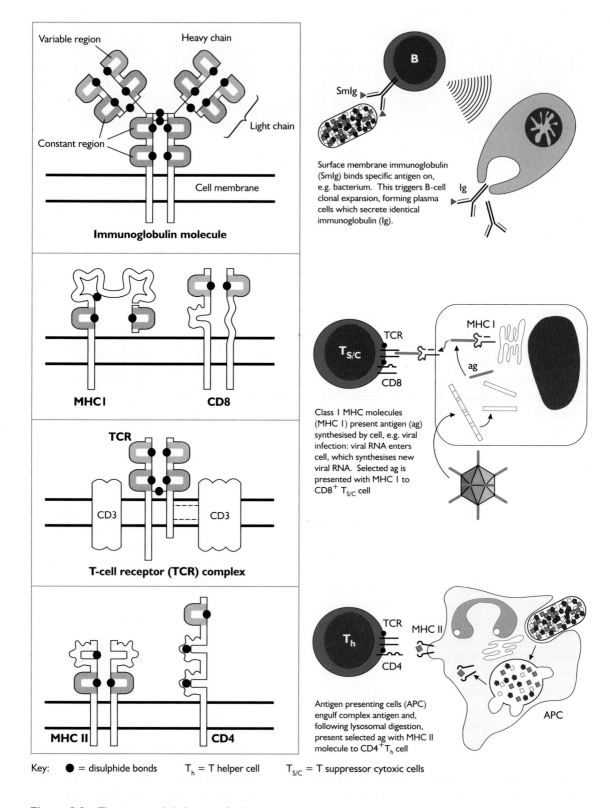

Figure 2.2 The immunoglobulin superfamily

ment and controlling the immunoglobulin class that is produced. The cytotoxicity of T cells takes three forms. Cytotoxic (CD8+) cells recognise foreign antigens on other cells, especially virus-infected cells. Natural killer (NK) cells are cytotoxic to cells without the need for specific antigen–receptor binding, and killer (K) cells are cytotoxic to cells coated with specific antibody (antibody-dependent cell-mediated cytotoxicity).

T cells have a variety of surface molecules, some of which are common to many T cell types (e.g. CD3), while others are limited to the various subtypes (e.g. CD4 and CD8). These molecules are involved in antigen recognition by combining with the T cell receptor.

cell–cell recognition, the so-called **immunoglobulin gene superfamily** (Fig. 2.2).

T cell recognition of antigen involves various superfamily members. MHC (major histocompatibility complex) molecules are important because T cells do not react with free, native antigens (that is the job for the immunoglobulin molecules) but instead bind to antigens that have been processed by special antigen-presenting cells or macrophages and are then displayed on the cell surface along-side MHC molecules. Helper cells with CD4 included in the TCR complex recognise processed antigen combined with class II MHC molecules (Figure 2.3), whereas cytotoxic T cells with CD8

HOW IS ANTIGEN RECOGNISED?

Although diagrams generally depict antibody molecules as simple bent dinner forks, they have a complex three-dimensional structure with many 'folds'. Antigen binds to the variable region, where there are **hypervariable regions** forming a potential 'pocket' for antigen attachment. This has a shape dependent on the outer electron clouds of its atoms, which determines the antigen *shape* that it recognises. The important point is that this inter-action depends on the antigen and antibody having complementary profiles; no covalent bonding is involved, so the chemical composition is not crucial. The shapes do not have to be a perfect fit, but a close fit gives the strongest binding.

T cell recognition of antigen is similar although more complicated, with a T cell receptor complex of several molecules interacting with antigen. The **T cell receptor (TCR)** of the majority of T cells is composed of an alpha chain and a beta chain with constant and variable regions analogous to those of immunoglobulins. In fact, the similarities between the TCR and immunoglobulin structure go even deeper as the genetic mechanisms for producing the necessary enormous diversity are almost identical. Nature has found this approach so useful that a common structure, the **immunoglobulin homology unit**, is the basic build-ing block for a range of molecules involved in

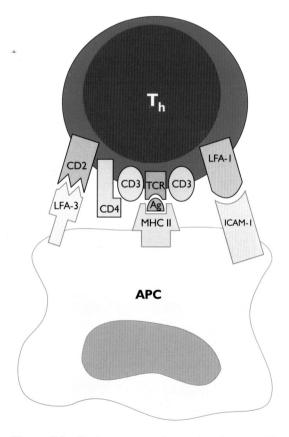

Figure 2.3 Surface receptor interactions between T$_h$ (helper T cells) and antigen-presenting cells (APCs). Many of the molecules involved (MHC II, T cell receptor [TCR], CD2, 3 and 4, and adhesion molecule ICAM) are members of the immunoglobulin gene superfamily

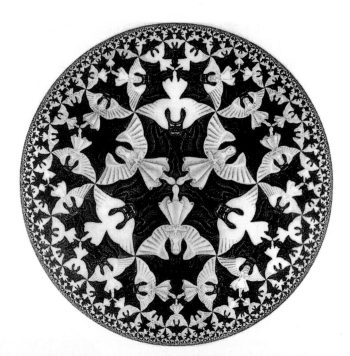

Figure 2.4

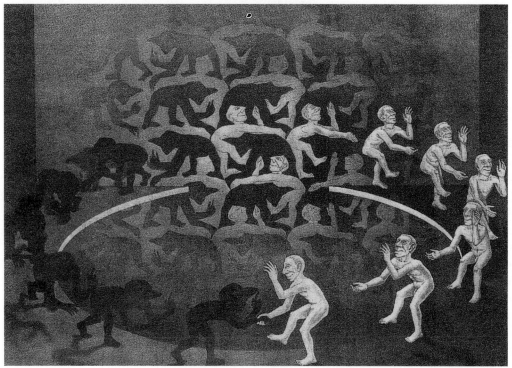

Figures 2.4 and 2.5 Escher's pictures **Circle Limit IV** (Figure 2.4) and **Encounter** (Figure 2.5) illustrate some concepts in molecular recognition. For maximum effect, the pairs of molecules should have complementary shapes so that there is a close three-dimensional fit. The two molecules may have no other similarities, as occurs in most antigen–antibody pairs; this is analogous to Escher's angels and devils. Alternatively, the pair of molecules may have structural homology and common genetic ancestry, as do the immunoglobulin gene superfamily. This may be likened to Escher's human figures in **Encounter**. M.C. Esher's 'Circle Limit IV' and 'Encounter' © 1997 Cordon Art-Baarn-Holland. All rights reserved.

molecules bind to processed antigen associated with class I molecules (Figure 2.2). Once the antigen and MHC molecule are bound to the TCR and subset molecule, the T cell is activated by a signal that passes via the CD3 molecule to the cell's interior.

Each person has an (almost) unique set of MHC molecules that are present on most cells and are inherited. This is relevant to transplantation, in which it is best to have a good 'match' between the donor and the recipient to minimise the risk of rejection. An identical twin will provide an excellent match, and some siblings are a good match, but other people's organs carry MHC antigens that will be identified by the recipient's immune system as foreign, the tissue then being rejected. The human MHC system is also called the HLA (human leucocyte antigen) system and is coded for on chromosome 6, where there are six loci: three for class I antigens (A, B and C) and three for class II antigens (DP, DQ and DR). Class I molecules are expressed on virtually all nucleated cells, while class II molecules are restricted to antigen-presenting cells, macrophages and B cells but can be expressed on many other cell types if they are stimulated with γ-interferon.

HOW DO B CELLS PRODUCE THE CORRECT ANTIBODY?

A B cell has no choice in the matter! Each B cell has the genetic code for a single antibody, and it displays this antibody on its own cell surface. This means that only B cells with the correct antibody will bind to the new antigen and be stimulated to proliferate. It is really the antigen that chooses the B cell best equipped to fight it. Of course, this requires an enormous number of B cells with different genetic codes, so that the body has a B cell equipped to fight any new foreign antigen. (There are at least 10^8 different immunoglobulin molecules in the serum.) Nature discovered a brilliant way of producing this variety of codes, which we shall describe below, and then used a similar approach for T cell receptor molecules.

Give examples of the immunoglobulin superfamily
Immunoglobulins
MHC class I and II antigens
T cell receptor
CD 2, 3, 4 and 8 antigens
Adhesion molecules, e.g. ICAM and VCAM

GENERATION OF DIVERSITY IN THE IMMUNE SYSTEM

It would have been possible to produce millions of subtly different receptors by joining polypeptide fragments in different combinations after translation, but nature has elected to alter the genetic code within lymphocytes and then translate each chain from the mRNA as a continuous polypeptide (possibly because it makes the deletion of autoreactive lymphocytes easier). The system is broadly similar for the immunoglobulin light chains and heavy chains, and for the α, β, γ and δ chains of the T cell receptor. The genes for each chain are not a continuous structure in non-lymphoid cells but are groups of exons separated by long non-coding introns.

There are four groups of exons, and, in lymphoid cells during maturation, one gene from each of three of the groups is rearranged so that they lie adjacent to each other. The four groups encode for variable (V), diversity (D), joining (J) and constant (C) regions. There is great diversity within the V, D and J groups, but the constant region genes are limited in number, with only a single gene for each subclass of molecule, e.g. for heavy chains Cμ, Cγ, Cα, Cδ, Cε (Fig. 2.6).

It is easy to see how an enormous variety of molecules can be produced in this way. For example, the mouse immunoglobulin heavy chain molecule genome is produced from a choice of 500 V gene segments, 15 D gene segments and 4 J gene segments. This gives a possible repertoire of 500×15×4 combinations for the heavy chain. That chain will be combined into an immunoglobulin

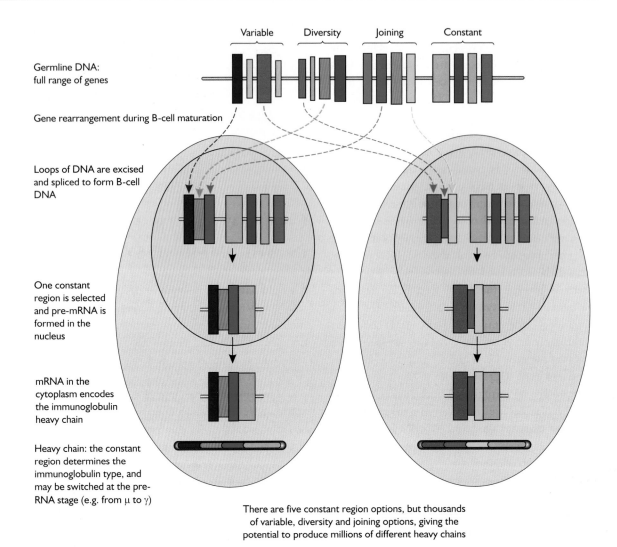

Germline DNA:
full range of genes

Variable   Diversity   Joining   Constant

Gene rearrangement during B-cell maturation

Loops of DNA are excised
and spliced to form B-cell
DNA

One constant
region is selected
and pre-mRNA is
formed in the
nucleus

mRNA in the
cytoplasm encodes
the immunoglobulin
heavy chain

Heavy chain: the constant
region determines the
immunoglobulin type, and
may be switched at the pre-
RNA stage (e.g. from μ to γ)

There are five constant region options, but thousands
of variable, diversity and joining options, giving the
potential to produce millions of different heavy chains

Figure 2.6 Gene rearrangement in the B cell heavy chain. This example shows two different heavy chains being produced

molecule, in humans, approximately 10^8 different immunoglobulins being produced in this way. Only the V, D and J region genes are rearranged to lie together in the DNA, the C region genes remaining separate. This means that the transcribed RNA in the *nucleus* has a VDJ section distant from the C section, so the remaining intron has to be excised to produce mRNA with consecutive V, D, J and C areas. Why is the C region treated differently? Probably because a lymphocyte that has recognised an antigen with the variable region on its surface molecule may need to produce molecules with different constant regions. This occurs in plasma cells that switch their immunoglobulin production

from IgM to IgG; the antigen is the same and the variable regions are the same, but the constant region has changed. If the alternative C region genes had been removed by the gene rearrangement that occurs in early B cell maturation, this would not be possible.

It must be emphasised that the V, D, J and C groups of genes are different for each type of molecule (i.e. heavy chain, light chain, TCRα, TCRβ, etc.), so the genes for each chain are rearranged independently. Only the genes on one of a pair of chromosomes is rearranged, the locus on the paired chromosome being inhibited (**allelic exclusion**).

Table 2.2 Immunoglobulin types

	Complement fixation by		Macrophage/ polymorph binding	Mast cell/ basophil binding	Cross placenta	Function
	Classical pathway	Alternative pathway				
IgG	++	−	++	−	++	Combats microorganisms and toxins. Most abundant Ig in blood and extravascular fluid
IgA	−	+−	+−	−	−	Most important immunoglobulin for protecting mucosal surfaces. Combines with secretory component to avoid being digested
IgM	+	−	−	−	−	Important in early response to infection as it is a powerful agglutinator
IgD	−	−	−	−	−	?Function. Present on the surface of some lymphocytes and may control lymphocyte activation/suppression
IgE	−	−	+−	+−	−	Involved in mast cell degranulation, thereby protecting body surfaces. Important in allergy and parasitic infections

WHAT DOES IMMUNOGLOBULIN DO?

Most importantly, immunoglobulin recognises antigen through the **variable regions** on the molecule. After that, the **constant regions** initiate the biological functions, such as complement fixation and opsonisation, appropriate for the immunoglobulin class. Each immunoglobulin molecule is formed from two identical **heavy chains** and two identical **light chains** joined by interchain disulphide links. There are two types of light chain (**kappa** and **lambda**) and five types of heavy chain (**G, A, M, D** and **E**). The light chains can combine with any type of heavy chain and do not influence biological function, whereas each heavy chain type supports different biological functions (Table 2.2).

Binding of antigen to antibody can lead to a variety of effects. Cross-linking of antigenic parti-

cles or cells will produce **precipitation** or **agglutination**, while binding of antibody to an active site on a virus or toxin can result in **neutralisation**. Other components of the immune response can become involved, for example when antibody fixes complement to produce **lysis** or enhanced **phagocytosis**. Antibody can also promote **cell-mediated cytotoxicity** involving K cells, so-called antibody-dependent cell-mediated cytotoxicity (ADCC).

TOLERANCE AND AUTOIMMUNE DISEASE

This ability of the body to mount an immune response against foreign antigens raises a very important question. How does the immune system distinguish between an antigen that is foreign and one that is normally present on the cells in the body?

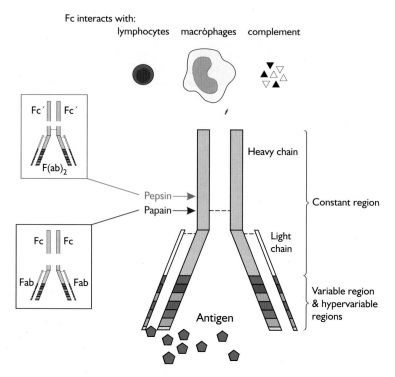

Fc interacts with:
lymphocytes   macrophages   complement

Fc′   Fc′
F(ab)₂

Fc   Fc
Fab   Fab

Pepsin→
Papain→

Heavy chain

Constant region

Light chain

Variable region & hypervariable regions

Antigen

The constant parts of the heavy & light chains interact with other cells and mediators. The variable regions form 3-dimensional antigen recognition sites.

Digestion with pepsin cleaves the Ig molecule into Fc′ & F(ab)₂ fragments, whilst papain digestion produces Fc & Fab, due to the positions of the disulphide bonds (–––)

Figure 2.7   The immunoglobulin molecule

This is achieved by selection in the thymus during fetal life. Stem cells in the bone marrow produce prothymocytes, which are attracted to the thymus by the chemotactic agent thymotaxin. Here, they mature along various pathways, producing cells that recognise 'self' antigens as well as foreign antigen, but the self-reacting T cells are believed to be eliminated or inactivated. The alternative view is that tolerance results from specific suppressor cells inhibiting immune responses against self antigens (Fig. 2.8).

This mechanism induces **tolerance** so that antigens that are exposed to the immune system during fetal life are not capable of eliciting a response in later life. Hence nature has devised a neat system of differentiating self from non-self. Or has it?

Parts of the body that are not exposed to the immune system during fetal life can produce a

response later on – lens protein and spermatozoa are just two examples. Even antigens exposed during fetal life may provoke immune activation much later in life, leading to a group of disorders called **autoimmune diseases**. It is assumed that, in autoimmune diseases, either the self antigen is modified, a new exogenous antigen closely resembles the self antigen or some changes in the immune system bypass the need for helper cells.

Autoimmune diseases include many clinically important and potentially life-threatening conditions such as Hashimoto's thyroiditis (antibodies to thyroglobulin and thyroid epithelium), myasthenia gravis (antibodies to the acetylcholine receptors of the neuromuscular junction), pernicious anaemia (antibodies to intrinsic factor and gastric parietal cells) and systemic lupus erythematosus (SLE) (numerous antibodies, especially antinuclear antibodies). As you can see, the first three are **organ**

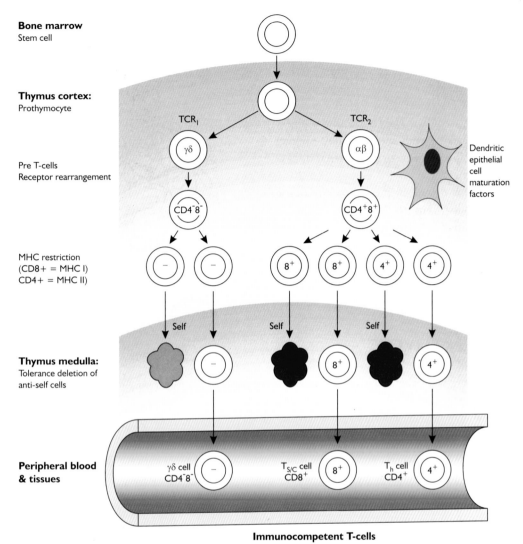

Bone marrow
Stem cell

Thymus cortex:
Prothymocyte

TCR₁ — TCR_1

TCR₂ — TCR_2

$\gamma\delta$

$\alpha\beta$

Dendritic epithelial cell maturation factors

Pre T-cells
Receptor rearrangement

$CD4^-8^-$

$CD4^+8^+$

MHC restriction
(CD8+ = MHC I)
CD4+ = MHC II)

$-$ $-$ 8^+ 8^+ 4^+ 4^+

Self Self Self

Thymus medulla:
Tolerance deletion of
anti-self cells

$-$ 8^+ 4^+

Peripheral blood & tissues

$\gamma\delta$ cell
$CD4^-8^-$ $-$

$T_{S/C}$ cell
$CD8^+$ 8^+

T_h cell
$CD4^+$ 4^+

Immunocompetent T-cells

Prothymocytes proliferate in the thymic cortex and undergo rearrangement of the genes for the T cell receptor molecule. The pre-T cells express either the gamma (γ) and delta (δ) chains (TCR_1) or the alpha (α) and beta (β) chains (TCR_2). At the next stage of maturation, the TCR_2 cells exhibit surface CD4 and CD8 molecules while the TCR_1 cells are CD4 and CD8 negative. $CD4^+$ cells give rise to helper/inducer cells which function best in collaboration with class II MHC molecules. This is termed MHC restriction. $CD8^+$ cells interact best with class I MHC molecules and have suppressor/cytoxic actions. Thymocytes that could attack 'self' antigens are removed in the thymic medulla. $\gamma\delta$T cells are a small subset of T cells with a large granular appearance. In humans, they are evenly distributed through the immune system and have cytoxic activity.

Figure 2.8 T cell maturation

specific while SLE is **non-organ specific**. We will briefly describe SLE to illustrate the wide-ranging effects of producing antibodies against the self.

Systemic lupus erythematosus is a systemic disorder in which there is chronic, relapsing and remitting damage to the skin, joints, kidneys and almost any organ. Like most immune disorders, it has a higher incidence in women. In America, it is also more common in blacks, and it tends to occur in the second and third decades of life. Patients may present with a characteristic 'butterfly' rash on the face, or with more subtle symptoms. Many present after their kidneys have been damaged beyond repair, i.e. with chronic renal failure. The fundamental feature of the disease is inflammation of the small arterioles and arteries, i.e. a vasculitis, often related to the deposition of antigen–antibody complexes in the vessel walls. Involvement of the glomerular capillaries in the kidney produces a variety of types of glomerulonephritis. The other sites of involvement are the joints (synovitis), heart (non-infectious endocarditis, named after Libman Sacks, and pericarditis), lungs (pleuritis and effusions) and CNS (focal neurological symptoms resulting from vasculitis). The course of the illness is extremely variable and unpredictable, ranging from mild skin involvement to severe renal disease leading to death.

In autoimmune disorders, the immune response is well controlled, but the initiating event of antigen recognition is wrong. There is another group of disorders in which antigen recognition proceeds normally but the response is exaggerated. These are called hypersensitivity reactions.

HYPERSENSITIVITY

Even today, there is public suspicion about some immunisation programmes because a tiny minority of children who are immunised suffer from adverse effects. The occurrence of these occasional idiosyncratic reactions should not deter one from protecting the vast majority of the population from serious disease. However, we should not believe that the immune system is all good: the immune mechanisms that exist to defend the host may also do harm. This phenomenon of damage caused by the immune system while trying to combat an injury is referred to as **hypersensitivity**.

Four main types of hypersensitivity reaction have been described by Gell and Coombs, and they are a useful way of dividing up the types of immune response that can occur, although more than one type is often involved.

TYPE I: ANAPHYLACTIC HYPERSENSITIVITY

This operates in atopic allergies such as asthma, eczema, hay fever and reactions to certain food where there is an immediate reaction. An extrinsic allergen (e.g. grass pollen, house dust mite faeces

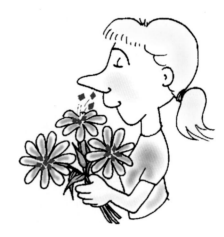

First exposure: nasal and bronchial mucosa exposed to pollen

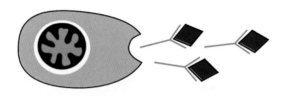

Soluble pollen antigen stimulates production of IgE antibodies

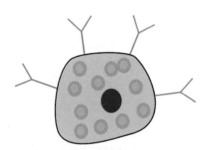

Fc component of IgE attaches to receptor on mucosal mast cell

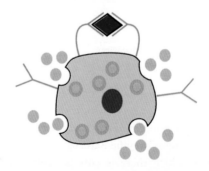

Second exposure to pollen: cross-linking of IgE molecules on mast cell stimulates release of primary and secondary inflammatory mediators

Figure 2.9 Type I hypersensitivity

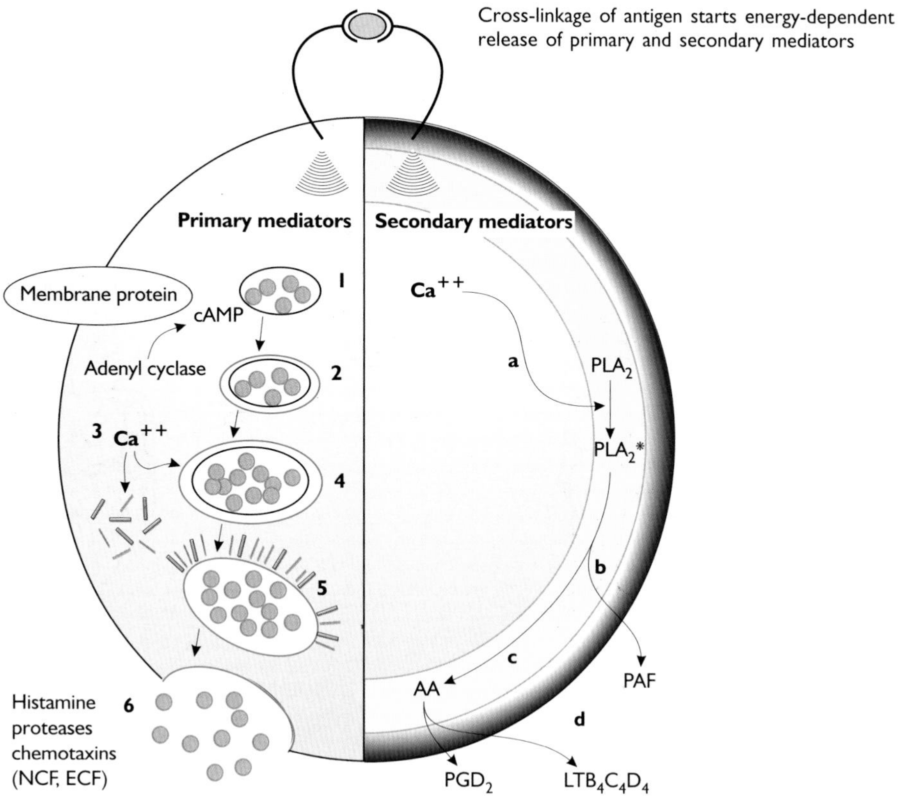

Cross-linkage of antigen starts energy-dependent release of primary and secondary mediators

Primary mediators

1. Increased cAMP produced
2. Phosphorylation of perigranular protein
3. Ca^{++}-dependant enzymes initiate microtubule & microfilament assembly
4. Ca^{++} & water enter granule, which swells
5. Granule moved toward membrane by microtubules and filaments
6. Discharge of pre-formed mediators invokes inflammatory response in 5–30 mins, lasting approximately 1 hour

Secondary mediators

a. Ca^{++}-mediated activation of membrane phospholipase A_2 (PLA_2)
b. Platelet activating factor (PAF) formed
c. Arachidonic acid (AA) formed
d. AA metabolites and PAF produce sustained response starting 8–12 hours after

Figure 2.10 Mast cell activation, stimulated by antibody cross-linkage

or seafood) binds to IgE on the surface of mast cells in the mucosa of the bronchial tree, nose, gut or conjunctivae, leading to the release of chemical mediators. These generally act locally, but they can also produce life-threatening systemic effects. Effects include constriction of smooth muscle in the bronchi and bronchioles, producing wheezing and dilatation, and increased permeability of capillaries, resulting in increased nasal and bronchial secretions, red watery eyes, skin rashes and diarrhoea.

TYPE II: ANTIBODY-DEPENDENT CYTOTOXIC HYPERSENSITIVITY

It is essential that any blood that is transfused into a patient is first cross-matched to ensure that the recipient does not possess antibodies to antigens on the donor red blood cells. This is because the donor red cells will become coated with antibody, which may promote phagocytosis as a result of opsonisation through the Fc, or may fix complement to

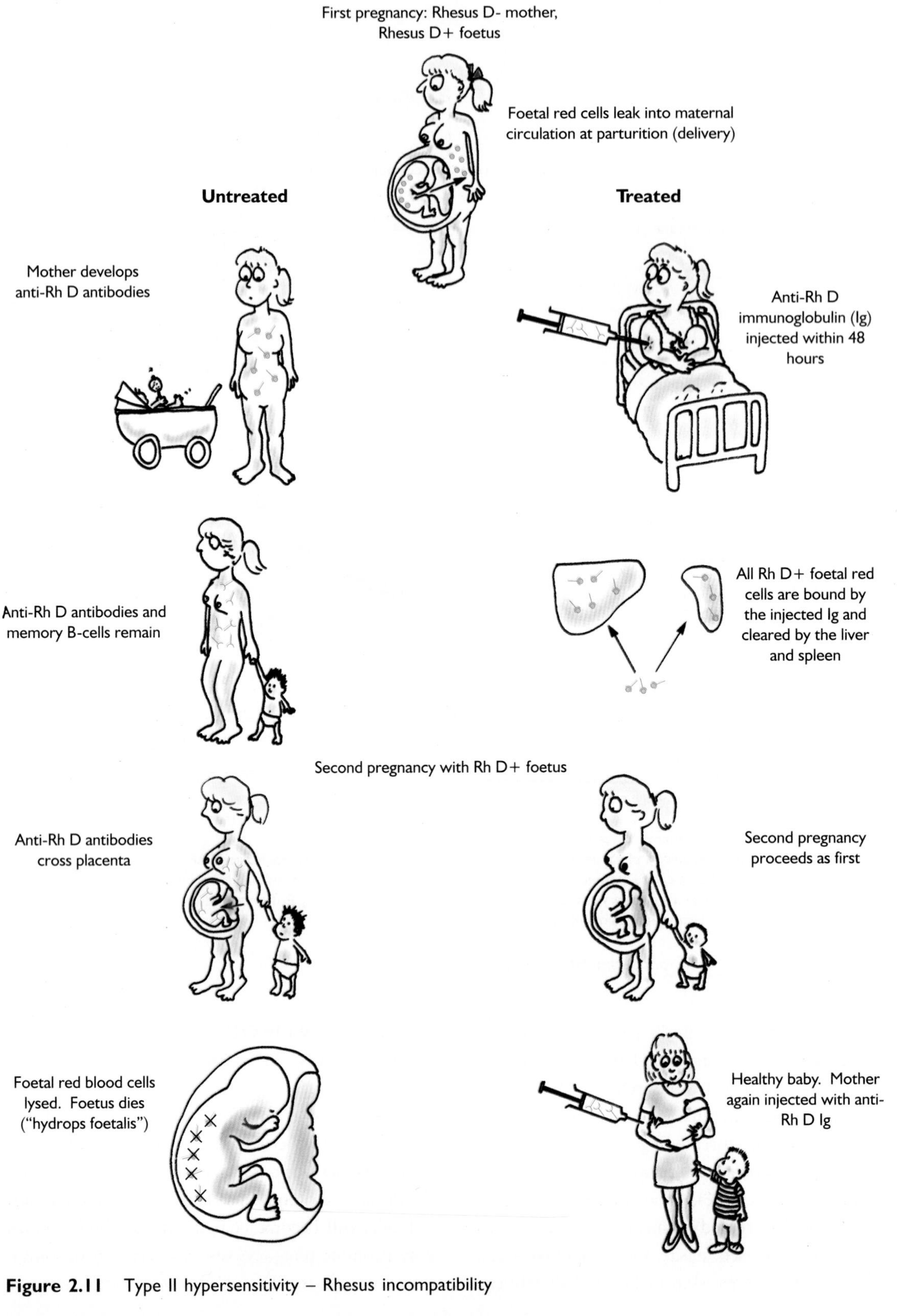

First pregnancy: Rhesus D- mother,
Rhesus D+ foetus

Foetal red cells leak into maternal
circulation at parturition (delivery)

Untreated

Treated

Mother develops
anti-Rh D antibodies

Anti-Rh D
immunoglobulin (Ig)
injected within 48
hours

Anti-Rh D antibodies and
memory B-cells remain

All Rh D+ foetal red
cells are bound by
the injected Ig and
cleared by the liver
and spleen

Second pregnancy with Rh D+ foetus

Anti-Rh D antibodies
cross placenta

Second pregnancy
proceeds as first

Foetal red blood cells
lysed. Foetus dies
("hydrops foetalis")

Healthy baby. Mother
again injected with anti-
Rh D Ig

Figure 2.11   Type II hypersensitivity – Rhesus incompatibility

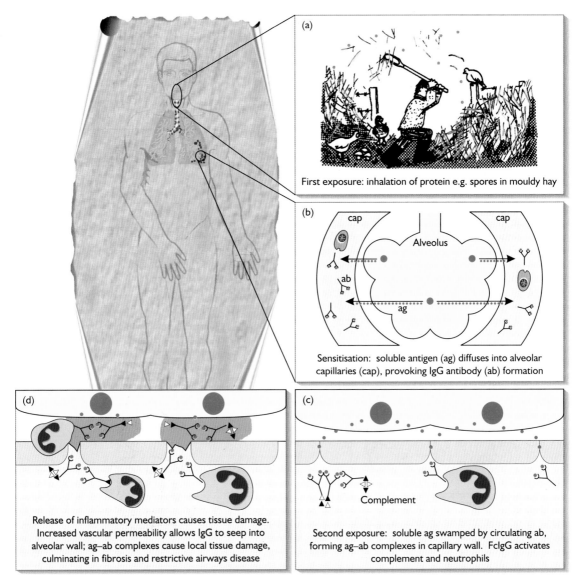

Figure 2.12 Type III hypersensitivity – extrinsic allergic alveolitis

produce cell membrane damage through C8 and C9 or phagocytosis through C3. Type II reactions are also involved in rhesus incompatibility (in which rhesus antibodies from a Rh– mother cross the placenta to damage the red cells of a Rh+ baby), some autoimmune diseases (e.g. Hashimoto's thyroiditis and autoimmune haemolytic anaemia) and some drug reactions (e.g. chlorpromazine-induced haemolytic anaemia and quinidine-induced agranulocytosis). NK cells, which are not restricted by HLA type, can kill through ADCC, which may be important for killing large parasites or tumour cells.

TYPE III: IMMUNE COMPLEX MEDIATED HYPERSENSITIVITY

Immune complexes can be soluble so that they circulate in the blood, giving rise to **serum sickness**, or they can be insoluble and precipitated where antigen first encounters antibody – the

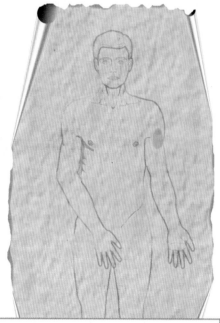

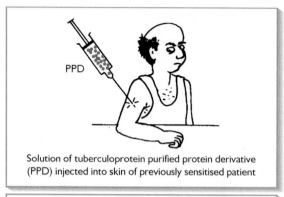

Solution of tuberculoprotein purified protein derivative (PPD) injected into skin of previously sensitised patient

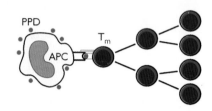

PPD antigen presented by antigen presenting cell (APC) to CD4 memory T-cell (T_m). Activated T_m cells undergo clonal expansion & secrete lymphokines and macrophage chemotactic factors

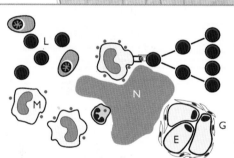

Cellular response includes recruited lymphocytes (L), & macrophages (M). Tissue damage and necrosis (N) occurs due to release of inflammatory mediators. Macrophages may become epithelioid cells (E) which aggregate to form granulomata (G)

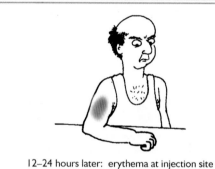

12–24 hours later: erythema at injection site

Figure 2.13 Type IV hypersensitivity – Mantoux test reaction

Arthus reaction. Both types of complex can activate macrophages, aggregate platelets and initiate the complement cascade. Circulating immune complexes can lodge in the vessels of many organs to give a **vasculitis**, principally affecting the kidney (glomerulonephritis), skin and joints. The Arthus reaction is most common in the lung, when an exogenous antigen is inhaled and precipitated locally. The antigens are generally animal or plant proteins that cause **extrinsic allergic alveolitis** and are often associated with specific occupations (Table 2.3).

Table 2.3 Some causes of extrinsic allergic alveolitis

Agent	Disease
Aspergillus fumigatus	Farmer's lung
Thermophilic actinomycetes	Farmer's lung
Avian protein	Bird fancier's disease
Fox fur proteins	Furrier's lung
Penicillium casei	Cheese washer's lung
Wood dust	Wood worker's lung

TYPE IV: CELL-MEDIATED (DELAYED-TYPE) HYPERSENSITIVITY

Unlike the other forms of hypersensitivity, which involve antibody, type IV requires T lymphocytes. Over several hours, these recruit and activate other T cells and macrophages to produce tissue damage and granulomata. This reaction can occur as a response to many viruses, fungi, bacteria and insect bites, and is often responsible for contact dermatitis related to simple chemicals. It is also important in the rejection of transplanted tissue and graft-versus-host reactions.

The Mantoux test, or tuberculin test, uses this reaction to see whether a person has some T cell immunity to tuberculosis. It involves injecting a small amount of extract of *Mycobacterium tuberculosis* into the skin and observing whether a localised red induration occurs over the next 48 hours as T cells and macrophages mount a type IV reaction.

TYPE V: STIMULATORY HYPERSENSITIVITY

There is another type of hypersensitivity reaction that is sometimes called type V and is sometimes included with type II. In this reaction, antibodies bind to non-immune cells (i.e. as in a type II reaction), but there is no cytotoxic effect. Instead, the antibody binding disturbs the normal function. For example, thyroid cells normally produce thyroxine when stimulated by thyroid stimulating hormone (TSH) from the pituitary. However, in patients with Grave's disease, there is an antibody that binds to thyroid cells and mimics the action of TSH, leading to excess thyroxine production (thyrotoxicosis). Myasthenia gravis is an example in which the antibody binds to the acetylcholine receptor, but instead of causing stimulation, it

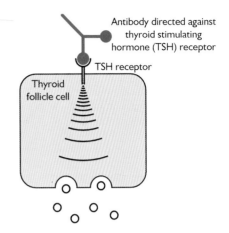

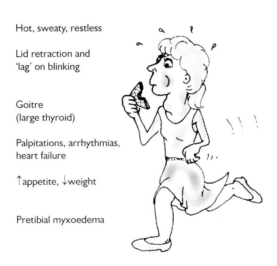

Some effects of excess circulating thyroid hormones

Figure 2.14 Type V hypersensitivity – Graves' disease

prevents the normal neurotransmitter binding and has an inhibitory effect.

This type of hypersensitivity was grouped with type II reactions in the original Gell and Coombs classification, but more modern authors usually separate it because there is no cytotoxic effect.

CHAPTER 3

INFECTIONS

- John Snow and the Broad Street pump
- What are the major routes of transmission?
- How do we defend against infections?
- Immunisation
- How do microorganisms attack us?
- How do microorganisms evade our defences?
- How do microbes invade the tissues?
- Mechanisms of cell and tissue damage
- How do bacteria develop antibiotic resistance?
- How is resistance passed to other bacteria?
- How can we prevent or overcome bacterial resistance?
- How do viruses develop resistance to antiviral agents?

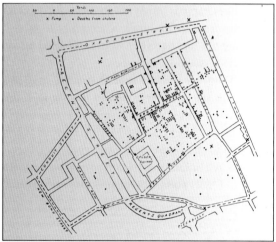

Deaths from cholera (•) in Broad Street, Golden Square, London, and the Neighbourhood, 19 August to 30 September 1854. Water pumps are denoted by an x. Courtesy of the Wellcome Institute for the History of Medicine

In Chapter 1, we listed the main causes of inflammation and emphasised that the largest group of causes was the infectious agents. Now is a good opportunity to discuss infectious agents in more depth, to consider the various weapons used by the microorganisms, the defence mechanisms that the body has evolved to combat bugs and the antibiotics available to give the body a helping hand. But first, some history.

JOHN SNOW AND THE BROAD STREET PUMP

It is quite possible to go through the entire medical curriculum without ever hearing the name of John Snow. He was a man of simple habits and seemed to lack the charisma that is vital in attracting attention on the world stage, yet his contributions to medicine were certainly 'world class'. John Snow (1813–58) made a significant contribution to anaesthesia and to the understanding of the transmission of cholera. He is perhaps best remembered for having anaesthetised Queen Victoria in 1853 and 1857, giving credibility to the use of pain relief during childbirth.

It was his contribution to the understanding of cholera that is relevant here. Snow's involvement with cholera evolved over a number of years. His first encounter with the disease was in Newcastle-upon-Tyne during the epidemic of 1831–32, when he had just started his training in medical practice. But it was during the next epidemic of 1848–49 that he made his seminal contribution.

By now, Snow was in London, where he began to unravel the mode of transmission of the disease. Snow's work was a masterpiece in epidemiological investigation. A slow and thorough assessment of where new cases of cholera were being diagnosed, the marked difference in the incidence and mortality of cholera in the south of London (8 deaths per 1000 inhabitants) compared with other areas (1–4 deaths per 1000 inhabitants) and the source of the water supply led him to his hypothesis that cholera was spread by water, and that social condition and hygiene were of paramount importance. Even before the identification of bacteria, he postulated that the transmission was a result of a *living* organism that had the ability to multiply. Although there was no treatment for cholera, it became apparent that the way to stop the epidemic was good sanitation and good hygiene. Snow is, of course, remembered for urging the removal of the handle of the pump that supplied contaminated water in Broad Street in London during the epidemic of 1854.

If you find epidemiological studies dull, Snow's biography is well worth a read. It demonstrates eloquently how epidemiological studies can have such a dramatic effect on public health.

WHAT ARE THE MAJOR ROUTES OF TRANSMISSION?

Infections have a reservoir that acts as a source of pathogens, the most common reservoir for human infections being infected humans, although some diseases involve animal reservoirs or soil organisms. It is not difficult to work out the main routes of spread from an infected human to another human. The bugs in the respiratory tract will be coughed out as aerosols, become **airborne** and are inhaled by others.

Direct mucosal contact is important in sexually transmitted diseases (HIV, herpes simplex, hepatitis B, papilloma virus, chlamydia and syphilis) and viruses infecting the salivary glands (herpes and mumps).

Contagious: when microbes are transmitted directly from person to person via contact or aerosol

Zoonosis: when animals are an important reservoir of infection for a human disease

Vertical transmission: microbes transferred from parent to offspring, generally across the placenta but also via milk, direct contact, sperm and ova

Horizontal transmission: transfer of organisms from one individual to another other than by vertical transmission

Commensals: harmless microbes living in or on a host and sharing the available nutrients

Symbiosis: microbes living in a host to mutual advantage, e.g. microflora in the rumen of cows, which are responsible for the release of nutrients from cellulose

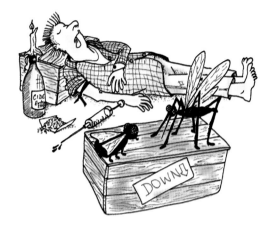

If this sort of thing goes on there'll be no more jobs for insect vectors

Figure 3.1

The gut pathogens will be excreted in the faeces and can re-enter the gut by faeces contaminating water or food supplies (**orofaecal route**). Contamination of food generally results either from lack of human handwashing or from failing to cover food so that flies with dirty feet are the guilty agents.

We are perhaps being unfair on the ignorant, uninfected fly that has inadvertently carried bacteria from faeces to food, because there is a much more guilty group of arthropods. These are the insects that are themselves infected and transfer the organism to humans by puncturing the skin (as in malaria and yellow fever: see below). This is one way by which **blood-borne** spread can occur. The insect sucks up infected blood from a human or animal and transfers it to another human or animal when it next bites. Comparable methods of spread are via hypodermic needles shared by drug addicts (e.g. hepatitis B) or through use of contaminated blood products (e.g. HIV and hepatitis C in haemophiliacs).

How do we defend against infections?

The first line of defence is preventing the multiplication and spread of organisms. Open sewers, overcrowded living conditions, a lack of clean drinking water, poor food storage and preparation, inadequate personal hygiene and unprotected sexual contact are a recipe for disaster. Since this is not a text on public health medicine or politics, we will not dwell on these points, but remember that it is estimated that each year in Asia, Africa and Latin America, 4–6 million die from diarrhoea and 1–2 million from malaria, that one-third of the world's population is subclinically infected with tuberculosis, and 3 million die, 12 million have HIV worldwide – all problems that are more likely to be solved by engineers and politicians than the latest advances in molecular biology.

Let us assume that we have normal healthy individuals; they are not malnourished, not on immunosuppressive drugs nor just recovering from an operation. What are their natural defences or, to look at it from the bug's point of view, what are the possible routes into the body? The surface of the body is covered by skin that is a tough waterproof layer that should be impervious to bugs. Unfortunately, there are holes in it. Most of the holes lead down into sweat ducts, hair shafts and other skin appendage structures that still have an epithelial lining, albeit a more delicate one. Bugs can live down these holes without causing particular problems unless the environment is upset, which disturbs the delicate balance between host and bug. This occurs for example in scarring acne, when the composition of the secretion is altered in the sebaceous glands, leading to blockage of the gland, proliferation of bacteria behind the blockage and breaching of the epithelial line of defence to provoke inflammation in the surrounding.

Diabetics are particularly prone to skin infections because, if their blood glucose levels are hard to control, their body fluids can be high in glucose, which provides an excellent culture medium for bacteria. They often have poor circulation, so bacteria can flourish relatively undisturbed by any immune response. The problem may be compounded by traumatic damage to the skin if they also have diabetes-induced peripheral nerve damage and might not notice, for example, the early stages of blisters or small abrasions. In fact, we are all likely to have some small cuts and grazes in our skin covering, but we know that when this defence is down, we must be extra vigilant and keep the area clean and dry and not do further damage to destroy the temporary and delicate protective layer of scab.

This becomes even more important when there is a large cut, as may follow an operation. Now the bacteria have a really good chance of success because they have a band of helpers (called doctors and medical students) who move rapidly from one patient to the next in the postoperative surgical wards, generously ensuring that all patients have the opportunity to acquire each other's skin flora. The combination of overcrowding (i.e. many sick people living in a closed environment), difficulty with personal hygiene (just try having a bed bath!)

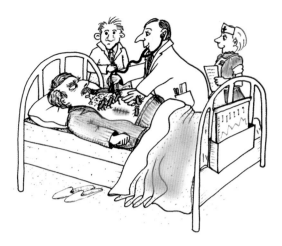

It's OK — this chap never washes his hands

Figure 3.2

and unprotected (non-sexual) contact with a large number of strangers describes both a postoperative surgical ward and a bacterium's idea of heaven. This is such an important topic that we will devote a later section to the problems of antibiotic resistance in hospital-acquired infections, but for now, let us go back to our defences.

There is a certain number of larger holes in the skin leading to areas covered by much more permeable epithelium. From the top down these are the eyes, nasal cavity, mouth, anus, urethra and vagina, each with its own defence system. The eye drops its portcullis and floods the moat because it is determined to repel invaders before they can produce any tissue damage. This is because the main parts of the eye must be transparent and able to transmit light without distortion. A scarred cornea can render the eye useless, so anything worse than a little inflammation of the conjunctiva can be devastating. Therefore the eye's defences include a nerve reflex to close the eyelids as danger approaches and a lacrimal gland to wash away particles, chemicals and bugs in a matter of seconds. In addition, tears contain lysozyme capable of degrading bacterial cell walls. If you have ever had even the smallest scratch to the surface of your eye, you will know that the desire to close the eyelids and the flow of tears keeps going until the epithelial covering is re-established.

Fortunately, this generally takes less than 24 hours.

The nose can be considered with the respiratory tract since both are covered predominantly by respiratory epithelium characterised by the presence of mucus-secreting cells and cilia. Cilia are tiny hair-like structures that beat in a synchronous fashion to move particles up the respiratory tract. This is made easier by the layer of mucus that lines the respiratory tract, thus providing a barrier against infectious agents, trapping the particles and acting as a conveyor belt propelled by the underlying cilia. This is called the mucociliary clearance mechanism and is severely damaged by smoking. The airways also have a nervous mechanism of defence in coughs and sneezes that push material out. This is good for the individual (and a super method of spread for air-borne bugs) but is potentially hazardous for those in the vicinity. If the microbes get past this barrier, there is a second line of defence involving the macrophages in the alveoli, often termed the sentries of the lung.

The mouth and anus are the ends of the gastrointestinal tract, both being defended by non-keratinising stratified squamous epithelium and a layer of mucus from local glands. The mouth has teeth and an enzyme (amylase), which, it could be argued, have a defensive role, although their main purpose is clearly related to digestion. There are similar dual-purpose roles for the acid and enzymes in the stomach or the secretions of the small intestine: their main role is digestive but they may also be harmful to many microorganisms. The gut, like the respiratory tract, has a layer of protective mucus. The gut is, of course, not sterile. It is colonised by a range of bugs that often live in peaceful coexistence unless something upsets the balance. This commonly occurs when a course of antibiotics destroys one type of bacteria, thus allowing another to overproliferate and cause problems, so-called antibiotic-associated or pseudomembranous colitis. *Clostridium difficile* is a bacterium that proliferates and secretes a toxin to produce bloody diarrhoea.

The urinary tract should have a one-way flow of urine from kidney to urethra along tubes lined by a multilayered transitional epithelium. There is no mucus barrier here, but it should not be needed as the urine formed in the kidney is sterile. The defences are the high volume of urine flushing the system, the physical barrier of the empty urethra and the composition of urine. The urinary composition varies, and it may have an acidic or alkaline pH, favouring some bacterial strains over others. Hopefully, the natural variations in pH will prevent bacteria becoming established and proliferating. Again, diabetics may have particular problems if the urine contains glucose to nourish the bacteria.

The genital tract of the female starts its defences with the vagina, lined by non-keratinising stratified squamous epithelium with mucus, and friendly colonies of Doderlein's bacillus, a lactobacillus that metabolises glycogen to lactic acid to produce a pH of 5, which inhibits colonisation by most other bacteria. Unfortunately, the glycogen is only present from puberty to menopause, when the vaginal epithelium is stimulated by oestrogens. At other ages, the vagina is alkaline and liable to infection with pathogenic Staphylococci and Streptococci. The uterus and tubes are specialised for their reproductive role, but it is possible that the monthly shedding of the endometrium may be a useful defence against infection and that the stereocilia in the tube, while wafting the ovum down, produce currents that might help to prevent bacteria ascending. The main defence, however, is the mucus in the normal cervix.

Secretory IgA antibodies are an important defence against infections on mucosal surfaces. IgA is an immunoglobulin dimer that acquires an extra secretory piece as it crosses the mucosal epithelium to reach the lumen. In the gut, there are about 20–30 times as many IgA- as IgG-producing cells. IgA defends both the luminal and subepithelial zones. Antigens penetrating the epithelium can combine with IgA to form immune complexes, which enter the blood and are transported to the liver, where a secretory piece is added by hepatic cells. The complex is then excreted in the bile. In addition, intestinal B cells can be stimulated by antigens and then migrate via the lymphatics and blood to localise in other areas, such as mammary glands or salivary glands, so that specific IgA

defends these sites. In fact, the various components of the immune system (macrophages, lymphocytes, complement, etc.) are an essential mechanism of defence and are termed **innate immunity**.

Amazingly, despite all these defences, bugs do sometimes break through, so we need a second line of defence involving the inflammatory response and the immune system – so-called **adaptive immunity**. We have already covered this in some depth in Chapters 1 and 2, so here we shall concentrate on how we can improve our defences by immunisation.

IMMUNISATION

It would be a crime to consider immunisation without pausing for a moment to think about its history and the man responsible for developing its

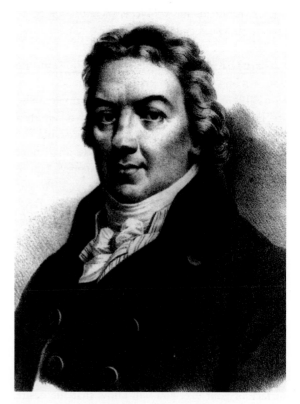

Figure 3.3 Edward Jenner (1749–1823) (Courtesy of the Wellcome Institute for the History of Medicine)

use. This man was Edward Jenner (1749–1823), a pupil of John Hunter. Jenner lived with Hunter for the first 2 years after coming to London, and the friendship they developed continued after Jenner left London to start in general practice in Berkeley, Gloucestershire. Jenner was profoundly influenced by Hunter's interest in natural history and in his methods of scientific investigation. To one of Jenner's questions, Hunter is said to have replied, 'I think your solution is just; but why think? why not try the experiment?'

Even before Jenner, it had been noticed that an attack of smallpox protected against further disease. It was known that the epidemics varied in severity and that it was best to contract a mild form of smallpox as this resulted in lifelong protection. This knowledge was widespread: in India, children were wrapped in clothing from patients with smallpox; in China, scabs from smallpox patients were ground and the powder was blown into the nostrils; in Turkey, female slaves were injected under the skin with dried preparations of pus from smallpox patients: inoculated slaves fetched a high price, while pock-marked slaves were worth nothing. Lady Mary Wortley Montagu, the wife of the British Ambassador in Constantinople, was aware of these techniques and took the risk of having her own children inoculated. When she returned to England in 1718, she tried to convince her friend, the Prince of Wales, that he should do the same. He was worried about experimenting on the royal children but, when six orphan children were successfully immunised against smallpox, he consented, and the royal children were inoculated. Medical ethics have made some advances since those days!

Jenner and others had noticed that cows suffered from a pustular disease resembling smallpox called 'variolae vaccinae' – cowpox. It was known that it could be transmitted to humans and that, apart from local symptoms, there were no ill-effects. There was a widespread belief that those who had suffered from cowpox became immune to smallpox, and a farmer in Dorset, Trevor Jesty, tried it out on his own children. The idea of using the cowpox virus to induce immunity to smallpox thrilled Jenner, but, rather than jumping to conclu-

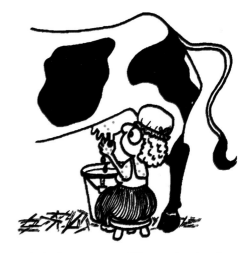

Figure 3.4 Jenner successfully inoculated against smallpox with cowpox. (From Lakhani, S 1992: Early Clinical Pathologists: Edward Jenner. *J Clin Path* 45. Reproduced with kind permission of the BMJ Publishing Group)

sions, he followed Hunter's example and experimented. On 14 May 1796, Jenner inoculated a boy of 8 named James Phipps with cowpox. The boy's illness took a predictable course and he recovered. On 1 July, Jenner inoculated the boy with smallpox and no reaction occurred, either on this occasion or on a subsequent occasion a few months later.

Jenner described this experiment to the Royal Society, but it was rejected. He continued to make his observations and, in 1798, published his work entitled *An inquiry into the causes and effects of the variolae vaccinae*. Hence inoculation with smallpox was replaced by inoculation with cowpox. The word '**vaccination**' came into use, and the number of smallpox cases dropped in the UK as a series of laws (the Vaccination Acts of 1840, 1841, 1853, 1861, 1867 and 1871) made vaccination free and compulsory, parents being liable to repeated fines until their children were vaccinated. Compulsion was withdrawn in 1948 and smallpox was eradicated globally by 1980, the last naturally occurring case being in Somalia in October 1977.

Immunisation may be active or passive. **Active immunity** involves using inactivated or attenuated live organisms or their products; the effect is reasonably longlasting and calls up an adaptive immune response. **Passive immunity** results from injecting human immunoglobulin and the effect is immediate, although it lasts only 1–2 weeks.

ACTIVE IMMUNISATION

First exposure to an antigen provokes a primary response in which IgM is the major antibody. Further exposure to the antigen produces a secondary response that occurs faster and produces higher levels of antibody, whose class is predominantly IgG. In addition to humoral immunity, cell-mediated immunity is also induced. The aim of active immunisation is to give sufficient doses of antigen to ensure that, after completing the course of immunisation, the person can mount a rapid effective response if exposed to the disease. The number of doses, the time intervals and the need for booster doses varies with the vaccine, the natural history of the disease and the likelihood of encountering the infection.

The UK's present immunisation schedule for children is shown in Table 3.1, and the recommendation for adults who are unimmunised or in a high-risk group is given in Table 3.2.

Live attenuated viral vaccines, such as those for polio, measles, mumps and rubella, generally produce the most longlasting immune responses, oral polio vaccine having the advantage of having maximal effect on local gut immunity, the natural portal of entry for wild polio. Non-live vaccines may be more effective when combined with adjuvants to enhance the immune response. For example, aluminium phosphate and aluminium hydroxide are used in DTP vaccine.

PASSIVE IMMUNISATION

Passive immunity relies on using either pooled plasma containing a variety of immunoglobulins to local infectious agents or specific immunoglobulin obtained from convalescent patients or recently immunised donors. Specific immunoglobulins are available for tetanus, hepatitis B, rabies and varicella zoster. They are most commonly used for postexposure prophylaxis.

Table 3.1 UK immunisation schedule for children

Vaccine	Age
DTP, polio and Hib	2m, 3m and 4m (primary course)
MMR (measles, mumps, rubella)	12–15m
Booster D/T and polio	3–5y
BCG (Bacillus Calmette–Guérin for tuberculosis)	10–14y or infancy
Booster D/T and polio	13–18y

D = diphtheria; T = tetanus; P = pertussis/whooping cough; Hib = *Haemophilus influenzae* type B (meningitis).

Table 3.2 Vaccination of adults

Vaccine	Examples of relevant groups
Rubella	Seronegative women
D/T and polio	Previously unimmunised individuals
Hepatitis B	Healthcare workers, haemophiliacs, intravenous drug users, prison inmates
Hepatitis A	Travellers, haemophiliacs, liver disease patients, some health workers
Influenza Pneumococcus	Elderly patients at risk of pneumonia
Anthrax	Occupational workers, e.g. abattoir
Tick-borne encephalitis	Travellers to forests of central and eastern Europe and Scandinavia
Typhoid Yellow fever Japanese encephalitis	Travellers to high-risk areas
Cholera	No longer a requirement anywhere in the world

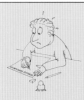

List the common types of vaccine

Live attenuated organisms
  Polio (oral: Sabin)
  Measles
  Mumps
  Rubella
  Tuberculosis (BCG)

Inactivated organisms
  Polio (subcutaneous: Salk)
  Pertussis
  Typhoid
  Hepatitis A
  Influenza (variable subtype depending on prevailing strain)

Toxoid (toxin inactivated by formaldehyde)
  Tetanus
  Diphtheria

Components of the organism
  Haemophilus influenza type B (HiB) (capsular polysaccharide)
  Hepatitis B (surface protein: recombinant)
  Pneumococcus (capsular polysaccharide)

List important pathogens for which there are no vaccines
Rhinoviruses (colds)
HIV/AIDS
Cytomegalovirus (CMV)
Epstein–Barr virus (EBV)
Gonorrhoea
Syphilis
Leprosy
Trachoma
Malaria
All parasitic and protozoal infections

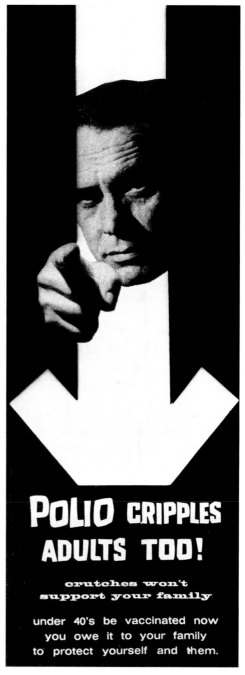

Figure 3.5 Elaborate bookmarks were made from silk in the 1860s but became more common as they were made from paper by the 1880s. They were a popular method of advertising and in the 1940s were used for conveying public messages on subjects such as health and road safety (Courtesy of Kirkdale Bookshop, London)

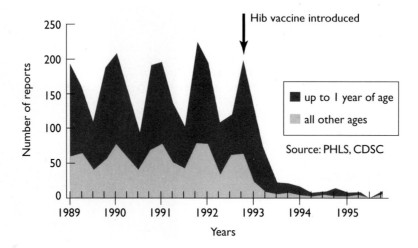

Figure 3.6 Laboratory reports of *Haemophilus influenzae* type b by age, England and Wales (1989–95) (PHLS and CDSC data). (From Salisbury, DM and Begg, NT 1996: Immunisation against infectious disease. Reproduced with permission of the Controller of Her Majesty's Stationery Office)

HOW DO MICROORGANISMS ATTACK US?

In any battle, it is important to know your enemy's strengths and weaknesses, so you need to know the different types of microorganisms and their preferred method of attack. It is beyond the scope of this book to detail even all of the most common infectious diseases, so we shall select diseases and microorganisms to illustrate particular mechanisms.

The stages of an attack can be divided into entry, spread and the specific method of damage, but first we should carry out a brief overview of the types of microorganisms.

BACTERIA

Bacteria (0.1–1.0 μm in size) lack nuclei and endoplasmic reticulum but are able to synthesise their own DNA, RNA and proteins. The bacterial chromosome is a single copy of a double strand of DNA (i.e. is haploid). Any bacteria can proliferate outside host cells through binary fission, but some are also capable of intracellular division, such as mycobacteria proliferating inside macrophages.

Bacteria are subdivided into **Gram-positive** and **Gram-negative** depending on the staining characteristics of their relatively rigid cell walls. Gram-positive walls have two layers, an inner cytoplasmic membrane composed of a phospholipid bilayer with embedded proteins similar to the cell wall of human cells, and an outer thick **peptidoglycan** layer. Gram-negative walls have three layers: an inner cytoplasmic membrane, a thin peptidoglycan layer and an outer membrane with lipopolysaccharide (LPS).

The next subdivision of bacteria is by shape: they can be spherical (**cocci**), rod-shaped (**bacilli**), short rods that are almost spherical (**coccobacilli**), spiral, comma or S-shaped, or of very variable shape (**pleomorphic**).

Finally, we should consider the different metabolic requirements of bacteria that influence where they live. The most important factor is how they handle oxygen; this separates them into **obligate aerobes, facultative anaerobes, microaerophilic bacteria** and **obligate anaerobes**.

Some other groups require a brief mention. Acid-fast bacteria are the various types of **mycobacteria** and nocardia. The mycobacterial wall is different in that it has a high lipid content, several of the lipids being important in mycobacterial virulence (see below).

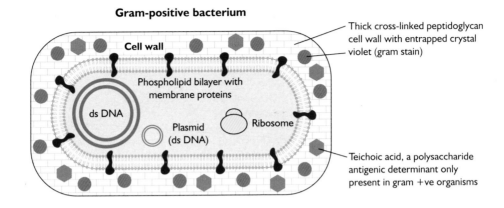

Gram-positive bacterium

Cell wall

Thick cross-linked peptidoglycan cell wall with entrapped crystal violet (gram stain)

Phospholipid bilayer with membrane proteins

ds DNA

Plasmid (ds DNA)

Ribosome

Teichoic acid, a polysaccharide antigenic determinant only present in gram +ve organisms

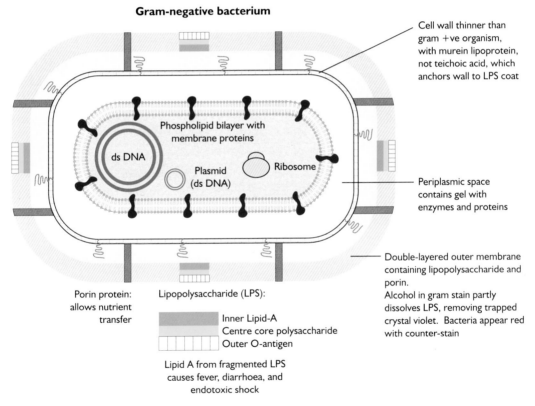

Gram-negative bacterium

Cell wall thinner than gram +ve organism, with murein lipoprotein, not teichoic acid, which anchors wall to LPS coat

Phospholipid bilayer with membrane proteins

ds DNA

Plasmid (ds DNA)

Ribosome

Periplasmic space contains gel with enzymes and proteins

Double-layered outer membrane containing lipopolysaccharide and porin.
Alcohol in gram stain partly dissolves LPS, removing trapped crystal violet. Bacteria appear red with counter-stain

Porin protein: allows nutrient transfer

Lipopolysaccharide (LPS):

Inner Lipid-A
Centre core polysaccharide
Outer O-antigen

Lipid A from fragmented LPS causes fever, diarrhoea, and endotoxic shock

Figure 3.7 Generalised diagram of the biochemistry and cell wall of Gram-positive and Gram-negative organisms

Mycoplasma lack a peptidoglycan wall and are smaller than some of the larger viruses but are capable of self-replication. They cannot be classified by shape because they lack any semi-rigid wall to give them a fixed shape. **Rickettsia** are obligate intracellular pathogenic bacteria that are often transmitted through the bites of infected lice, ticks and fleas and are thus called **arthropod-borne zoonoses**. They are particularly likely to invade and damage endothelial cells, with potentially devastating haemorrhagic effects. **Chlamydia** are also obligate intracellular pathogenic bacteria but are generally found in epithelial cells. They can cause pneumonia, urethritis and trachoma, a

Give examples of aerobic and anaerobic bacteria

	Gram-positive	Gram-negative	Acid fast
Obligate aerobes	*Bacillus cereus*	Neisseria	Mycobacteria
Facultative anaerobes	*Bacillus anthracis* Staphylococcus	E. coli Salmonella	
Microaerophilic bacteria	Streptococcus	Spirochaetes	
Obligate anaerobes	Clostridia	Bacteroides	

Give examples of morphologically distinct Gram-positive and Gram-negative bacteria

Morphology	Gram-positive	Gram-negative
Cocci (spherical)	Streptococci (in chains) Staphylococci (in clusters)	Neisseria
Bacilli (rod-shaped)	Corynebacteria Clostridia Bacillus Listeria	Haemophilus Bordetella Klebsiella, Proteus, Shigella, E. coli, Vibrio, Salmonella
Spiral		Treponema, Borrelia, Leptospira (spirochaetes). Helicobacter, Campylobacter
Pleomorphic		Chlamydia, Rickettsia (intracellular obligates)
Branching	Actinomyces, Nocardia	

major cause of blindness. Their life cycle has two phases: an *elementary body* that survives extracellularly, so is the method of transmission but is unable to divide, and a *reticulate body*, which multiplies within the host's cells.

VIRUSES

Viruses (30–400 nm in size) depend on the host cell for replication and are thus obligate intracellular parasites. They are classified as DNA or RNA viruses depending on the nucleic content of their core and are subdivided according to the shape of their protein coat (**capsid**) into spherical (**icosahedral**) or cylindrical (**helical**) types. They lack organelles and ribosomes but may have some structural proteins and enzymes inside their capsid. Outside the capsid, there may be an **envelope** of cytoplasmic membrane acquired by the virus from the host as it pushes through the host's membrane. Some viruses are naked or **non-enveloped**, and their release from the cell involves disrupting the cell membrane and generally causing the host cell's death.

The DNA or RNA can be **double stranded** or **single stranded**, and the RNA can be **positive** or **negative**. A positive RNA strand can be translated

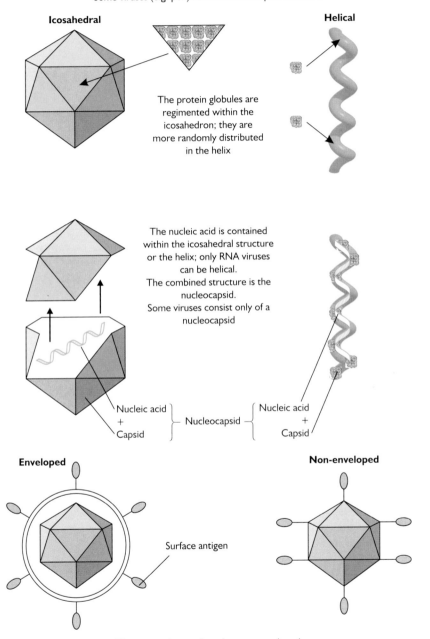

Globular protein is arranged to form the viral capsid in either an icosahedral or helical array: this is called the capsid. Some viruses (e.g. pox) have a more complex structure

Icosahedral

Helical

The protein globules are regimented within the icosahedron; they are more randomly distributed in the helix

The nucleic acid is contained within the icosahedral structure or the helix; only RNA viruses can be helical.
The combined structure is the nucleocapsid.
Some viruses consist only of a nucleocapsid

Nucleic acid + Capsid } Nucleocapsid { Nucleic acid + Capsid

Enveloped

Non-enveloped

Surface antigen

Viruses may be enveloped or non-enveloped.
The envelope is derived from the lipid bilayer peeled off the surface of infected host cells as the virus exits.

Non-enveloped viruses usually exit by causing cell lysis and thereby host cell destruction

Figure 3.8 Viral types

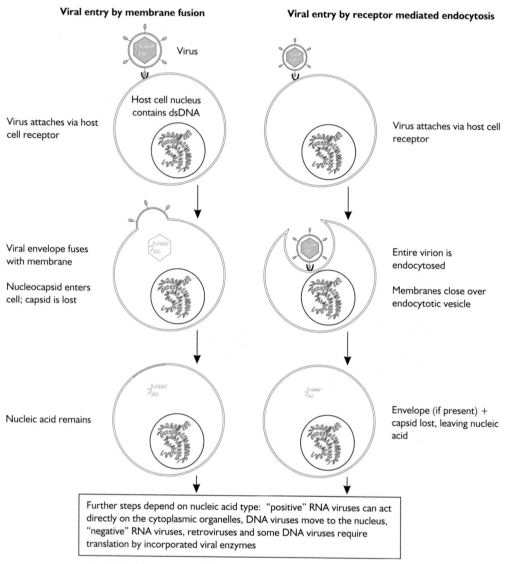

Viral entry by membrane fusion

Virus

Virus attaches via host cell receptor

Host cell nucleus contains dsDNA

Viral envelope fuses with membrane

Nucleocapsid enters cell; capsid is lost

Nucleic acid remains

Viral entry by receptor mediated endocytosis

Virus attaches via host cell receptor

Entire virion is endocytosed

Membranes close over endocytotic vesicle

Envelope (if present) + capsid lost, leaving nucleic acid

Further steps depend on nucleic acid type: "positive" RNA viruses can act directly on the cytoplasmic organelles, DNA viruses move to the nucleus, "negative" RNA viruses, retroviruses and some DNA viruses require translation by incorporated viral enzymes

Bacteriophages inject their RNA or DNA directly - see fig 3.13

Figure 3.9 Entry of viruses into host cells

immediately by the host's ribosomes, while a negative strand first requires transcribing to give a positive strand. This transcription requires an enzyme – RNA-dependent RNA polymerase not present in human cells; hence it has to be included in the viral particle. HIV is a retrovirus with reverse transcriptase and integrase enzymes. The viral RNA is reverse-transcribed into DNA in the cytoplasm. Double-stranded DNA is formed and transported into the nucleus, where it is integrated into the host DNA.

The main groups and some examples are shown in Table 3.3.

PROTOZOA

Protozoa are free-living, single-celled eukaryotes with nuclei, endoplasmic reticulum, mitochondria and organelles. They ingest nutrients through a cytosome and can reproduce sexually and asexually. Most are able to form cysts when in hostile environments.

Table 3.3 Outline classification of viruses

Nucleic acid	Symmetry	Envelope	Strand	Family	Example
RNA	Icosahedral	No	SS+	Picorna	Polio, Coxsackie
			DS	Reo	Rotavirus
		Yes	SS+	Toga	Rubella (rubivirus)
				Flavi	Yellow fever
	Helical	Yes	SS+	Corona	Colds
			SS–	Orthomyxo	Influenza A, B and C
				Paramyxo	Mumps, measles
				Rhabdo	Rabies
	Complex	Complex	SS+	Retro	HIV, HTLV
DNA	Icosahedral	No	SS linear	Parvo	Aplastic anaemia
			DS circular	Papova	Papilloma virus
			DS linear	Adeno	Colds
		Yes	DS linear	Herpes	Herpes simplex
					Varicella zoster
					Cytomegalovirus
					Epstein–Barr virus
			DS circular	Hepadna	Hepatitis B
	Complex	Complex	DS linear	Pox	Smallpox

SS = single strand; DS = double strand.

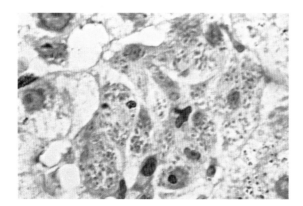

Figure 3.10   Leishmania

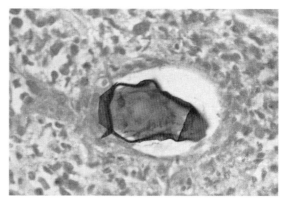

Figure 3.11   Schistosome

OTHER ORGANISMS

Helminths

Helminths, or worms, can usually be seen by the naked eye. They may be round (**nematodes**) or flat (**platyhelminths**).

Fungi

Fungi are eukaryotic cells requiring an aerobic environment. Athlete's foot is common, but life-threatening fungal infection is relatively rare unless a person is immunosuppressed.

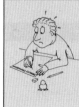

Give examples of protozoa that cause human disease

Organism	Disease
*†*Toxoplasma gondii*	Cerebral,ocular, lymphoid and lung damage
Plasmodium (falciparum, vivax, ovale and malariae)	Malaria
Leishmania (various)	Cutaneous and visceral leishmaniasis
Trypanosoma (various)	Sleeping sickness and Chagas' disease
*†*Pneumocystis carinii*	Interstitial pneumonia
Entamoeba histolytica *Giardia lamblia* * Cryptosporidia * Isospora	Diarrhoea
* Acanthamoeba *Naegleri fowleri*	Amoebic meningitis
Trichomonas	Vaginal discharge

People with defective immune systems are more liable to have significant problems with the organisms marked *. The problems often relate to reactivation because the immune defences are reduced rather than there being a primary infection †.

Give examples of helminths that cause human disease

Helminth	Disease
Platyhelminths	
Schistosoma (various)	Schistosomiasis (liver, lung, gut and bladder damage)
Echinococcus	Hydatid disease
Taenia solium, *Taenia saginata* and *Diphyllobothrium latum*	Tapeworm infestation from pig, cow and fish
Nematodes	
Necator, Trichuris	Hookworm, whipworm (gut infestation)
Wucheria, Onchocerca	Elephantiasis, river blindness, filariasis

Subcellular infectious agents of uncertain significance

This is a short section, but we should flag up our ignorance concerning certain diseases and some

'infectious' particles. There is great interest in transmissible spongiform encephalopathies, which can produce progressive and fatal brain damage in humans (kuru), sheep (scrapie) and cows (bovine spongiform encephalopathy or 'mad cow' disease).

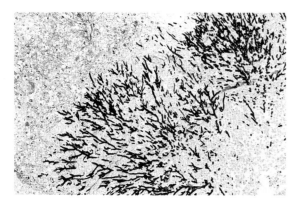

Figure 3.12 Aspergillus

They are experimentally and naturally transmissible with no viruses or bacteria detectable, and **prion proteins** have been proposed as the cause. These are naturally occuring proteins in most mammals that may be induced to change shape if a mutant or foreign prion protein enters the cell. It is still speculation, but the suggestion is that 'infected' animals have abnormally folded proteins in nerve cells that lead to cell death and the release of prions that enter adjacent cells. It appears that strains can vary in virulence. This all sounds similar to the case of viruses, but the particle is protein without any evidence of nucleic acid.

HOW DO MICROORGANISMS EVADE OUR DEFENCES?

Our defences can be thought of as first-line defences, such as a skin covering or the lining of

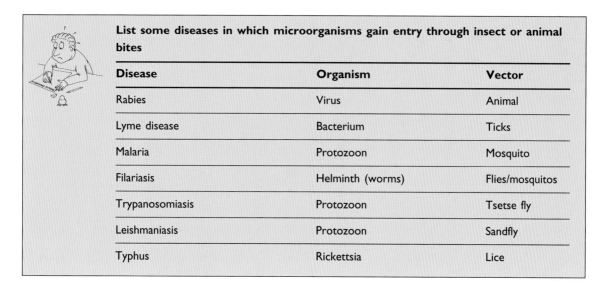

Give examples of fungi that cause human disease	
Fungus	**Disease**
Microsporum, Trichophyton (dermatophytes)	Ring worm, athlete's foot, etc.
Histoplasma capsulatum	Pneumonia or disseminated disease
Aspergillus (various)	Pneumonia or disseminated disease
Candida Cryptococcus Coccidioides	Disseminated disease in immunosuppressed individuals

List some diseases in which microorganisms gain entry through insect or animal bites		
Disease	**Organism**	**Vector**
Rabies	Virus	Animal
Lyme disease	Bacterium	Ticks
Malaria	Protozoon	Mosquito
Filariasis	Helminth (worms)	Flies/mosquitos
Trypanosomiasis	Protozoon	Tsetse fly
Leishmaniasis	Protozoon	Sandfly
Typhus	Rickettsia	Lice

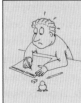

Discuss the mechanisms used by microbes to evade the immune system

Mechanism	Example
Shedding of antigens	*Schistosoma mansoni*
Changing antigens during infection	Neisseria altering pilins African trypanosomiasis
Many antigenic variants so no protective cross-immunity	*Rhinovirus* Influenza virus
Resistance to phagocytosis	Carbohydrate capsules of pneumococcus, Meningococcus and Haemophilus
Interference with antibodies or complement	Protein A molecules of Staphylococcus blocking Fc portion of immunoglobulin Digestion by proteases of Neisseria, Streptococcus and Haemophilus
Resistance to complement-mediated lysis	K antigens on some *E. coli*
Resistance to macrophage killing	Legionella, Mycobacterium and Toxoplasma inhibit acidification
Inaccessible to immune system	Gut luminal proliferation of *Clostridium difficile* Papilloma virus or fungi in superficial layer of skin Direct viral transfer between adjacent cells
Specific damage to immune cells	Pseudomonas secretes a leucotoxin to kill neutrophils
Mimicry of host antigens	Group A Streptococci and myocardium
Interference with MHC presentation of antigens	*Herpes simplex* inhibits peptide transporter CMV blocks MHC I presentation and expresses MHC I mimic
Bind to and inhibit cytokines	Vaccinia virus produces soluble interferon receptor
Immunosuppression	HIV, Epstein–Barr virus

the gut, and the second-line defences of the immune system.

Entry through intact skin is most easily achieved if there is an animal vector designed for the purpose. Many microorganisms associate with biting insects that pierce human skin and thus provide the route in. The rabies virus relies on larger animals, such as infected dogs or bats, to bite humans. In these examples, the microorganism itself does not have special characteristics for skin penetration, but some, such as the helminth larvae of hookworm or Schistosoma, have lytic proteases to allow them to digest and burrow through intact skin.

The digestive tract's acid and enzymes can be evaded by protective coverings, as in bacterial spores, protozoan cysts and thick-walled helminth eggs. Some parasites' eggs (e.g. those of Giardia) actually need stomach acid as a stimulus to cause them to hatch into the trophozoites that infect the intestine. Many of the non-enveloped viruses (hepatitis A, *Rotavirus*, *Reovirus* and Norwalk agents) are resistant to digestive juices, and bacteria can 'hide' in food to avoid the acidity. *Helicobacter pylori* is the only pathogen that survives in the stomach acid. It does this by producing a urease that converts urea to ammonia, thereby changing the pH of its microenvironment.

The respiratory tract's mucociliary defence may be impaired by hosts' own actions if they smoke or aspirate stomach acid. The mucin layer may be degraded by neuraminidase-producing microorganisms, and mucosal cilia can be paralysed by toxins produced by Haemophilus and Bordetella. Even if the mucociliary mechanisms are working well, some viruses can still avoid being expelled by having specific methods for adhesion to the epithelial surface, such as haemaglutinins on the influenza virus. Once the defences are damaged, for example by a bad cold or flu, bacterial pneumonias are common.

Many microorganisms avoid our second line of defences by not attempting to pass through the epithelial surface, instead being content to grow on the top. Skin fungi (dermatophytes, e.g. candida) and skin viruses (papilloma viruses causing warts) live in the superficial layers. Gut pathogens, such as *Vibrio cholera*, multiply in the mucus layer, releasing exotoxins that cause watery diarrhoea. Some bacteria cause us harm without even entering the body if they produce exotoxins that contaminate food (as in Staphylococci)

So the first line of defence has been breached, but the immune system and inflammatory mechanisms should still be able to defend us, shouldn't they? Thankfully, they normally do, but the microbes have some clever tricks to avoid them.

First, the immune system must spot the invader, so invaders change their surface antigens by shedding them, changing them during an infection or having numerous antigenic variants so that infective episodes do not produce useful immune memory. The next phase is killing the bugs by phagocytosis, complement-mediated lysis, antibody-mediated mechanisms or neutrophil activity.

Yes, you've guessed it: somewhere, there is a bug that will have evolved a way round each of these. A few examples are given in the 'written examination' box.

HOW DO MICROBES INVADE THE TISSUES?

Most bacteria are harmless, and those that cause human disease have evolved a series of weapons that can be coordinated through a group of genes. These weapons are called **virulence factors**. Having reached a suitable host site, the bacteria need to attach to the host cell; this is achieved through adhesion molecules (adhesins). These molecules can have a very broad specificity, such as hydrophobic lipoteichoic acids on some Gram-positive cells that can bind to all eukaryotic cells, or they can be very specific and determine **bacterial tropism**, i.e. direct the bacteria to the most favourable host environment. Adhesins can be like a glue over the whole surface of the cell or they can be on the tips of specialised projections called pili.

Unless the bacteria wants to remain on the surface, the next phase of virulence requires gaining entry to the cell or insinuating between the cells to lie in the tissue spaces. Bacteria produce a variety of enzymes (fibrinolysins, haemolysins, coagulases and hyaluronidases) capable of lysing

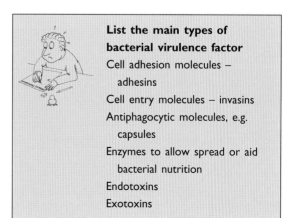

List the main types of bacterial virulence factor

Cell adhesion molecules – adhesins

Cell entry molecules – invasins

Antiphagocytic molecules, e.g. capsules

Enzymes to allow spread or aid bacterial nutrition

Endotoxins

Exotoxins

tissue components and possibly assisting invasion and spread. Some bacteria penetrate host cell walls, while others gain entry to the cell by encouraging endocytosis in the host cell. Once inside the cell in a phagosome, they can either use a haemolysin to digest the endocytotic vesicle and thus enter the cytoplasm, or they can replicate within the phagosome.

Pathogenic bacteria have evolved shared strategies for virulence in that they use similar modes of action or affect similar host target sites yet produce a range of different diseases. A good example is a family of bacterial proteins that are secreted by the bacteria and are targetted into the host's cell to modify or inactivate the cell in preparation for bacterial attachment or entry; in this way, the host's cell is prepared by the bacteria to the bacteria's advantage, truly a marvellous evolution of host–pathogen interaction. These types of secretory protein are called **Type III secretory proteins**, and they function as versatile weapons in the bacterial armoury, the proteins acting as multiple warhead missiles fired at the host's cells in a vanguard action against the hostile host. These bacterial protein systems are responsible for the pathogenicity of a range of bacteria that cause human diseases such as bubonic plague (*Yersinia pestis*) and diarrhoea (Shigella and Salmonella and *E. coli*) and can also be found in plant bacterial pathogens.

This suggests the acquisition of sets of genes encoding these protein systems and accounts for the evolution of pathogenic bacterial species. The genes for these protein warheads are clustered together in the genome as a sort of 'cassette' that can be swapped around between bacteria, acquired or deleted by the mechanisms of DNA exchange. Yersinia deploys Yersinia outer membrane proteins (YOPs) by this method to prevent phagocytosis by macrophages, whereas Salmonella and Shigella use it for the opposite purpose: to stimulate bacterial uptake by non-immune cells to create a safe intracellular haven for growth and spread and to avoid immune attack. Enteropathogenic *E. coli* use this system to alter host cell microfilaments to create an intracellular bundle of microfilaments that protrudes from the cell, upon which the bacteria attaches.

Other types of virulence determinants can be found in gene clusters or **pathogenicity islands**, found on mobile genetic elements such as plasmids, bacteriophages or transposons, and flanked by insertion sequences that direct their insertion or deletion from the genome. These can code for toxin complexes, type III secretory proteins or whole metabolic pathways that allow the synthesis of particular virulence determinants such as adhesins or polysaccharide capsules. These islands have been acquired during evolution from other bacteria, as evidenced by their percentage guanosine:cytosine ratios being different from those of the rest of the genome and are not found in non-pathogenic strains of closely related bacteria. Thus the cell biology of bacterial pathogenesis and the genetic structure of virulence genes show common strategies in host damage and present a model for the evolution of bacterial pathogens based on genetic exchange: bacterial genetic promiscuity rules OK.

Viruses also show tropism for particular cell types. Again, this is primarily determined by the surface receptors involved in adhesion; for example, the gp160 molecule on HIV binds to the CD4 molecule on helper T cells, *Rhinovirus* binds to ICAM-1 on mucosal cells, and the rabies virus attaches to the acetylcholine receptor on neurons.

Entry of the virus into the cell is similar in principle to bacterial mechanisms and involves one of three processes:

- translocation of the entire virus through the cell membrane
- fusion of the viral envelope with the cell membrane
- receptor-mediated endocytosis of the virus followed by fusion with the endosome membrane.

MECHANISMS OF CELL AND TISSUE DAMAGE

By now, you will have realised that, in any war, many innocent bystanders get hurt. The bugs need

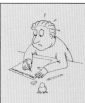

List the main sources and effects of bacterial toxins

Toxin	Bacteria	Effect
Endotoxin	Gram-negative lipopolysaccharide	Fever and inflammatory cell stimulation
Exotoxins		
Neurotoxins	*Clostridium tetani* *Clostridium botulinum*	Disordered neuromuscular transmission (tetanus and botulism)
Enterotoxins (infectious diarrhoea)	*Vibrio cholera, E. coli* *Bacillus cereus*	Diarrhoea
Enterotoxins (food poisoning)	*Staphylococcus aureus* *Bacillus cereus*	Diarrhoea and vomiting
Tissue-invasive toxins	*Staphylococcus aureus* *Streptococcus pyogenes* *Clostridium perfringens*	Tissue destruction by enzymes
Pyrogenic toxins	*Staphylococcus aureus* *Streptococcus pyogenes*	Toxic shock syndrome Scarlet fever
Verotoxins	*E. coli* (O157:H7)	Haemolytic uraemic syndrome
Miscellaneous	*Bordetella pertussis* *Corynebacterium diphtheria* *Clostridium difficile*	Whooping cough Diphtheria (heart and nerve damage) Pseudomembranous colitis

to survive, replicate and be shed to find new hosts. The normal flora or commensals manage this without causing damage, but the pathogens are greedy, have more weapons and provoke a conflict with the inflammatory and immune cells. Damage to the host cells occurs because of competition for nutrients, the release of inflammatory mediators and toxic substances by the host's inflammatory cells, the production of substances by the microbes that damage the host's tissues and direct cellular damage by bugs. Major bacterial weapons are endotoxin and exotoxins.

BACTERIAL ENDOTOXIN

Endotoxin is not secreted by living bacteria but is a cell wall component that is shed when the bacterium dies. It is lipid A, which is part of the LPS in the outer cell wall of Gram-negative bacte-

ria, and it causes fever and macrophage and B cell activation by inducing host cytokines. Only Gram-negative bacteria have endotoxin, the one exception being the Gram-positive *Listeria monocytogenes*.

Endotoxin is a potent stimulator of a wide range of immune responses. The recognition of LPS by the immune system spells drastic danger and warrants an immediate and dramatic response, which is often detrimental to the host itself. Clinically, this manifests itself as fever and vascular collapse or shock. Macrophages are stimulated by LPS to produce TNF and IL-1, which have many effects, including acting directly on the hypothalamus to produce fever. LPS also stimulates, directly or indirectly, the complement and clotting pathways and platelets to produce disseminated intravascular coagulation (DIC), thrombosis and shock. Shock results from increased vascular permeability produced by mediators from mast cells and platelets, combined with TNF and LPS affecting endothelial cells. LPS also stimulates the liver to produce acute phase proteins and hypoglycaemia.

BACTERIAL EXOTOXINS

Exotoxins are proteins released by living bacteria, and there is a wide variety with different actions. **Neurotoxins** act on nerves or end plates to produce paralysis, **cytotoxins** damage a variety of cells, **tissue-invasive toxins** are often enzymes capable of digesting host tissues, and **pyrogenic toxins** stimulate cytokine release and cause rashes, fever and toxic shock syndrome.

A very important group are the **enterotoxins**, which act on the gastrointestinal tract to produce diarrhoea by inhibiting salt absorption, stimulating salt excretion or killing intestinal cells. There are two broad categories: **infectious diarrhoea** and **food poisoning** with preformed toxin. In infectious diarrhoea, the bacteria proliferate in the gut, continuously releasing enterotoxin. The symptoms do not occur immediately after ingestion but require a day or two for the bugs to become established in sufficient numbers. In food poisoning, the bacteria grow in the food, releasing their exotoxin, which acts very quickly after ingestion to produce diarrhoea, abdominal pain and vomiting, although the symptoms only last for 24 hours because no new toxin is created.

Bacterial exotoxins may be classified by their site of action:

1. Extracellular, e.g. the epidermolytic toxin from *Staphylococcus aureus* that causes scalded skin syndrome
2. At the cell membrane (not being transported into cell but causing changes in intracellular cGMP), e.g. *E. coli* heat stable enterotoxin (ST) causing travellers' diarrhoea and *Staph. aureus* TSST 1 toxin, leading to toxic shock syndrome.
3. On the cell membrane, causing pore formation or disruption of lipid by enzymic activity e.g. phospholipase C activity arises from *Clostridium perfringens*. Pore-forming toxins (thiol activating haemolysins) are streptolysin

(*Strep. pyogenes*), pneumolysin (*Strep. pneumoniae*), listeriolysin (*Listeria monocytogenes*), perfringolysin (*Cl. perfringens*; gas gangrene) and cerolysin (*Bacillus cereus*; food poisoning).

4. Type III toxins, acting intracellularly by translocating an enzymic component across the membrane (the A subunit), which modifies a target molecule in the cytoplasm. These can be grouped by the type of enzymic activity:
   (a) ADP-ribosylation: cholera, diphtheria and pertussis
   (b) N-glycosidases: shiga toxin
   (c) glucosyl transferases: *Cl. difficile* toxins A and B
   (d) Zn^{2+}-requiring endopeptidases: tetanus and botulism toxins.

GTP-binding proteins are often the target for ADP-ribosylation by type III bacterial exotoxins. These proteins are involved in signal transduction and the regulation of cellular function by either cAMP levels or kinase cascades, leading to transcription modification. For example:

- G proteins (stimulatory or inhibitory on adenyl cyclase) – cholera, pertussis, *E. coli* LT toxin
- elongation factor 2 (translational control) – diphtheria toxin
- rho proteins (small G proteins that regulate the actin cytoskeleton) – these can be inactivated by *Cl. difficile* A and B toxins and also activated by deamination by pertussis necrotising toxin.

The structure of these toxins consists either of A:B5 (enzyme active A subunit and five B subunits required for binding) or A:B type with A (enzyme active) and B (binding) domains on a single polypeptide chain. A:B5 types are seen in cholera and pertussis, and *E. coli* LT1 and LT2. A:B type occurs in diphtheria, botulism and tetanus.

An interesting phenomenon of toxin structure and function in human disease is seen in the neurotoxins of *Cl. tetani* and *Cl. botulinum*, which cause tetanus and botulism respectively. These diseases are purely a result of toxin-mediated action following infection and are quite different in pathology, yet the molecular action of the two toxins is identical. They are both endopeptidases specific for synaptobrevin, a protein found in the cytoplasm of synaptic vesicles. However, the

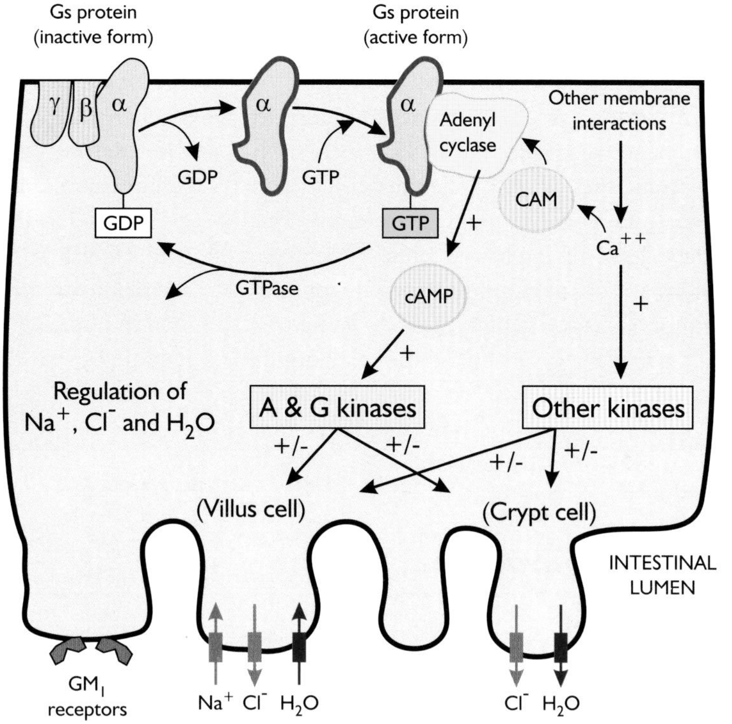

Gs protein
(inactive form)

Gs protein
(active form)

BASOLATERAL
MEMBRANE

Other membrane
interactions

Normal state

Activation of Gs proteins in
the basolateral intestinal cell
membrane by the addition of
GTP leads to the production
of cAMP via adenyl cyclase.
Together with calcium, cAMP
controls intracellular kinases
which regulate sodium,
chloride and water levels in
the cell. Any excess passes
into the intestinal lumen

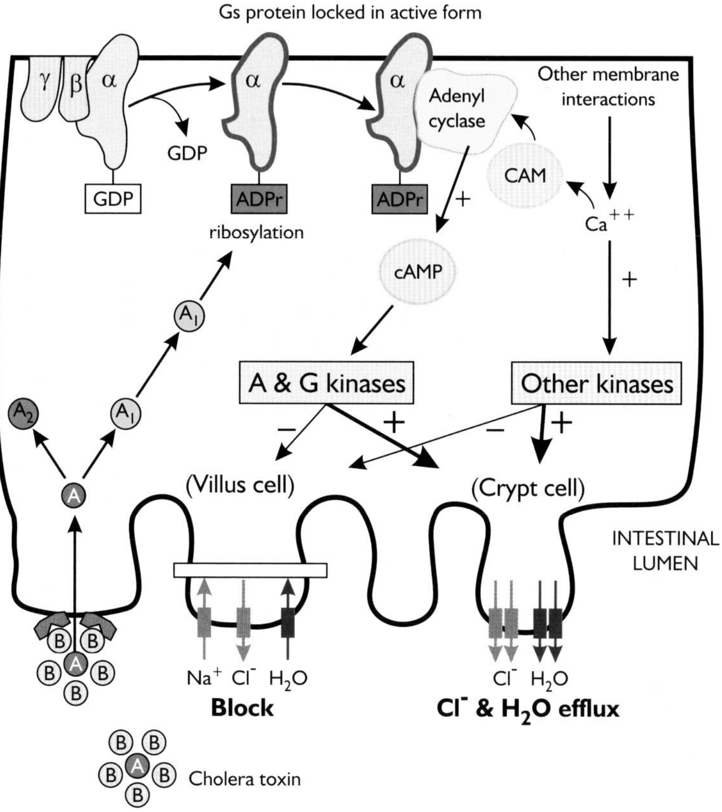

Regulation of
Na^+, Cl^- and H_2O

A & G kinases

Other kinases

(Villus cell)

(Crypt cell)

INTESTINAL
LUMEN

GM_1
receptors

Na^+ Cl^- H_2O

Cl^- H_2O

Gs protein locked in active form

5. The net result is an anti-
absorptive effect at the villus
cell and a secretory effect at
the crypt cell level, causing
severe diarrhoea

4. The altered subunit cannot
be 'switched off' by the
normal enzymic mechanism
and there is an uncontrolled
increase in cAMP

3. The A1 enzyme causes
ADP ribosylation of the
alpha subunit of the Gs
protein complex

2. The A unit is translocated
across the membrane and
splits to form an active
enzyme (A1 component)

1. Cholera toxin: one A and
5 B subunits, the latter
attaching via GM_1
ganglioside receptors on
the intestinal cell

Other membrane
interactions

ribosylation

cAMP

A & G kinases

Other kinases

(Villus cell)

(Crypt cell)

INTESTINAL
LUMEN

Na^+ Cl^- H_2O
Block

Cl^- H_2O
Cl^- & H_2O efflux

Cholera toxin

Figure 3.13   Intestinal cell in the normal state and affected by cholera toxin

binding (B) domains of the toxins show different specificities for cell receptors. Tetanus toxin binds to the gangliosides of the neuronal membrane, is internalised and moves by retroaxonal transport from peripheral nerves to the CNS, where it is released from the postsynaptic dendrites and localises in presynaptic nerve terminals. This blocks the release of inhibitory neurotransmitter, γ-aminobutyric acid to cause unopposed, continuous excitatory synaptic activity, leading to *spastic* paralysis. Botulism toxin binds the ganglioside receptors of cholinergic synapses and prevents the release of acetylcholine at the neuromuscular junctions, causing *flaccid* paralysis.

DIRECT CELL DAMAGE

Microorganisms can also damage cells directly, this being particularly true of viruses. You will recall that viruses are obligate intracellular organisms requiring the host cell's machinery for replication. We have already described the three main methods that viruses use for entering cells, so what happens once they are inside the cell?

First, the particle must uncoat and separate its genome from its structural components. It then uses specific enzymes of its own or ones present in the host cell to synthesise viral genome, enzyme and capsid proteins. These must be assembled and released, either directly (unencapsulated viruses) or by budding through the host cell's membrane (encapsulated viruses).

The virus can damage the host cell in a variety of ways:

- interference with host cell synthesis of DNA, RNA or proteins (e.g. polio virus modifying ribosomes so that they no longer recognise *host* mRNA)
- lysis of host cells (e.g. poliovirus lyses neurons)
- inserting proteins into the host cell membrane, thus provoking an immune attack by host cytotoxic lymphocytes (e.g. hepatitis B and liver cells)
- inserting proteins into the host cell membrane to cause direct damage or promote cell fusion (e.g. herpes, measles and HIV)

- transforming host cells to make them malignant (e.g. EBV, papilloma virus and HTLV-1)
- secondary effects of damage:
  – increased susceptibility to infection by damaging defences (e.g. viral damage to respiratory epithelium facilitates bacterial pneumonia, HIV depletes CD4+ T cells, allowing opportunistic infections)
  – death or atrophy of cells dependent on the viral-damaged cell (e.g. muscle cells after motorneuron damage by polio).

Viral infection can be:
- persistent – virions synthesised continuously, e.g. hepatitis B
- latent – virions temporarily inactive, e.g. herpes zoster in dorsal root ganglia
- abortive – incomplete viral replication

HOW DO BACTERIA DEVELOP ANTIBIOTIC RESISTANCE?

There is a wide range of antimicrobials that are beyond the scope of this book. The general principle is that of **selective toxicity**, i.e. you need to exploit differences between the microbe and the host so that you kill one without harming the other. Unfortunately, the bugs do not give up when we develop antibiotics but fight back. This is now a battle between the medics and the microbes. How does the bug develop resistance? How does it share its success with other bacteria? What can the pharmacologist and doctor do to prevent or overcome resistance?

Bacterial resistance can occur not only through spontaneous mutation but also commonly by the transfer of resistance from other bacteria. The mechanism may be in continuous operation (constitutive) or may be switched on in the presence of the antibiotic (inducible).

Enzymatic action against penicillin is common in both Gram-positive and Gram-negative bacteria, and may be coded for in the bacterial chromosome or on plasmids or transposons (see below). Altered bacterial membrane permeability in Gram-negative organisms by mutations in the **porins** (protein channels in the outer membrane) increases resistance to penicillins and some other antibiotics. Erythromycin and clindamycin resistance in Gram-positive organisms occurs by changing the ribosome, which is the target for the antibiotic. Drug-resistant enzymes can be produced when the antibiotic acts by blocking a metabolic pathway, e.g. trimethoprim.

HOW IS RESISTANCE PASSED TO OTHER BACTERIA?

The information for resistance is coded in the bacteria's DNA, so transfer of resistance involves the exchange of genetic fragments. This can occur in various ways:
• transformation
• transduction
• conjugation
• transposon insertions.
As well as antibiotic resistance, bacteria can also pass on information for exotoxins, enzymes and other virulence factors.

Transformation

Naked DNA fragments are released from a bacteria as it is lysed. These fragments then bind to the cell wall of another bacterium, are taken in and become incorporated into the recipient's DNA. This sounds simple, but it generally only occurs between closely related bacteria with similar DNA (i.e. extensive homology) and suitable binding sites on the cell wall.

Transduction

Bacteria can themselves be infected by viruses, called **bacteriophages**. These viruses bind to specific receptors on the bacterial surface and then push a tube through the wall and inject the viral nucleic acid. The virus (bacteriophage) can take over the bacterial cell's replication mechanism in the same way as viruses replicate in human cells. New capsid proteins, nucleic acid and enzymes are produced and assembled so that, when the bacterial cell lyses, the phages are released. This is what occurs with **virulent phages**, but there are also **temperate phages** that can insert their DNA into the host's DNA and lie dormant for long periods. These little time bombs eventually go off, replicate and lyse the host cell in a fashion similar to that of virulent phages, but the fact that they have inserted into the bacteria's DNA is relevant to our discussion of the transfer of resistance.

Generalised transduction involves virulent phages taking over the bacterial cell and accidentally packaging some bacterial DNA fragments instead of viral nucleic acid into one of the daughter phages. The mutant daughter phage will inject this bacterial DNA into the next cell it tries to infect, and the bacterial DNA may incorporate into the host cell DNA, comparable to the changes in transformation. The host cell survives happily because no viral nucleic acid is injected, and it may gain useful resistance or virulence factors depending on the source of the fragment of bacterial DNA.

Specialised transduction utilises temperate phages. When the phage DNA in the host genome (**prophage**) is reactivated, it is spliced out of the bacterial chromosome, replicated, translated and packaged into a capsid. The splicing may include taking some bacterial DNA immediately adjacent to the prophage, which will be incorporated into daughter phages. If the bacterial DNA confers resistance or virulence, this is a powerful method for sharing the information; it is called **lysogenic conversion**. The genes for exotoxin production by *Corynebacterium diphtheriae*, *Vibrio cholera* and *Strep. pyogenes* (scarlet fever) can spread in this way.

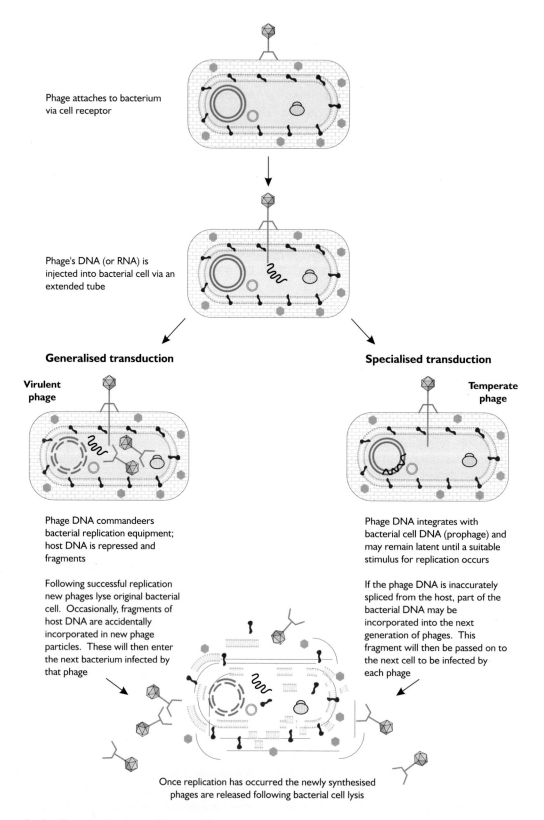

Phage attaches to bacterium via cell receptor

Phage's DNA (or RNA) is injected into bacterial cell via an extended tube

Generalised transduction

Virulent phage

Specialised transduction

Temperate phage

Phage DNA commandeers bacterial replication equipment; host DNA is repressed and fragments

Following successful replication new phages lyse original bacterial cell. Occasionally, fragments of host DNA are accidentally incorporated in new phage particles. These will then enter the next bacterium infected by that phage

Phage DNA integrates with bacterial cell DNA (prophage) and may remain latent until a suitable stimulus for replication occurs

If the phage DNA is inaccurately spliced from the host, part of the bacterial DNA may be incorporated into the next generation of phages. This fragment will then be passed on to the next cell to be infected by each phage

Once replication has occurred the newly synthesised phages are released following bacterial cell lysis

Figure 3.14 Transduction by viral bacteriophage

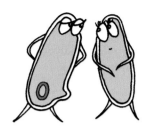

Plasmid determining, for example, penicillin resistance, is present in one bacterium (factor positive, F+ve). A sex pilus forms in the F+ve cell

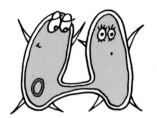

The sex pilus connects the F+ve and F-ve bacteria

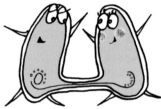

DNA from the plasmid is transferred. Complementary nucleotides are added, forming a complete plasmid in each bacterium

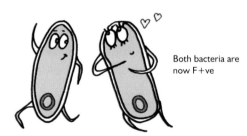

Both bacteria are now F+ve

Figure 3.15 Bacterial conjugation

Conjugation

Conjugation is the major mechanism for the transfer of antibiotic resistance and involves the exchange of plasmids. **Plasmids** are circular, double-stranded DNA pieces separate from the chromosome that carry a variety of genes, including some for drug resistance and some coding for the enzymes and proteins needed for conjugation. These are called self-transmissible or F plasmids,

and bacteria can be F⁺ or F⁻ depending on whether they contain the plasmid.

Bacterial sex involves a specialised **sex pilus** protruding from the surface of an F⁺ bacterium. This binds to and penetrates the cell membrane of a F⁻ bacterium and a single strand of the F plasmid DNA passes from one cell to the other.

The former F⁻ cell is now F⁺ and has the information for resistance and for conjugation with other cells. The plasmid DNA is not totally fixed but can acquire additional bacterial genes if it integrates into the bacterial chromosome in a fashion similar to that of a temperate bacteriophage, i.e. when it is spliced out of the host chromosome, it includes some of the adjacent bacterial DNA and is called an **F prime** (F′) plasmid. An alternative is that the bacterial chromosome with the incorporated plasmid is all transferred to the F⁻ cell during conjugation.

Plasmids encode medically important enzymes, such as penicillinase, and virulence factors, such as exotoxin and fimbriae.

Transposons

Transposons are also DNA fragments that can carry genes for resistance and virulence, but they differ in that they can insert into host DNA that is dissimilar (i.e. lacks homology), so spreading resistance across bacterial genera. They can insert into phages, plasmids and bacterial DNA.

How can we prevent or overcome bacterial resistance?

Life is a struggle, a struggle for survival, and the animal, plant or microorganism best adapted to a particular environment is most likely to flourish. Humans can have an enormous impact on the environment, and we must use this ability with care. In this context, we are concerned that we might alter the microbes' environment in order to give the resistant bacteria a survival advantage. In the extreme case, if everyone were taking a particular antibiotic, only microbes resistant to that drug would survive, so that specific environmental niche would become populated with resistant bugs and the antibiotic would be useless. This is the fear with tuberculosis as the incidence of dormant multiple drug-resistant tuberculosis increases. Of course, we do not have everyone taking the same antibiotic, and we have to hope that the non-resistant bugs will predominate when the antibiotic is stopped.

Problems occur when antibiotics are widely used, particularly in a hospital setting, and the resistant bug gains a clear advantage. We shall consider methicillin-resistant *Staph. aureus* (MRSA) as an important example of how man and microbe each develop strategies to defy the other. *Staphylococcus aureus* is a Gram-positive coccus that was originally sensitive to penicillin. By the 1950s the bug had developed enzymes (β-lactamases) to destroy penicillin. Man then produced a penicillin analogue called methicillin, with a side chain that reduced the binding to the enzyme. Further development led to the widely used flucloxacillin, so man had the upper hand until the late 1970s and early 80s, when *Staph. aureus* strains resistant to multiple antibiotics, including methicillin and gentamycin, emerged. These bugs are an enormous problem in hospitals, particularly on surgical wards where wound infections are a major concern. The only effective drug against such Staphylococci is vancomycin, which is somewhat toxic and requires intravenous administration. The recent identification of vancomycin-resistant enterococci in a patient with MRSA has set the scene for the nightmare scenario in which resistance to vancomycin may be transferred from the enterococci to the MRSA, both of which may be found in the gut or surgical wounds. A truly 'superbug' MRSA would then be unstoppable. It is just a matter of time, since nothing we have done with antibiotics suggests we can contain such an event.

There are three main strategies for trying to avoid or overcome bacterial resistance:
- the control of antibiotic use
- the modification of existing antibiotics or the development of new antibiotics capable of bypassing the bacteria's method of resistance
- the use of combinations of antibiotics employing different mechanisms.

The best approach is preventative. If antibiotics are used less and are only used appropriately, resistant strains are less likely to evolve. This means that there should be great caution about using antibiotics as growth promoters in animal feeds for fear that this will result in resistant bugs that may be transferred to humans. In humans, antibiotics should not be used unnecessarily, and care should be taken to avoid incomplete treatment. Incomplete treatment is a problem in tuberculosis, in which lengthy treatment with multiple drugs may be necessary to eradicate the organisms but patient compliance may be poor. Incomplete treatment will allow the most resistant bug to survive, regrow and spread to other susceptible individuals. Multiple drug-resistant tuberculosis strains now represent more than 20% of cases in parts of New York and are now being found in Europe and the UK. Common sense also demands that, particularly in hospitals, the transfer of bugs from one patient to another must be minimised, which requires special attention to the disinfection of endoscopes, bronchoscopes, etc., which cannot be autoclaved.

The second strategy involves developing new drugs or modifying existing ones. The idea is that once the mechanism for bacterial resistance is understood, it should be possible to redesign the molecule to get around the problem. We have already mentioned the example of methicillin, with its side chain to prevent it from binding to the enzyme β-lactamase. Another example involves the tetracyclines, which have little effect on bugs that have developed a highly efficient mechanism for excreting the drug from the bacterial cell through specific 'efflux proteins'. A new group of tetracyclines called glycylcyclines have an altered side chain that prevents their excretion via efflux proteins.

The third approach is to use combinations of antibiotics. Sometimes the combinations have been developed empirically, but there are examples of deliberately designing combinations to overcome resistance. This is the case with clavulanic acid, which is only a weak antibiotic but binds irreversibly to many β-lactamases and can thus protect β-lactam antibiotics from destruction. This is used clinically as Augmentin, which is a combination of amoxycillin and clavulanic acid.

How do viruses develop resistance to antiviral agents?

Viruses also become resistant to antiviral agents through the selection of naturally occurring mutants, which have amino acid changes at the active site or binding site of the antiviral agent. This is only normally seen in immunocompromised hosts, in whom the number of viral particles (viral load) is high, thus increasing the chances of a natural mutant occurring. Viruses have small genomes (HIV = 9 kb; herpes = 500 kb; bacteria = 3 Mb; human = 4000 Mb), so the chance of a mutant occurring is dependent on the number of virions and the size of the genome. HIV is a good example of this, in terms of both drug resistance and immune evasion.

The first part of HIV replication is the conversion of its RNA genome into DNA prior to integration into the host cell chromosome as proviral DNA. This reaction is unique to retroviruses and is mediated by the virally encoded RNA-dependent DNA polymerase – reverse transcriptase (RT).

RT is the target for the antiviral drug AZT used in the treatment of AIDS. AZT is an analogue of thymidine with an azide group at the 3′ OH group of the ribose moeity. When incorporated into the DNA by RT, AZT causes chain termination and stops DNA synthesis, thus halting the viral life cycle. Fortunately, AZT has higher affinity for RT than for cell-encoded DNA polymerases, hence its

selective toxicity. AZT-resistant HIV mutants have amino acid substitutions in the active site, so AZT no longer binds. The RT of HIV does not possess any proofreading activity, as seen in cellular DNA polymerases, and has an error rate of 10^{-4}; i.e. it makes a mistake every 10 000 bases, which is about once every time a genome is copied. Thus, if 10^8 virions were made, there would be a chance for each base to be changed in the viral progeny (genome size = 9000 bases). During HIV infection, about 10^9 virions are made and destroyed by the immune system every day, so it is easy to see that a random mutation in the active site of RT is highly likely. The use of AZT selects out the resistant mutant, which continues to replicate and spread within the body; thus AZT resistance can emerge readily in a few months or less. Combined anti-HIV chemotherapy is now used that includes several anti-RT compounds and a protease inhibitor, because it is much less likely that any one virus will acquire mutations in two or three separate sites to affect the binding and activity of all of the inhibitors. HIV also uses this natural mutation rate to its advantage to change the amino acid sequences of its exterior glycoprotein (gp120), which binds the cell CD4 receptor. The V3 region of gp120 shows epitope changes in isolates from the same patient infected with HIV, and these have been shown to permit escape from a cytotoxic T cell immune response. Thus the RT error rate provides a mechanism for generating immune escape mutants and drug resistance.

It is hardly surprising that chronic infection is still a challenge, and the next chapter is devoted to the topic of chronic inflammation, which includes conditions of infective and immune aetiology.

ACKNOWLEDGEMENT

Special thanks are due to Dr Philip Butcher of the Microbiology Department at St George's Hospital Medical School for assisting in the writing of this chapter.

CHAPTER 4

CHRONIC AND GRANULOMATOUS INFLAMMATION

- Tuberculosis
- Sarcoidosis
- Macrophages in specific diseases

Chronic inflammation differs from acute inflammation in a number of respects. Apart from the generally longer duration of the process, the main features of chronic inflammation are:

- a mononuclear cell infiltrate composed of macrophages, lymphocytes and plasma cells
- tissue destruction
- granulation tissue formation, i.e. the proliferation of fibroblasts and small blood vessels (this is not the same as a granuloma)
- fibrosis.

Granulomatous inflammation is a special type of chronic inflammation, characterised by the presence of granulomata. A granuloma is a collection of macrophages frequently surrounded by a rim of lymphocytes. These macrophages are usually modified to become larger with more abundant pink cytoplasm and are referred to as 'epithelioid' cells.

The factors influencing granuloma formation are largely unknown, but a variety of cytokines appears to be involved. Animal experiments suggest that IL-1 is important in the initiation of granulomata and that TNF is responsible for their maintainance. IL-2 has been shown to increase their size, and IL-5 attracts eosinophils to the granulomata seen in parasitic disease. IL-6 is believed to have an important role in tuberculous granulomata.

Chronic inflammatory disorders are some of the most common, fascinating, devastating and

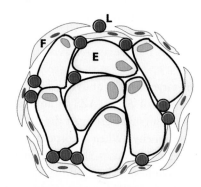

Group of epithelioid cells (E), with variable numbers of lymphocytes (L) and fibroblasts (F)

Figure 4.1   Non-caseating granuloma

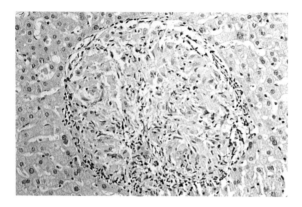

Figure 4.2 Non-caseating granuloma from a patient with sarcoidosis

mysterious diseases to affect mankind. They include tuberculosis, sarcoidosis, syphilis, leprosy, Crohn's disease, rheumatoid arthritis, systemic lupus erythematosus and the pneumoconioses. Despite the availability of treatment and some information on prevention, tuberculosis remains a significant worldwide problem. For this reason (and because it turns up in examinations with frightening regularity), we shall discuss this disorder as an example of a chronic granulomatous inflammatory disease.

TUBERCULOSIS

The great German bacteriologist Robert Koch was the first to show that tuberculosis is an infective disease, a fact we now take for granted. Koch's original investigations (1876) were performed with anthrax, which he demonstrated to be the cause of what was then known as 'splenic fever'. It was clear to Koch that, in order to implicate a particular organism as the cause of a disease, he must:

- demonstrate the organism in the lesions in all cases of that disease
- be able to isolate the organism and cultivate it in pure culture outside the host
- produce the same disease by injecting the pure culture into a healthy subject.

These three criteria are known as **Koch's postulates**.

On 24 March 1882 Koch announced the discovery of the tubercle bacillus to the Berlin Physiological Society. His work proved that 'pulmonary consumption' was not a disorder of nutrition but an infective disease that ran a chronic course. Although Koch is best remembered for his contribution to tuberculosis, he did not confine his interests to that disease. He discovered the cholera vibrio that had created havoc from India to Egypt, investigated bubonic plague in India, researched diseases caused by the tsetse fly in East Africa and studied malaria in Java.

Tuberculosis is a worldwide problem and is caused by *Mycobacterium tuberculosis*, sometimes called the 'Koch Bacillus'. Two strains – *M. tuberculosis hominis* and *M. tuberculosis bovis* – infect humans. Bovine tuberculosis is passed from cattle to humans in milk so that it enters through the gastrointestinal tract to produce abdominal tuberculosis. It is uncommon in developed countries now that dairy herds are generally free of mycobacteria and milk is pasteurised. Infection with *M. hominis* is the common form and produces pulmonary tuberculosis.

Tuberculosis is more common in the young and the very old, and there are definite racial and ethnic differences in incidence. It is more common in Asians, American Indians, Africans, the Irish and Eskimos. It also flourishes in socially deprived areas, poverty and malnutrition appearing to be important predisposing factors. There is a higher incidence in males and in people suffering from alcoholism, chronic lung diseases and conditions causing immunosuppresion, e.g. cancer and AIDS. Patients with tuberculosis may present with a cough producing bloodstained sputum, or more subtly, with night sweats, weight loss and vague symptoms of ill-health.

Mycobacterium tuberculosis is a slender, rod-shaped organism, approximately 4 μm in length. It is not visible on haemotoxylin and eosin stained sections but can be stained using the Ziehl-Neelsen method. This reaction relies on the fact that, once stained, the organisms are resistant to decolourisation with acid and alcohol (hence the term acid and alcohol fast bacilli: AAFB). Mycobacteria grow very slowly in culture and may not be apparent for

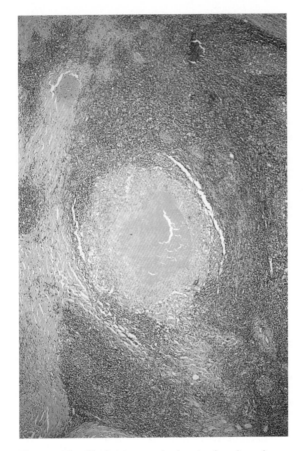

Figure 4.3 Photomicrograph showing lymph node with caseous necrosis

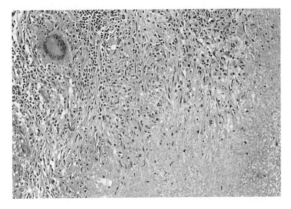

Figure 4.4 Higher power view to show necrosis and Langhan-type giant cell

6 weeks. Observing the bacilli in excised tissues will allow faster diagnosis and treatment, but they will not be seen in sections unless there are approxi-

mately one million bacteria per millilitre of tissue. Using a polymerase chain reaction (see p. 301) to detect mycobacterial nucleic acid is both reasonably fast and more sensitive but technically more difficult and not generally available.

Mycobacterium tuberculosis does not possess any toxins with which to harm its host; however, a number of cell membrane glycolipids and proteins, including bacterial stress proteins, act to provoke a hypersensitivity reaction. It is the hypersensitivity reaction that causes the tissue destruction that is so characteristic of this disease.

PRIMARY TUBERCULOSIS

This occurs in individuals who have never previously been infected with *M. tuberculosis*.

Inhalation of the organism produces a small lesion (approximately 1 cm in diameter), usually in the subpleural region in the lower part of the upper lobe or the upper part of the lower lobe. This is referred to as the **Ghon focus**. Lesions occur in these sites because the bacterium is a strict aerobe and prefers these well-oxygenated regions. When the tissue is first invaded by the Mycobacteria, there is no hypersensitivity reaction but instead an initial acute, non-specific, inflammatory response with neutrophils predominating. This is rapidly followed by an influx of macrophages that ingest the bacilli and present their antigens to T lymphocytes, leading to the proliferation of a clone of T cells and the emergence of specific hypersensitivity. The lymphocytes release lymphokines, which attract more macrophages. These accumulate to form the characteristic granuloma, containing a mixture of macrophages, including epithelioid cells and Langhan-type giant cells. Tissue destruction leads to necrosis in the centre of the granuloma, called **caseous necrosis** because, macroscopically, the necrotic area resembles cheesy material. Tubercle bacilli, either free or contained in macrophages, may drain to the regional lymph nodes and set up granulomatous inflammation, causing massive lymph node enlargement. The combination of the Ghon focus and the regional nodes is called the **primary complex**.

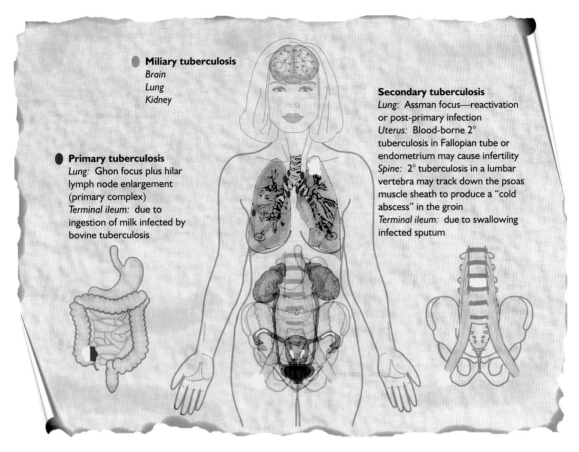

Miliary tuberculosis
Brain
Lung
Kidney

Secondary tuberculosis
Lung: Assman focus—reactivation or post-primary infection
Uterus: Blood-borne 2° tuberculosis in Fallopian tube or endometrium may cause infertility
Spine: 2° tuberculosis in a lumbar vertebra may track down the psoas muscle sheath to produce a "cold abscess" in the groin
Terminal ileum: due to swallowing infected sputum

Primary tuberculosis
Lung: Ghon focus plus hilar lymph node enlargement (primary complex)
Terminal ileum: due to ingestion of milk infected by bovine tuberculosis

Figure 4.5 Tuberculosis

Thus the development of hypersensitivity not only results in tissue destruction but also improves the body's resistance to the Mycobacterium by promoting phagocytosis and reducing the intracellular replication of bacilli. It is not known why the granulomatous response to mycobacteria produces caseation whereas most other granulomatous reactions do not. Another puzzle is why the attraction of macrophages in most inflammatory responses produces a dispersed infiltrate, while in granulomatous reactions they form well-demarcated collections – granulomata.

To return to our patient with tuberculosis and a Ghon focus; the next phase is that, in the majority of cases, this primary complex will heal. There will be replacement of the caseous necrosis by a small fibrous scar, and the lesion will be walled off. Calcification may also occur in these lesions. Despite this, the organisms may survive and lead to **reactivation infection** at a later date, especially if the host defences become lowered, as can occur with cancer.

There are, however, a number of alternative outcomes. If the hypersensitivity reaction is severe, it will lead to a florid inflammatory response, and the patient may present with a systemic illness. If the caseous necrosis is extensive, the tissue destruction may erode major bronchi and allow the airborne spread of organisms to produce satellite lesions in either lung. Alternatively, tubercle bacilli may enter the blood stream. If they enter a small pulmonary arteriole, the bacilli will lodge in lung tissue. However, if they enter a pulmonary vein, the bacilli may disseminate throughout the systemic circulation. If this occurs, numerous small granulomata may be encountered in almost any organ, including the meninges, kidneys and adrenals. This type of disease is called **miliary** tuberculosis, so called because the lesions look like millet seeds. Fortunately, systemic spread is not a common event in primary disease.

SECONDARY TUBERCULOSIS

Secondary, or post-primary, tuberculosis refers to infection occurring in a patient previously sensitised to mycobacteria. Most of these cases result from **reactivation** of latent mycobacteria following an asymptomatic primary infection. The latency period can vary tremendously, and reactivation may not occur for many decades. Occasionally, there is reinfection from an exogenous source.

Secondary infection tends to affect the subapical region of the upper lobe, and although the reasons for this are far from clear, it is believed to be due to the higher oxygen concentration in this area. (If you remember, tubercle bacilli are obligate aerobes.) This focus of reactivation is called the **Assman focus**. There are three possible outcomes of the secondary infection: healing, cavitation or spread.

Owing to the previous infection, the host will have some degree of immunity, and if this is sufficient, the infection will heal with **scarring** and subsequent **calcification**. Intervention with antituberculous drugs will also enhance and modify the healing process. If, on the other hand, the degree of hypersensitivity is high and/or the organisms are particularly virulent, there may be considerable lung parenchymal tissue destruction and caseous necrosis, which can lead to the formation of a **cavity**. The infected caseous material may spread through destroyed tissue, or via bronchi to adjacent parts of the lung, and extend the local disease. The pleura may become involved, with the production of an effusion that may contain caseous and necrotic material – **tuberculous empyema**. Infected sputum may be swallowed, spreading the disease to the gastrointestinal tract. Systemic spread to produce miliary tuberculosis is more common in post-primary tuberculosis because tissue destruction is greater.

The natural history of the disease will depend on the host's immunity, hypersensitivity and

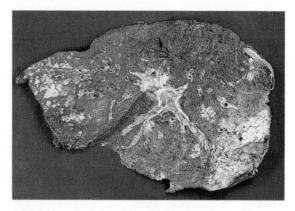

Figure 4.6 Cut surface of the lung showing white areas of caseation due to tuberculosis in the upper and lower lobes

factors such as nutritional status, associated disease and intervention with drugs. Tuberculosis is a treatable disease, yet, despite this, it remains a major problem in underdeveloped countries, and

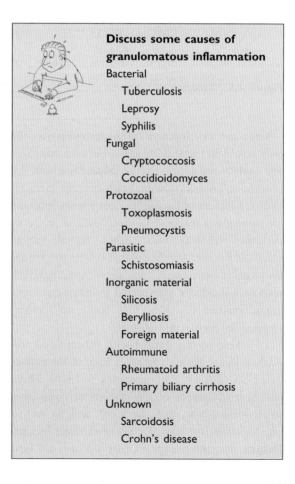

Discuss some causes of granulomatous inflammation
Bacterial
    Tuberculosis
    Leprosy
    Syphilis
Fungal
    Cryptococcosis
    Coccidioidomyces
Protozoal
    Toxoplasmosis
    Pneumocystis
Parasitic
    Schistosomiasis
Inorganic material
    Silicosis
    Berylliosis
    Foreign material
Autoimmune
    Rheumatoid arthritis
    Primary biliary cirrhosis
Unknown
    Sarcoidosis
    Crohn's disease

there is a worrying trend towards the development of antibiotic-resistant strains in the developed countries.

Some of the other causes of granulomatous inflammation are listed in the 'written examination' box. Many result from infections, some are of autoimmune aetiology, and sometimes we do not know the cause, as in the case of sarcoid.

SARCOIDOSIS

Sarcoidosis is a baffling systemic disease of unknown aetiology characterised by the presence of granulomata, which, unlike those of tuberculosis, do not exhibit caseous necrosis so are termed 'non-caseating granulomas'.

Sarcoidosis is a systemic disorder of variable severity, hence presenting in numerous ways. Patients are often asymptomatic, and diagnosis is only made at post mortem. Almost every organ in the body may be affected, the most common being lung, liver, spleen, skin and salivary glands, with the heart, kidneys and central nervous system being slightly less commonly affected. Most patients present with respiratory symptoms (shortness of breath, haemoptysis and chest pains), but some have a more rapid course with fever, erythema nodosum and polyarthritis. Patients may also present with the signs and symptoms of hypercalcaemia, and lytic bone lesions, especially

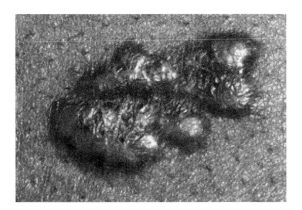

Figure 4.7 Raised skin lesion in sarcoidosis. Microscopy would show epithelioid granulomata

in the phalanges, are strong supportive evidence for the disease.

A tissue biopsy may be essential to make the diagnosis of granulomatous disease and can be helpful in elucidating the cause. The only way to be certain of the cause is either to see it under the microscope, for instance with fungal hyphae, or to culture the organism. However, some macrophage variants are more common in specific conditions.

MACROPHAGES IN SPECIFIC DISEASE

Epithelioid cells occur in all types of granulomatous disease. They have some resemblance to epithelial cells as they possess abundant pink cytoplasm, packed with endoplasmic reticulum, Golgi apparatus and vesicles. Thus the cells are well adapted to synthesise macrophage products, such as arachidonic acid metabolites, complement, coagulation factors and cytokines. However, they are less mobile and less proficient at phagocytosis than are ordinary macrophages. The **multinucleate giant macrophages** principally form by the fusion of epithelioid cells. Each may have 50 or more nuclei, and it is the arrangement of these nuclei that distinguishes the types. The **Langhan giant cell** is typical of tuberculosis or sarcoid and has its nuclei arranged as a horseshoe at the periphery. The **foreign body giant cell** is, predictably, associated with foreign material, which is sometimes identifiable in the cytoplasm. Its nuclei are randomly arranged throughout the cell. Foreign body giant cells are also seen in parasitic infections.

These are the most important macrophage variants, but, for completeness, we will mention two others. These are the **Warthin-Finkeldey** cell, pathognomonic of measles and characterised by the presence of eosinophilic nuclear and cytoplasmic inclusions, and **Touton giant cells**, which have a central cluster of nuclei surrounded by foamy lipid-laden cytoplasm. Touton cells occur in xanthomata, which are benign tumorous collections of lipid-laden macrophages in the skin.

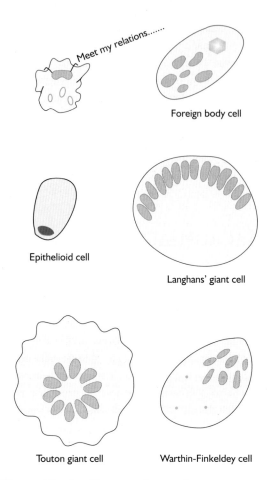

Meet my relations.......

Foreign body cell

Epithelioid cell

Langhans' giant cell

Touton giant cell

Warthin-Finkeldey cell

Figure 4.8 Specific types of macrophage

What roles can macrophages play in chronic inflammation?
- Antigen presentation to T cells and B cells, leading to clonal expansion
- Scavenging abnormal cells, particles, large molecules, immune complexes, etc.
- Chemotactic factors for other leucocytes
- Stimulating endothelium for adhesion molecule activation and granulation tissue formation
- Fusion with other macrophages to form giant cells
- Phagocytosis and the killing of some organisms
- Harbouring of some organisms
- Exocytosis for attacking parasites or damaging tissues

List the macrophage products involved in tissue injury

Toxic oxygen metabolites

Nitric oxide

Proteases

Eicosanoids

Coagulation factors

Neutrophil chemotactic factors

Having learnt about acute inflammation, chronic inflammation and the immune system, you will appreciate the complex interplay between cells and mediators. It is a veritable orchestra, but who is the conductor? As yet we do not know – perhaps there is not one – but a key player is undoubtedly the macrophage, and it is useful to summarise inflammation and repair by reviewing macrophage function.

Macrophages are involved in all stages of these processes, with their ability to phagocytose particles, process and present antigens and secrete an array of mediators. Macrophages are derived from stem cells in the bone marrow that also give rise to polymorphonuclear leucocyte precursors. The marrow cells produce monocytes that circulate in the blood for a day or two before migrating into the tissues, where they are called macrophages or (a more old-fashioned term) histiocytes. As well as entering areas of inflammation and damage, there are also relatively fixed macrophages lining the endothelial aspects of vessels in the liver (Kupfer cells), spleen, bone marrow and lymph nodes – the so-called **reticuloendothelial system**.

Just like neutrophils in acute inflammation, macrophages emigrate and activate under the influence of chemotactic factors, adhesion molecules, cytokines, etc. An activated macrophage increases its size and its lysosomal enzyme content and speeds up its metabolism and ability to phagocytose and kill microbes. A crucially important function is their ability to scavenge and phagocytose in areas of damage. Macrophages possess scavenger receptor molecules, which are important in self/non-self discrimination and appear able to bind to a wide range of modified molecules. Most important of these is modified low density lipoprotein (LDL), but modified albumin and probably also other molecules can also be bound and phagocytosed. Unlike LDL receptors on other tissue cells, these surface receptors are not downregulated as the LDL content of the cytoplasm increases. This means that macrophages keep taking up lipid, etc. and become foamy macrophages, seen in areas of tissue damage and atheromatous plaques (see p. 144).

Macrophages are also important because they synthesise and secrete factors that promote granulation tissue formation and enhance healing and repair. For example, macrophage-derived growth factor stimulates endothelial cells for new vessel formation, and fibroblasts for collagen and extracellular matrix production.

In acute insults, macrophages will assist in healing and repair and then depart. However, in chronic inflammation, they are potentially harmful because they produce a variety of substances that keep the inflammation going, attract and stimulate other inflammatory cells and contribute towards tissue injury and fibrosis. Their continued presence is due principally to continued emigration from the blood, a reduction in movement out of the tissues and some local proliferation.

CHAPTER 5

HEALING AND REPAIR

- Cell capacity for regeneration
- Wound healing
- Growth factors
- Modifying factors
- Improving wound healing
- Clinicopathological case study
- Further reading

When injury takes place and the process of inflammation is set in motion, the elements of repair and healing are also activated. For convenience, we discuss these after acute and chronic inflammation, but the process actually begins early on.

If your patient, injured while at work as the target half of a circus knife-throwing act, asks how long it will be before he or she can take the bandages off and return to the arena, what must you consider before answering? Briefly, the processes that take place during and after the injury are:

- **removal** of dead and foreign material
- **regeneration** of injured tissue from cells of the same type
- **replacement** of damaged tissue by new connective tissue.

Ideally, adequate tissue repair will occur within 3 weeks – we have, in Chapter 1, already seen an example of this in lobar pneumonia. The infection causes an inflammatory response that leads to cells and debris accumulating in alveoli. When these are removed by the macrophages and the lymphatics, we again have normal intact alveoli that can

participate in gas exchange. This process of restoring the tissue to pristine condition is called **resolution**. Resolution requires that the inflammatory process deals quickly with the insult, the tissue has not lost its basic scaffolding and any damaged specialised cells are capable of regeneration.

What happens if part of this system fails? In this case, other mechanisms must operate, and, although healing may still take place, the result will not be perfect. If the exudate is not cleared, it will be **organised**; this means that there is an ingrowth of capillaries and fibroblasts, called **granulation tissue**, which leads to the production of fibrous connective tissue, i.e. a scar.

CELL CAPACITY FOR REGENERATION

What happens when injury causes loss of normal tissue and leaves a defect, for example a cut in the skin? In this situation, the end result depends on

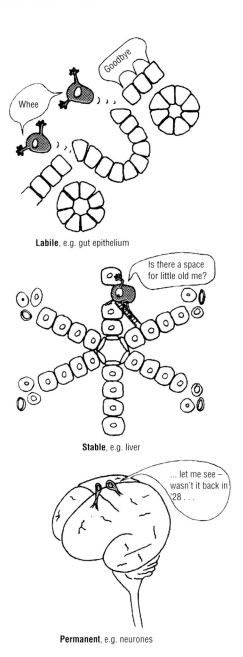

Figure 5.1 Cell capacity for regeneration

cells have a set life span. **Stable** cells normally divide extremely slowly but can proliferate rapidly if required: if you remove half the liver, the cells will regenerate and return it to its original size. Other examples of stable cells are fibroblasts, vascular endothelial cells, smooth muscle cells, osteoblasts and renal tubular epithelial cells. **Permanent** cells cannot divide but may be capable of some individual cell repair if the nucleus and synthetic apparatus are intact. Examples include neurons and cardiac muscle cells. If a permanent cell is damaged but not destroyed, as in injury to a nerve axon, there may be regrowth of the damaged portion. However, if the whole cell is destroyed, it must be replaced by a small scar because its neighbouring cells are incapable of proliferating to replace it.

WOUND HEALING

The size of the defect is very important as any destruction of the tissue scaffold will result in scarring. Figure 5.3 illustrates the healing of a large skin wound.

The damage to the small blood vessels causes haemorrhage, which helps to 'glue' the edges together and provides the protective dry surface scab (a). First, neutrophils migrate from the vessels to the damaged area, and epidermal cells proliferate at the surface. Within 24–48 hours, the epidermal cells grow underneath the scab to form a thin but complete layer. Meanwhile, there is an influx of macrophages, a proliferation of fibroblasts and an ingrowth of many fine capillaries (granulation tissue) (b). At this stage, there is a temporary matrix of type III collagen. Epithelial migration halts by contact inhibition and a definitive matrix (type I collagen) is laid down. The vessels and inflammatory cells reduce in number (c). By day 5, bundles of collagen have been laid down across the damaged tissue to form a scar, and the epidermis has returned to normal thickness (d).

The scar is initially red, because of the increase in small vessels, but it will blanch over the next few weeks as the vessels regress and the collagen

the size of the defect and the capacity of the tissue to regenerate. Not all tissues of the body have the same capacity to regenerate, and cells can be divided into three major types: labile, stable and permanent.

The **labile** cells include epithelial and blood cells; these divide and proliferate throughout life and the

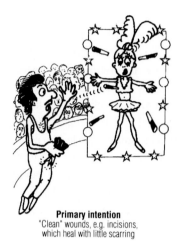

Primary intention
"Clean" wounds, e.g. incisions,
which heal with little scarring

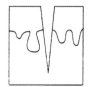 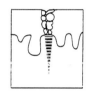

Figure 5.2 Healing by primary intention

thickens. If the cut is fine and there is good wound apposition, the scar tissue is limited and the cosmetic result good, but how strong is the repair? Immediately after surgery, the wound has around 70 per cent of the strength of normal skin, but this is principally conferred by the sutures. When these are removed, after 7–10 days, the wound strength drops to 10 per cent of normal, a point to emphasise to patients. Strength then increases rapidly over the next month to reach a maximum at around 3 months, when a well-healed scar will have 70–80 per cent of the tensile strength of uninjured skin. Interestingly, the strength does not correlate with the amount of collagen but may be related to the type, type I being stronger than the type III deposited early in the repair process.

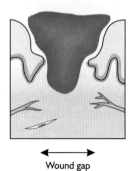

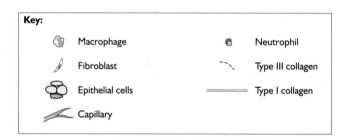

Key:

Macrophage		Neutrophil	
Fibroblast		Type III collagen	
Epithelial cells		Type I collagen	
Capillary			

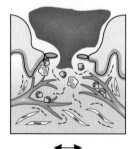 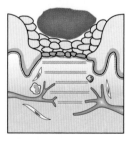 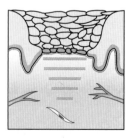

Wound gap   Wound gap

a. Fibrin clot

b. Day 1–2: cellular infiltrate, temporary matrix, wound contraction, epithelial migration, clot dissolution

c. Day 3–4: surface intact, new basement membrane, definitive matrix

d. Day 5: scar

Figure 5.3 Healing by secondary intention

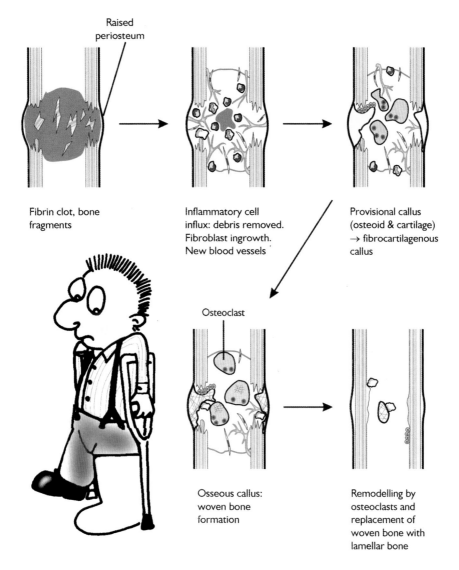

Figure 5.4   Bone healing

HEALING BY PRIMARY AND SECONDARY INTENTION

When the wound is sharp and clean, the healing is termed healing by primary intention. One in which there is a large tissue defect heals by secondary intention. The processes are the same as described above, but the sharp wound heals with little scarring, whereas with large wound defects there is a more intense inflammatory reaction and a larger amount of granulation tissue. There is also contraction of the wound, an intriguing phenom-

enon thought to be produced by myofibroblasts, which, as the name implies, have features of both fibroblasts and smooth muscle cells.

Granulation tissue production is a fascinating process common to all forms of repair. Fibroblast growth factors (FGFs; see also later) stimulate the endothelial cells of capillaries and postcapillary venules to secrete proteases that digest the surrounding basement membrane. The endothelial cells then proliferate to produce a bud of cells protruding through the gap in the wall towards the source of the stimulus. At first, the bud of endothelial cells is solid, but it eventually canalises to allow the flow of blood, although quite how the circulatory loop is completed is not known.

Most wounds, whether of skin or internal organs, will heal in this way, an interesting exception being bone. This breaks the rules and does not heal with a fibrous scar. Even if the 'scaffold' is completely distorted, as with a traumatic fracture, it will remodel to resemble the original structure and function. If it did not, the bone would remain flexible at the breakpoint.

HEALING OF BONE

Figure 5.4 outlines the stages from fracture to healing and remodelling.

Following a fracture, there is bleeding from the damaged blood vessels so that blood and fibrin clot accumulate within the gap, leading to elevation of the periosteum. Just as in soft tissues, this is organised by the formation of granulation tissue and the phagocytosis of debris and necrotic bone. It differs in that osteoid (non-calcified bone matrix) and cartilage appear after a few days; this is termed the **provisional** or **procallus**. Over the next week, the amount of fibrous tissue and number of bone spicules increase (**fibrocartilaginous callus**) and immobilise the fracture. The bone content continues to expand (**osseous callus**), and **remodelling** by osteoblasts and osteoclasts will occur according to the stresses acting on the bone. The collagen fibres in the osteoid are initially arranged in an irregular fashion, called **woven** bone. When the normal 'onion-skin' pattern has been restored, it is referred to as **lamellar** bone. Finally, as the internal callus is removed, marrow cells will return.

If the alignment is perfect, it may not be possible to see the site of the previous fracture, but if malaligned, complicated, infected or not properly immobilised, the end result is not perfect. Remodelling of bone is not confined to the healing of fractures. It occurs during normal growth and in pathological conditions unrelated to bone fractures, such as osteomalacia or Paget's disease.

The redoubtable Scot John Hunter investigated the healing of tendons. It is said that he ruptured his Achilles tendon while dancing, but since he did it at 4 am, this seems unlikely. By his own account, he did it while jumping, but why he was jumping at this hour is also a mystery! Either way, true to his nature, he did not let the opportunity go to waste: he observed the healing of his own tendon and later undertook experiments in dogs to show that they heal by formation of dense scar tissue.

GROWTH FACTORS

Just as there is a wide range of chemical mediators coordinating inflammation, so there are a number of factors controlling growth. These operate in normal growth, in benign and malignant tumours, in inflammation and in healing and repair.

Platelet-derived growth factor (PDGF) is, not surprisingly, stored and released from platelet alpha granules but can also be produced by macrophages, smooth muscle cells, endothelium and some tumour cells. It stimulates macrophages, fibroblasts and smooth muscle cells. **Fibroblast growth factors** (FGFs) and **vascular endothelial growth factor** (VEGF) are groups of substances crucial for new blood vessel formation and are produced by activated macrophages. **Transforming growth factor beta** (TGF-β) is released by wound macrophages and has a key role in stimulating collagen and matrix protein production by fibroblasts. Dermal cells produce **keratinocyte growth factor** to stimulate re-epithelialisation.

Repair is really just a continuation of inflammation, so it is not surprising that the macrophage plays such a central role in both. In repair, it is capable of phagocytosis, enzyme release and the secretion of growth factors (PDGF, FGF, IL-1, TNF, TGF-β and VEGF) and growth inhibitors (prostaglandins).

MODIFYING FACTORS

The scenario of healing and repair that we have described above is an ideal one. There are several factors that can modify the response.

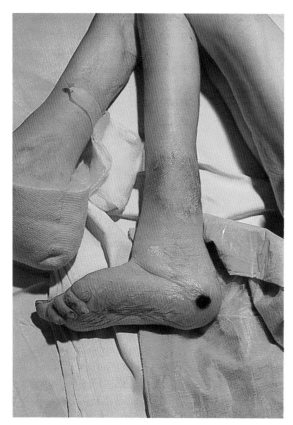

Figure 5.5 Poor blood supply, oedema of the lower limbs, poor nutrition and infection may all contribute to the failure to heal of a pressure sore in a bedridden patient

Blood supply

At the very beginning, we mentioned that the microvasculature is of fundamental importance to the inflammatory response. Similarly, it is vital to healing. Without adequate perfusion, a small injury would lead to massive tissue destruction. It is the inadequate blood supply that may cause delay in wound healing in the elderly.

Infection and foreign material

The presence of infection or foreign material will delay healing by fuelling the process of inflammation. Infection in a fracture will delay union and healing. The foreign material does not have to be exogenous: the damaged tissue itself may act as 'foreign' material. Sutures are essential for limiting the size of the defect and holding the sides of the wound together; however, their presence stimulates continuing inflammation and provides an entry route for bacteria.

Mobility

It is not difficult to imagine that if the ends of a broken bone are continually moved, they will not mend. The situation is not restricted to bone and applies in varying degrees to all tissues.

Nutrition

The role of nutritional factors in healing has long been recognised. In parts of the world where malnutrition is widespread, impaired wound healing is a common phenomenon, probably exacerbated by infection. Vitamin C deficiency (scurvy) results in the impaired synthesis of normal collagen, as does a protein-poor diet. The trace element zinc is also important, and deficiency may occur in patients with severe burns and those receiving long-term parenteral nutrition.

Steroids, chemotherapy and radiotherapy

It is well known that steroids damp down the inflammatory response and are of great use in diseases where the inflammatory response is causing more harm than good. The effect on healing may be a secondary phenomenon related to this effect on inflammation. This is probably due to a reduction in macrophages entering the wound and hence a reduction in macrophage-derived factors important in healing. There may also be a direct effect on fibroblasts to reduce collagen production.

Chemotherapy and radiotherapy also reduce the number of circulating monocytes and so probably cause a reduction in wound macrophages.

IMPROVING WOUND HEALING

The discussion of factors modifying wound healing emphasises that a clean, uninfected, immobile wound with the sides closely apposed in a healthy patient is most likely to heal quickly and neatly. There are several new approaches to wound healing that are under investigation. Wound healing may be improved by the local use of ultrasound or laser therapy, which are thought to increase vascular permeability. Synthetic growth factors, applied topically, may stimulate the healing of chronically ulcerated sites, and there has been particular interest in the topical application of keratinocyte growth factor and TGF-β. Stubborn bone fractures may be persuaded to unite by the passage of electrical currents through the bone.

Before we finish, we should not forget the **complications of healing**. While a cleanly incised wound from an appendicectomy may only cause minor embarrassment to the vain, **scarring** resulting from severe burns may limit movement across joints as a result of **contractures**. A scar in the heart, following the death of muscle fibres from a myocardial infarction, may dilate to produce an **aneurysm**. This may become the site of thrombus formation and may also produce cardiac arrhythmias, both of which may cause death. Repeated inflammation of the liver because of alcohol ingestion or viral infection may produce scar tissue that distorts the normal architecture and produces **cirrhosis**.

CLINICOPATHOLOGICAL CASE STUDY

With such a vast array of different mechanisms and the complex interplay that takes place between them, it is easy to lose sight of the whole process as it applies to disease. We will therefore take the example of lobar pneumonia to present a clinicopathological correlation that summarises the processes and clinical relevance of inflammation. The format used for the clinical details is based on the history-taking approach taught in most clinical medical schools.

CLINICOPATHOLOGICAL CASE STUDY

Clinical
A 60-year-old man presented to the accident and emergency department complaining of a productive cough, fever, rigors and general malaise. The onset of symptoms was sudden and he had been perfectly well 2 days previously.
He had no past medical history of note and he was not on any medication.

Systemic enquiry
Respiratory system – he was coughing up rusty coloured sputum and also complained of chest pain on inspiration.
Allergies – nil known.

Pathology
The symptoms are due to local respiratory irritation from the inflammatory process and the fever is secondary to the production of pyrogens.

Inflammation causes vasodilatation, followed by the margination and emigration of cells. Together with increased permeability, this leads to a purulent exudate within the alveoli, which is coughed up as sputum.

The chest pain results from friction between two inflamed pleural surfaces, which are roughened and adherent owing to the inflammatory exudate. This is also responsible for the pleural rub heard on auscultation.

CLINICOPATHOLOGICAL CASE STUDY

Examination

Temperature 39.4°C (normal 37°C)
Pulse 90/min regular (normal approx. 70/min)
Respiratory rate 30/min (normal approx. 14/min)

Pyrogens cause a rise in body temperature by resetting the thermoregulatory centre in the hypothalamus. A rise in temperature will also increase the metabolic rate and therefore cause an increase in cardiac output. Decreased gas transfer plus the rise in temperature will lead to an increase in the respiratory rate.

Examination also revealed a dull percussion note in the right lower zone and auscultation confirmed decreased air entry and bronchial breathing. There was also a pleural rub over the affected area.

The decreased air entry due to the inflammatory exudate within the alveoli is responsible for the dull percussion note and the findings on auscultation.

Investigations

Full blood count – white cell count 18×10^9/l with 95% neutrophils (normal 4–11×10^9/l with approx. 65% neutrophils)

Cytokines cause bone marrow stimulation and hence a leucocytosis.

Chest X-ray – opaque right lower lobe
Sputum culture – *Streptococcus pneumoniae*

Airless alveoli full of exudate appear white on X-ray. Streptococcus pneumoniae is the most common organism causing lobar pneumonia. With effective treatment, there will be complete reversal of all the clinical and radiological signs as the exudate is cleared away from the alveoli. This ideal process may not occur, and healing may take place by scarring. Lobar pneumonia differs from the more common bronchopneumonia in that the latter tends to be patchy and caused by a variety of organisms, e.g. Haemophilus influenzae.

A diagnosis of lobar pneumonia was made and he was started on a course of penicillin. He did not have a history of allergy to this drug.

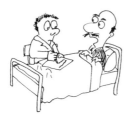

We thus come to the end of Part 1, which has considered the processes of inflammation and healing and looked at the mechanisms involved and their clinical relevance. It should be clear that it is important not to divide the phenomenon into different pieces, as in a jigsaw, but to think of them as interlacing connections. In any one situation, it is the unique combination of these connections that produces the final picture. The idea that it is connections rather than individual objects that are important is well recognised in atomic physics. As Heisenberg (of Heisenberg's uncertainty principle) said:

'[In modern physics], one has now divided the world not into different groups of objects but into different groups of connections... *What can be distinguished is the kind of connection which is primarily important in a certain phenomenon...*The world thus appears as a complicated tissue of events, in which connections of different kinds alternate or overlap or combine and thereby determine the texture of the whole.'

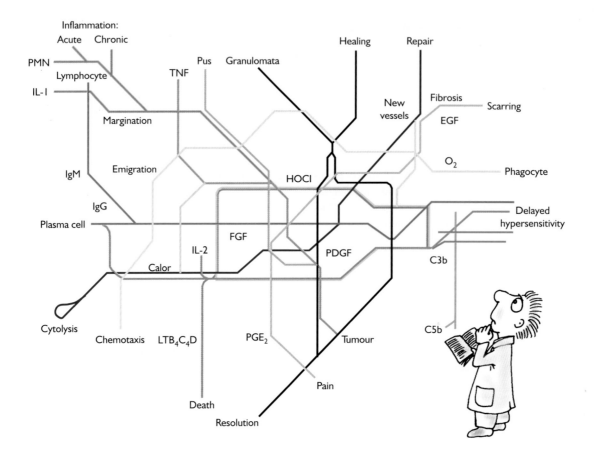

FURTHER READING

Cotran, R.S., Kumar, V., Robbins, S.L. 1994: Inflammation and repair. In *Robbins' Pathologic Basis of Disease*, 5th edn. Philadelphia: W.B. Saunders, Ch. 3.

Mitchinson, M.J. 1996: *Essentials of Pathology*. Oxford: Blackwell Science.

Prusiner, S.B. 1995: The prion diseases. *Scientific American* Jan, 30–37.

Salisbury, D.M., Begg, N.T. 1996: *Immunisation against Infectious Disease*. London: HMSO.

Samuelson, J., von Lichtenburg F. 1994: Infectious diseases. In *Robbins' Pathologic Basis of Disease*, 5th edn. Philadelphia: W.B. Saunders, Ch. 5.

Whaley, K., Burt, A.D. 1992: Inflammation, healing and repair. In *Muir's Textbook of Pathology*, 13th edn. London: Edward Arnold, Ch. 4.

PART 2

CIRCULATORY DISORDERS

CHAPTER 6

VASCULAR OCCLUSION AND THROMBOSIS

- Introduction
- Vascular occlusion
- Thrombosis
- Normal haemostatic mechanisms
- Applying Virchow's triad
- Arterial thrombosis
- Venous thrombosis
- Natural history and complications of thrombosis

> When I first applied my mind to observation from the many dissections of Living Creatures as they came to hand, that by that means I might find out the use of the motion of the Heart and things conducible in Creatures; I straightwayes found it a thing hard to be attained, and full of difficulty, so with Fracastorius I did almost believe, that the motion of the heart was known to God alone.
>
> William Harvey

INTRODUCTION

It is extraordinary to think that diseases whose effects are as diverse as those of gangrene, strokes, heart attacks and divers' 'bends' are all disorders of the circulatory system. The general features of circulatory disorders are almost the opposite of the cardinal features of inflammation – for 'calor, rubor, tumor and dolor' read 'coldness, pallor/cyanosis, pain and loss of sensation'.

Why is this? The drop in temperature and change in colour are easily understood, since blood carries body heat from the core and dissipates it in the extremities, and it is the red colour of the oxygenated haemoglobin pigment in the red blood cells that makes pale-skinned persons look pink. Anything decreasing blood flow to a finger or toe

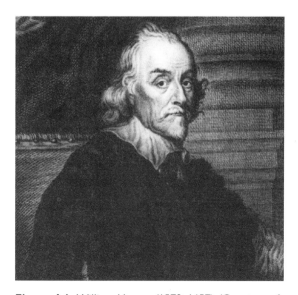

Figure 6.1 William Harvey (1578–1657) (Courtesy of the Wellcome Institute for the History of Medicine)

will decrease the tissue perfusion by warm blood, making it cold and pale, and any delay in the delivery of red blood cells to the affected digit will mean that more of the haemoglobin will have given up its oxygen load, leaving blue-coloured deoxyhaemoglobin (**cyanosis**).

Pain is a variable phenomenon, depending on the tissue affected and the type of injury; for example, a 'heart attack', or myocardial infarction, caused by sudden blockage of a coronary artery, is usually associated with intense central chest pain, often radiating down the left arm, while a gradual 'furring up' of the arteries supplying the legs causes severe pain on walking, which disappears when the demand for oxygen by the leg muscles is removed by rest (**intermittent claudication**). In comparison, a 'stroke', in which the blood supply to part of the brain is suddenly interrupted, will generally cause weakness or paralysis but no pain.

Loss of sensation also varies according to the type of vascular disease and the tissue or organ affected: a stroke may destroy a sensory pathway to the brain, leading to a large area of numbness that may involve half the body, while blockage of the blood flow to a toe would cause numbness in just the area supplied by the vessel because of ischaemic damage to the local sensory nerves.

You will have gathered from the preceding discussion that the term 'circulatory disorders' encompasses a spectrum of symptoms and signs related to an abnormality in the blood supply. Circulatory disorders may be **local** or **systemic** and may gradually develop over months or years, or strike suddenly and catastrophically. They may result from a problem in the vessels, the blood or the heart.

Perhaps the easiest way to look at these diseases is to relate them to a domestic plumbing system, the main components of which are the pipes and the pump. Pipes may gradually 'fur up' (**atherosclerosis**) or become blocked (**vascular occlusion**). In plumbing, the blockage may be water freezing in the winter, while our cardiovascular equivalent is **thrombosis**. Sometimes small fragments of thrombus may break off and be carried around the system until they lodge in a pipe with a diameter too small to let them through (**embolism**).

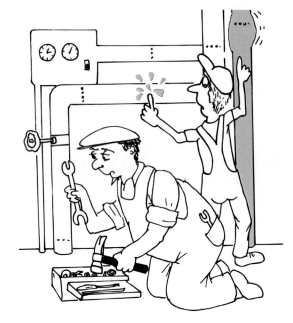

Figure 6.2

Burst pipes (**haemorrhage**) are a nuisance and can be extremely damaging. One can sometimes spot the area at risk, because the pipe may bulge alarmingly before it bursts (**aneurysm**). Pump failure for whatever reason is fairly disastrous; in the heart, this may be due to valve disease, myocardial infarction, infection, congenital abnormality, etc.

Some solutions to these problems have been found. Thus affected segments of piping can be replaced (arterial bypass grafts), pumps can be tinkered with (valve grafts) or replaced (heart transplants), high pressure causing strain on the system can be relieved (antihypertensive drugs), and it is sometimes possible to remove some of the 'scale' that furs up the pipes (reaming out of arteries using balloon catheters or, more recently, lasers). Of course, these are usually only partial solutions, and there is no doubt that prevention is the best medicine.

It would be unjust to discuss circulatory disorders without a brief mention of the historical figures involved. Had you been alive in the sixteenth century, you would have been taught that blood was produced by the liver and then carried in the veins to the organs, where it was

Embolus: an intravascular solid, liquid or gaseous mass carried in the blood from its origin to lodge in another site

Thrombus: a solid mass of blood formed within the cardiovascular system involving the interaction of endothelial cells, platelets and the coagulation cascade

Blood clot: a solid mass of blood formed by the action of the coagulation cascade

Infarct: a localised area of ischaemic tissue necrosis generally caused by an impaired blood supply

Haematoma: an extravascular accumulation of clotted blood

Haemorrhage: discharge of blood from the vascular compartment into the extravascular body spaces or to the exterior

Petechiae, purpura, ecchymoses: small haemorrhages

Hyperaemia: an increased volume of intravascular blood in an affected tissue, which may result from increased flow (active hyperaemia) or reduced drainage (passive hyperaemia = congestion)

The left ventricle received this blood, which mixed with the 'pneuma' (air) coming to the heart through the pulmonary veins. The blood, fortified by the 'pneuma', was then ejected via the aorta towards the peripheral organs.

In 1628 this theory was challenged when William Harvey published his famous work *De motu cordis*, describing the dual **circulation** of the blood, but even in the sixteenth century people were starting to doubt Galen's theory. There were several problems with the theory. First, nobody had managed to identify 'interseptal' pores, so Michael Servetius, the Spanish theologian and physician, suggested that blood travelled from the right to the left ventricle by circulating through the lungs, an idea for which he died a martyr's death after being denounced by John Calvin for holding heretical opinions. Second, Galen's theory proposed a mixture of air and blood in the left side of the heart, which was a difficult concept to accept once the structure of the heart valves had been established. Leonardo da Vinci had drawn these accurately, but it was Andrea Caselapino who, in 1571, correctly described the valves' actions, going on to use the term 'circulatio'. Thus Harvey, who studied in Padua from 1600 to 1602, would have been familiar with the Italians' ideas and was able to reach his own conclusions by 'standing on the shoulders of these giants'. Even Harvey was left with a problem: he could not demonstrate the connections between the arterial and venous sides of the circulation. The discovery of the capillaries had to wait for Marcello Malpighi's microscopic analysis of frog lung in 1661.

VASCULAR OCCLUSION

To return to the present day, we shall first consider the problems of vascular occlusion.

Vascular occlusion may be arterial or venous, the effect of any occlusion depending on:

- the type of tissue involved
- how quickly the occlusion develops
- the availability of collateral circulation.

consumed; this was Galen's theory of the **regeneration** of the blood. The portion of blood from the liver that entered the right side of the heart divided into two streams. One route was through the pulmonary artery to bathe the lungs and the other was across the heart through 'interseptal pores'.

Collateral vessels provide an alternative route for the blood and are sometimes able to compensate completely, especially if the occlusion develops slowly. The venous system has more collaterals than the arterial system. For example, there are anastomoses between the portal and systemic veins, around the lower end of the oesophagus, and also linking veins between the deep and superficial venous plexuses in the leg. This means that occlusion of a deep vein in the calf does not produce haemorrhagic infarction of the foot but only a mild oedema of the tissues and congestion of the superficial veins because of their increased flow.

Unfortunately, not all veins have a collateral system. If the central vein of the retina is occluded, as may happen in thrombosis of the cavernous sinus as a result of local infection, the tissue of the orbit becomes oedematous and congested so that the eye is pushed forward (proptosis), and there may be local haemorrhage as the small vessels rupture because of the increased pressure. In the worst cases, the venous pressure rises until it exceeds the arterial pressure and prevents arterial flow. This produces infarction, i.e. death of the tissue, and the infarcted tissue is red or purple and swollen because of the haemorrhagic oedema. The word 'infarction' actually comes from the Latin *farcire*, meaning to stuff, and it is thought originally to have been used for the appearance of venous infarcts stuffed with blood.

Arterial collaterals exist in various areas such as the gut, circle of Willis and, to some extent, the heart (see Figure 6.13). Arterial occlusion without the benefit of collaterals will produce ischaemic infarction, in which the tissue is pale without any swelling. Occasionally, arterial infarcts are haemorrhagic because there is reperfusion or some limited arterial flow, leading to leakage of blood from necrotic small vessels. In incomplete arterial occlusion, the effects depend on the tissue's demand for metabolites. Brain and heart tissue are highly susceptible to ischaemic injury, while bone and skeletal muscle are quite resistant. It is possible to reduce a tissue's demand by cooling the tissue, as is done in some types of surgery.

Vascular occlusion can result from:
- thrombosis
- embolism
- atherosclerosis
- external compression
- spasm.

We shall discuss the first three of these causes in some depth in this chapter, starting with thrombosis.

THROMBOSIS

Patients presenting with an **arterial thrombus** are generally middle-aged or elderly and may have circulatory problems due to atherosclerosis. Many will be smokers, and some may suffer from diabetes. Their symptoms and signs will depend entirely on which vessel is affected. In contrast, a patient with **venous thrombosis** may be any age but will generally be rather immobile or forced to be immobile, such as after an operation. Such patients frequently complain of pain in a calf muscle and often swelling of the foot and ankle. (If you recall the discussion in Chapter 1 about flow of fluid in and out of capillaries, you can work out why the area is oedematous: it is because the hydrostatic pressure at the venous end of the capillaries is raised secondary to the obstructed venous flow.)

But why should such people suddenly develop a thrombus? Much is known now about normal haemostatic mechanisms, but the most important factors influencing thrombus formation were described more than a century ago by Virchow.

Rudolf Ludwig Karl Virchow was born on 13 October 1821. As a child, he excelled at school, his examination reports being rather monotonous as they contained only three terms – 'excellent', 'very good' and 'most satisfactory'! Virchow attended medical school in Berlin in 1839 and, even before the existence of platelets and clotting factors was known, had suggested that the development of a thrombus depended on:
- alteration to the constituents of the blood

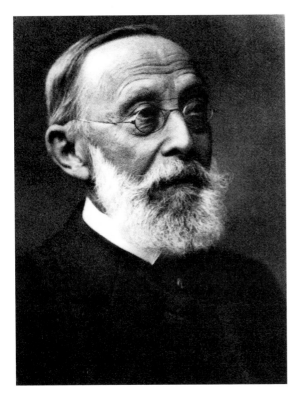

Figure 6.3 Rudolf Virchow (1821–1902) (Courtesy of the Wellcome Institute for the History of Medicine)

- damage to the endothelial layer of the blood vessel
- changes in the normal flow of blood.

These three factors are known as **Virchow's triad** and are the clues that allow us to understand what has happened to our patients with venous and arterial thrombosis. But first, we must revise the body's normal haemostatic mechanisms.

NORMAL HAEMOSTATIC MECHANISMS

The normal haemostatic mechanisms must be capable of stopping blood from leaking through damaged vessels and must also be finely controlled so that thrombus does not form in normal circumstances. There are three main components:

- platelets
- soluble blood proteins of the coagulation pathway
- the vessel wall.

Briefly, the sequence of events is as follows. Injury to the vessels causes an initial *vasoconstriction*, which helps to slow the blood flow. The damaged endothelium of the vessel exposes the subendothelial connective tissue, which attracts platelets and causes them to adhere to the damaged area to form the **primary haemostatic plug**. The adhesion of the platelets alters their physiology and causes them to release soluble factors, which, together with tissue factors, results in the formation of **fibrin** via the coagulation pathway. The fibrin acts to stabilise the platelet plug, and the process is termed **secondary haemostasis**.

If this were all that was involved in maintaining haemostasis, could we really survive the assault on our circulation? Of course not! If the above system were set in motion with nothing to check its progress, the whole circulation would soon come to a standstill and become one big mass of thrombus. This is avoided by the clearance, inhibition and inactivation of the coagulation factors as well as by the digestion of fibrin.

We will now consider both the normal physiology and pathology of each component in more detail.

BLOOD CONSTITUENTS IN NORMAL HAEMOSTASIS

The most important blood constituents involved in normal haemostasis and thrombosis are platelets and the numerous components of the coagulation pathway.

Platelets

Platelets are small (2 μm) cytoplasmic fragments produced by megakaryocytes in the bone marrow. They survive for 8–12 days in the peripheral circulation and contain a variety of granules (see

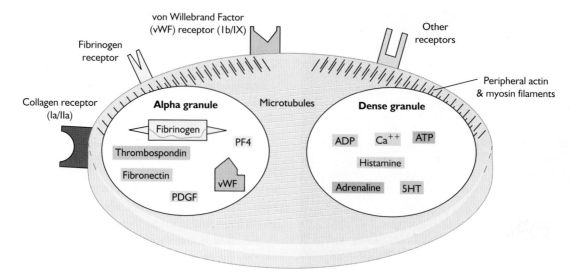

The resting platelet is disc shaped, maintained by microtubules and peripheral actin and myosin filaments. The alpha and dense granules contain various chemical mediators and the surface bears several different receptors, most importantly the collagen receptor (gp Ia/IIa) and the vWF receptor (gp Ib/IX)

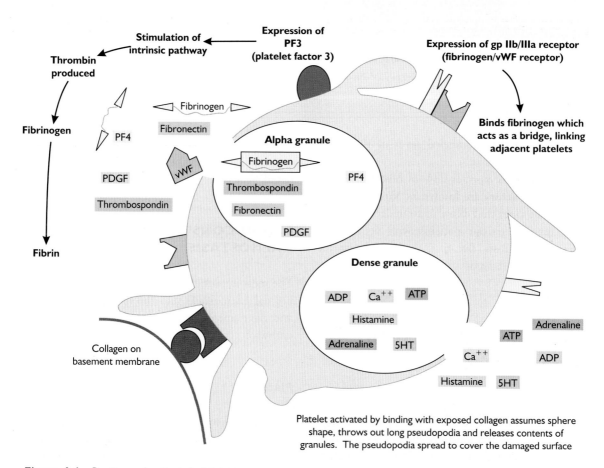

Platelet activated by binding with exposed collagen assumes sphere shape, throws out long pseudopodia and releases contents of granules. The pseudopodia spread to cover the damaged surface

Figure 6.4   Resting and activated platelets

(a) Adhesion, activation and release of granules

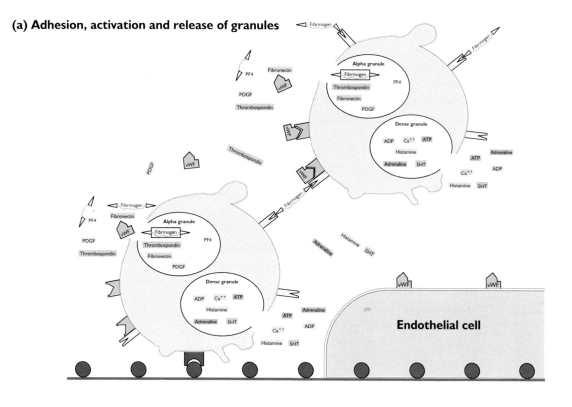

(b) Aggregation

Cross-linking of platelets by fibrinogen produces a mesh which traps rbc's and inflammatory cells. The thrombus is stabilised and anchored by contraction of the platelet microtubule assembly

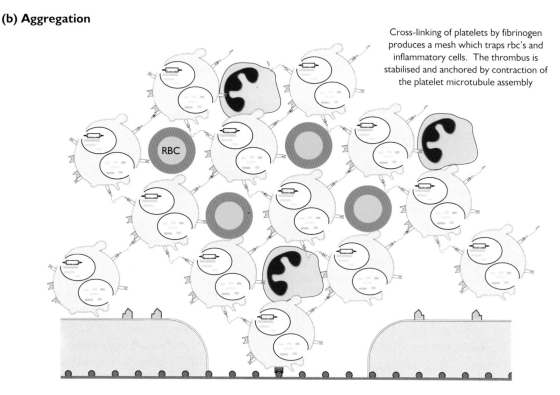

Figure 6.5 (a) Adhesion, activation and release of platelet granules. (b) Aggregation

Platelet granules

Alpha granules

  Fibrinogen

  von Willebrand factor

  Thrombospondin

  Platelet-derived growth factor

  Fibronectin

  Platelet factor 4 (an

    antiheparin)

Dense granules

  ADP/ATP

  Calcium

  Histamine

  Adrenaline

  Serotonin

Rare diseases due to platelet abnormalities

von Willebrand's disease	Lack of vW factor
Bernard–Soulier syndrome	Lack of gp Ib
'Grey platelet' syndrome	Lack of alpha granules
Wiskott–Aldrich syndrome	Lack of dense bodies

calcium, which is needed for the coagulation pathway, and adenosine diphosphate (ADP) and thromboxane (TXA_2), which induce platelet aggregation. **Platelet aggregation** involves the gp IIb/IIIa receptor complex mentioned above. This is expressed after activation and is most important in binding fibrinogen, which acts as a bridge to the adjacent platelet (Figure 6.5). Not surprisingly, there are 'loops' in this process to amplify the reaction. Most importantly, activated platelets express **platelet factor 3**, which stimulates the intrinsic pathway of the coagulation cascade (see below), resulting in the production of thrombin. **Thrombin** acts to stimulate platelets and thus enhances the reaction.

The platelet has another important facet to its character: it has mechanical properties. An unstimulated platelet has a disc shape maintained by microtubules and actin and myosin filaments at the periphery. On activation, the platelet is transformed into a sphere with long pseudopods that spread over the damaged surface; then, after aggregation, the internal filaments slide so that the platelet plug contracts to stabilize and anchor it.

Coagulation components

The components and pathway involved in coagulation are shown in Figure 6.6. This is the same system as the one mentioned in Chapter 1 when discussing inflammatory mediators. Then we were particularly interested in fibrin degradation products; now our interest focuses on **fibrin**, which is the final product of the pathway and acts to stabilise the plug of aggregated platelets.

The coagulation pathway has traditionally been divided into the extrinsic and intrinsic pathways, although a complex interplay occurs between them. The common pathway begins at factor X, which acts on prothrombin to produce thrombin, which itself has a variety of actions but most importantly converts fibrinogen to fibrin. Generally, each step in this cascade involves:

- an activated enzyme
- a substrate for a coagulation factor

above). Their role in thrombosis can be divided into three phases:

- adhesion
- secretion
- aggregation.

When the endothelium is damaged and collagen is exposed, the first event is **adhesion** of the platelets. This is achieved via platelet surface membrane receptors:

- **gp Ia/IIa**, which binds to collagen
- **gp Ib/IX**, which binds to von Willebrand factor (vWF or factor VIII-related antigen)
- **gp IIb/IIIa**, which binds to fibrinogen and vWF.

Following adhesion, the platelets release the contents of their granules. There are two main types of granules: alpha granules and dense bodies. The contents of the granules are listed in the box here. The most important secretory products are

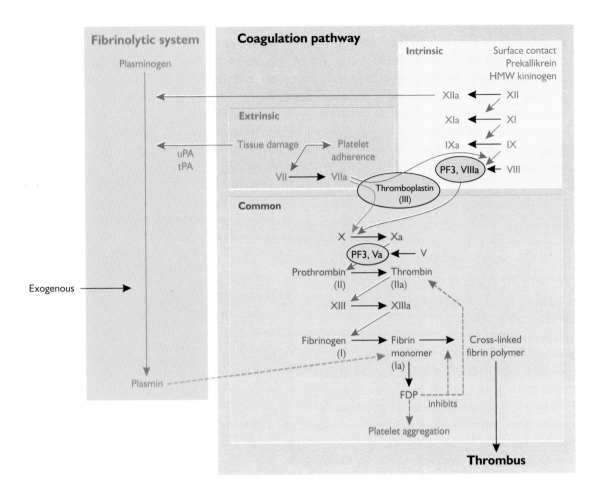

Figure 6.6 Interaction of coagulation and fibrinolytic pathways

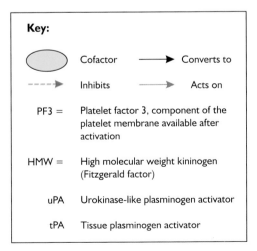

- a co-factor
- calcium ions (Factor IV)
- a phospholipid surface.

Some feedback loops are included in the figure but, for simplicity, the control mechanisms that inhibit or inactivate reactions have been omitted.

These mechanisms include:

- the depletion of local clotting factors
- the clearance of the activated clotting factors by the liver and mononuclear phagocyte system.
- neutralisation of the activated coagulation factors by forming a complex, e.g. antithrombin III, α_2-macroglobulin
- the proteolytic degradation of active coagulation factors, e.g. protein C
- fibrinolysis – this is of major importance (see Figure 6.6).

The most important enzyme capable of digesting fibrin is **plasmin**. This is produced from plasminogen either by a factor XII-dependent pathway, by therapeutic agents such as streptokinase or by tissue-derived plasminogen activators. Plasminogen activators (PAs) fall into two classes:

- urokinase-like PA (uPA)
- tissue-type PA (tPA).

They differ in that uPA activates plasminogen in the fluid phase, whereas tPA (principally produced by endothelial cells) is active only when attached to fibrin. Conveniently, some plasminogen is bound to fibrin as a thrombus is formed, so it is perfectly situated for conversion by tPA to plasmin, which can then digest the thrombus. Compounds capable of breaking down thrombi have enormous therapeutic potential for restoring blood flow before significant myocardial or cerebral infarction has occurred.

APPLYING VIRCHOW'S TRIAD

ALTERATION IN THE CONSTITUENTS OF THE BLOOD

Blood that clots more readily than usual is termed **hypercoagulable**. This may be caused by a variety of different mechanisms including:

- an increase in the number of red blood cells (polycythaemia)
- a loss of the plasma fraction of the blood (severe burns)

- increased numbers of platelets
- an increased amount or aggregation of plasma proteins (myeloma, cryoglobulinaemia)
- severe trauma
- disseminated cancer
- late pregnancy.

Hypercoagulability presumably results from either an increase in activated coagulation proteins, an increased risk of platelet aggregation or a decrease in antithrombotic proteins. However, the actual sequence of events leading to this state is not at present clear. Some mechanisms have been elucidated, such as deficiencies of protein C and a hereditary lack of antithrombin III.

Polycythaemia: an increase in the number of red cells that occurs as a normal compensatory mechanism if the person has chronic hypoxaemia because of chronic cardiorespiratory problems or because they live at high altitudes. It can also occur because of uncontrolled erythropoietin production by various tumours (e.g. renal cell carcinoma) or uncontrolled proliferation of the haemopoietic cells. This neoplastic proliferation is called polycythaemia rubra vera, and patients often present with thrombosis

CHANGES IN THE ENDOTHELIUM

Normal endothelium

The fact that the vascular tree is lined by endothelium means that the endothelial surface must be resistant to thrombus formation. The endothelium is quite remarkable, for it is capable of initiating both thrombogenic and antithrombogenic stimuli

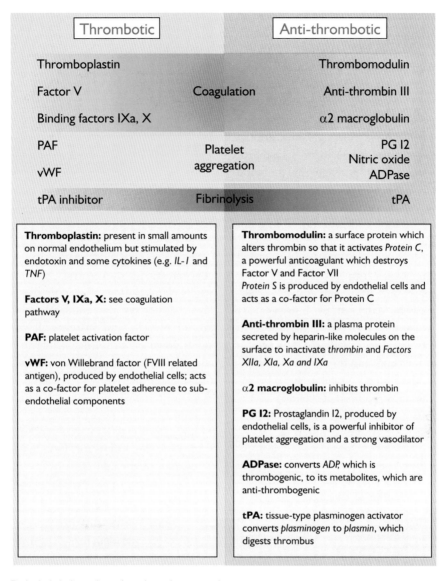

Thrombotic		Anti-thrombotic
Thromboplastin		Thrombomodulin
Factor V	Coagulation	Anti-thrombin III
Binding factors IXa, X		α2 macroglobulin
PAF	Platelet	PG I2
	aggregation	Nitric oxide
vWF		ADPase
tPA inhibitor	Fibrinolysis	tPA

Thromboplastin: present in small amounts on normal endothelium but stimulated by endotoxin and some cytokines (e.g. *IL-1* and *TNF*)

Factors V, IXa, X: see coagulation pathway

PAF: platelet activation factor

vWF: von Willebrand factor (FVIII related antigen), produced by endothelial cells; acts as a co-factor for platelet adherence to sub-endothelial components

Thrombomodulin: a surface protein which alters thrombin so that it activates *Protein C*, a powerful anticoagulant which destroys Factor V and Factor VII
Protein S is produced by endothelial cells and acts as a co-factor for Protein C

Anti-thrombin III: a plasma protein secreted by heparin-like molecules on the surface to inactivate *thrombin* and *Factors XIIa, XIa, Xa and IXa*

α2 macroglobulin: inhibits thrombin

PG I2: Prostaglandin I2, produced by endothelial cells, is a powerful inhibitor of platelet aggregation and a strong vasodilator

ADPase: converts *ADP*, which is thrombogenic, to its metabolites, which are anti-thrombogenic

tPA: tissue-type plasminogen activator converts *plasminogen* to *plasmin*, which digests thrombus

Figure 6.7 Endothelial thrombotic/antithrombotic mechanisms

(Figure 6.7). These two groups of actions are normally finely balanced in favour of preventing thrombus formation. Damage to the endothelium, however, will tip the balance towards thrombosis.

The endothelium also has another very important role, which is to prevent the elements of blood from coming into contact with the subendothelial connective tissue, which is highly thrombogenic. This tissue normally comprises collagen, elastin, fibronectin and glycosaminoglycans. **Collagen** is by far the most important of these constituents, activating the coagulation pathway as well as

being a strong stimulator of platelet aggregation. In vessels affected by atheroma, not only is the endothelium more readily damaged but also the subendothelial tissue consists of the components of atheroma, which are extremely thrombogenic.

Damage to the endothelium

Endothelial damage is of most significance in **arterial thrombosis**. There may be obvious loss of endothelial cells or more subtle metabolic damage to the cells. Endothelial cells may be lost where an atheromatous plaque has ulcerated or when vessels are damaged by surgery, infection, immune-mediated damage (arteritis), indwelling vascular catheters or the infusion of sclerosing chemicals in the treatment of varicose veins and haemorrhoids. Haemodynamic stress is believed to be important in producing metabolic damage to arterial endothelial cells in areas where there is turbulent flow or in patients with prolonged high blood pressure. Other potentially damaging agents include derivatives of cigarette smoke, bacterial toxins, immune complex deposition, transplant rejection and radiation.

In the heart, the endocardial surface is covered by endothelium, which can be damaged in a myocardial infarction. Also, the valve surface endothelium may be damaged by inflammatory endocarditis, which promotes thrombus formation on valve leaflets, resulting in altered function, a variety of heart murmurs and the danger of throwing emboli into the systemic circulation.

Clinically, the most important change is the endothelial damage related to atherosclerosis, which is discussed later in this chapter.

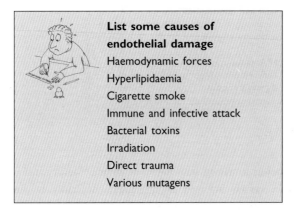

List some causes of endothelial damage

Haemodynamic forces

Hyperlipidaemia

Cigarette smoke

Immune and infective attack

Bacterial toxins

Irradiation

Direct trauma

Various mutagens

CHANGES IN THE NORMAL FLOW OF BLOOD

There are two principal ways in which normal flow can be disturbed: the normal lamellar flow pattern can be altered (**turbulence**) or the speed may be reduced (**stasis**), both leading to similar changes.

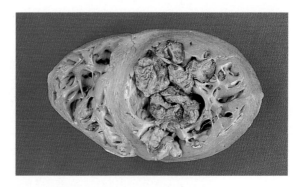

Figure 6.8 Apical section of heart with thrombus in left ventricle following myocardial infarction

During normal flow, red and white blood cells concentrate in the central, fast-moving stream, while platelets flow nearer to the periphery, the layer closest to the endothelium usually being devoid of cells and platelets. If the blood flow slows down or turbulence produces local counter-currents, several factors increase the likelihood of thrombus formation:

- platelets come into contact with the endothelium
- turbulence may damage endothelial cells
- there is no inflow of fresh blood containing clotting factor inhibitors

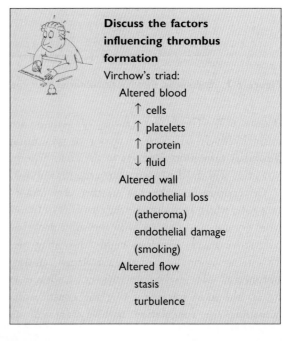

Discuss the factors influencing thrombus formation

Virchow's triad:

Altered blood

↑ cells

↑ platelets

↑ protein

↓ fluid

Altered wall

endothelial loss (atheroma)

endothelial damage (smoking)

Altered flow

stasis

turbulence

• there is no clearance of blood containing activated coagulation factors.

As you see, both turbulence and stasis operate in thrombosis, but turbulence is most important in arteries, whereas stasis is more important in veins.

ARTERIAL THROMBOSIS

Turbulence tends to occur where arteries branch, and over the irregular surface of an atheromatous plaque. It also occurs when cardiac valves have been damaged by inflammation, as may occur with rheumatic fever and infective endocarditis, or when they have been replaced by artificial valves.

Stasis is generally only important in arterial thrombosis if the heart or arteries have been damaged. Abnormal dilatations of large vessels (aneurysms) will produce pockets of stagnant blood, which will thrombose, and myocardial infarction may result in a localised area of damaged heart muscle, which does not move, or in an arrhythmia, which will affect the contraction of a whole chamber.

VENOUS THROMBOSIS

Thrombus formation, related to stasis of the blood, is more common in the venous circulation and occurs particularly in the legs or pelvic veins of immobile individuals. Why is stasis common in the leg vessels when the patient is immobilised? If you remember the physiology of venous return from the legs, you will recall that it is the contraction of skeletal muscles that pushes blood along the veins and the presence of valves that ensures the direction of flow. Understanding this has influenced patient management. Patients are encouraged to move their legs regularly when confined to bed, leg muscles are stimulated to contract during long operations, and it is no longer common to have patients bed-bound for weeks.

Thrombus formation often begins within the venous valve pockets. The initial cluster of

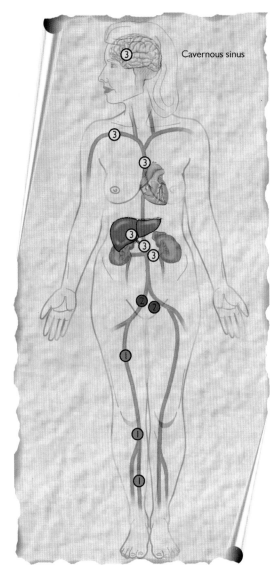

In order of frequency:	Associated factors
1. Leg veins	Immobility, post-surgery and hyper-coagulability states
2. Pelvic veins	Post-childbirth, puerperal sepsis, pelvic surgery and tumours
3. Others: Inferior vena cava	Extrinsic compression by tumour, extension from leg or iliac veins
Renal vein	Tumour extension from kidney
Portal/hepatic veins	Local sepsis, tumour compression
Cavernous sinus	Facial sepsis
Superior vena cava	Extrinsic compression by mediastinal tumour
Axillary vein	Trauma from rucksack, local surgery

Figure 6.9 Sites of venous thrombosis

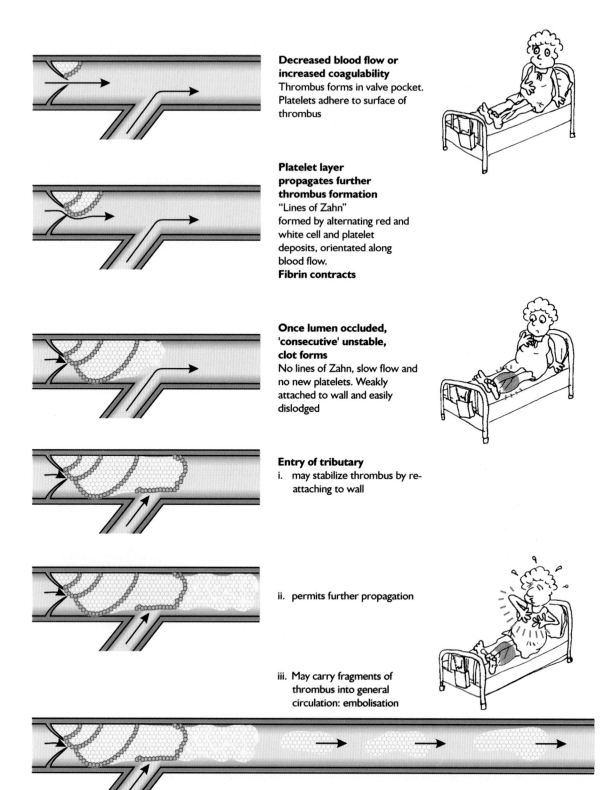

Decreased blood flow or increased coagulability
Thrombus forms in valve pocket. Platelets adhere to surface of thrombus

Platelet layer propagates further thrombus formation
"Lines of Zahn" formed by alternating red and white cell and platelet deposits, orientated along blood flow.
Fibrin contracts

Once lumen occluded, 'consecutive' unstable, clot forms
No lines of Zahn, slow flow and no new platelets. Weakly attached to wall and easily dislodged

Entry of tributary
i. may stabilize thrombus by re-attaching to wall

ii. permits further propagation

iii. May carry fragments of thrombus into general circulation: embolisation

Figure 6.10 Venous thrombosis and embolism

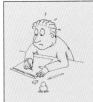

Compare and contrast arterial and venous thrombosis		
	Arterial	*Venous*
Patient risk factors	Presence of atheroma	Immobility
Pathogenesis	Turbulent flow	Stasis
	Damaged endothelium	Hypercoagulable blood
Symptoms	Sudden onset	Slow onset
Complications	Infarction	Pulmonary embolus
	Arterial embolism	

platelets activates the clotting cascade to produce a small thrombus. A second phase of platelet aggregation then occurs to cover the original thrombus and promote a further wave of coagulation. This process is repeated again and again to extend the thrombus– so-called **propagation**. The resultant thrombus has alternate layers of platelets and a red cell/white cell/fibrin mixture that produces a rippled effect, termed **lines of Zahn**. The direction of the lines relates to the pattern of blood flow in the vessel. These platelet layers anchor the thrombus to the adjacent endothelium, helping to stabilise it.

Once a vessel is completely occluded by thrombus, blood flow ceases and the stagnant column of blood clots without the production of any lines of Zahn. This is called consecutive clot and is particularly dangerous because it is only adherent to the vessel wall through its attachment to the original focus of thrombus. This makes it especially likely to break off and embolise to another area (see Fig. 6.10).

If the blood flow is slowed in the entire limb, a very large consecutive clot is formed along the length of the limb's venous system. Alternatively, the consecutive clot only extends to the point where the next venous tributary enters the main vessel. Here the blood may be flowing at a reasonable speed, but the presence of activated clotting factors will promote the adherence of a layer of platelets, which may result in a fresh wave of thrombosis from this point. The involvement of platelets, however, does mean that the clot will be anchored at the points where the tributaries enter and be slightly less likely to embolise. Lines of

Zahn can also be seen in arterial thrombus. These processes are illustrated in Figure 6.10.

It is also worth emphasising at this point that, like most phenomena in the body, the three major factors of Virchow's triad rarely work in isolation. In myocardial infarction, ischaemia damages the endocardium, but the affected myocardium also fails to move normally, hence causing local stasis of blood, which is also important in the formation of the thrombus within the ventricle. So, while it is imperative that one knows the basis for Virchow's triad, it is also important to remember that many factors interact to produce the final picture in any one patient.

NATURAL HISTORY AND COMPLICATIONS OF THROMBOSIS

Once a thrombus has formed, what are the possible outcomes? As you know, the body possesses many effective systems for regulating thrombus formation during normal haemostasis. The ideal solution is that these systems halt the thrombotic process and remove the debris to leave a normal blood vessel. This process is termed **resolution**. If the thrombus cannot be removed, it may be **organised** or **recanalised**. Alternatively, it may be cast off into the circulation, i.e. it may **embolize**.

Resolution is thought to occur commonly in the small veins of the lower limb. Interestingly, venous intima contains more plasminogen activator than

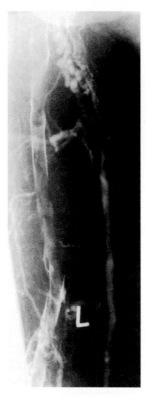

Figure 6.11 The femoral/popliteal vein (left) is occluded by thrombus so that the contrast medium only fills the edge of the vessel

does arterial intima, which may be the reason. Drugs with a thrombolytic action, such as streptokinase, can be given to patients early after thrombosis to promote dissolution of the clot and hence resolution. It is important that this drug is given within hours because the drug has much less effect on polymerised fibrin, which predominates later.

Organisation of a thrombus involves processes similar to those of the organisation of inflammation, described in Part 1. When the thrombus has formed, polymorphs and macrophages begin to degrade and digest the fibrin and cell debris. Later, granulation tissue grows into the base of the thrombus so that the thrombus is converted into a mass of small vessels separated by connective tissue. These vessels originate from the vasa vasorum of the adventitia of the blood vessel, and it is unlikely that the blood flowing through these is of much clinical importance (but see below for collateral circulation).

Alternatively, the thrombus may occlude only part of the vessel, so that, on cross-section, it is attached to one side of the lumen. Organisation of this mural thrombus also involves digestion by inflammatory cells, but it differs in that small vessels grow in from the luminal surface rather than from the outer layers. The thrombus ultimately shrinks and is covered by endothelial or smooth muscle cells, which produce PDGF. As we shall see, this is of interest because of its potential role in the formation of atheromatous plaques (see p. 144).

Recanalisation is a term used by clinicians to indicate that there is useful flow through a previously occluded vessel. Obviously, if streptokinase treatment has been successful, the thrombus will be dissolved, the original intimal lining will still exist and the clinician will see flow on the arteriogram; he will call this recanalisation, but we will not! A similar situation occurs if the clot retracts so that it is obstructing only part of the flow. The blood flow is, at least partially, restored but through the original lumen rather than through new channels.

To a pathologist, recanalisation involves the production of *new* endothelium-lined channels that convey blood through the occlusive thrombus. This is thought to occur by the production of clefts within the thrombus, resulting from a combination of local digestion and shrinkage. The clefts extend through the clot and become lined by endothelial cells derived from the adjacent intima. This can produce several channels separated by loose connective tissue. The amount of flow through such a segment will depend on the number and size of the conduits, but the vessel will not be 'as good as new' (Fig. 6.12).

This is a convenient moment to digress and discuss the way in which the cardiovascular system tries to compensate for a reduced flow through a vessel. Just as you might try to avoid a traffic jam by driving through the back roads, so the blood will search for alternative routes. The availability of such routes depends on the local anatomy. In the venous circulation, there are specific anastomoses between the systemic and portal systems around the rectum, oesophagus and umbilicus, but

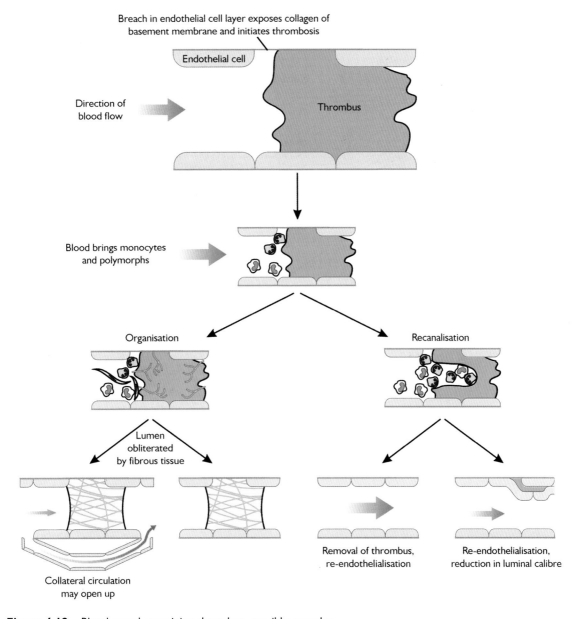

Figure 6.12 Blood vessel containing thrombus, possible sequelae

the penetrating veins linking the deep and superficial lower limb venous plexuses are of more relevance to our patient with a deep vein thrombosis. Thus, if a segment of the deep veins is occluded, the blood will bypass it by moving into the superficial plexus.

The arterial system has some well-characterised alternative routes, such as the arterial roundabout of the circle of Willis and the dual arterial supply of the lung. However, most organs do not have a dual supply and must rely on collateral vessels opening up if the main supplying vessel is occluded. If we take the heart and coronary arteries as an example, we can often see a collateral arterial circulation in a patient who has suffered a coronary artery thrombosis. The apparently new network of small vessels has always existed, but little blood would have flowed through these channels because it was easier to flow down the larger artery. Once thrombosis occurs, the resis-

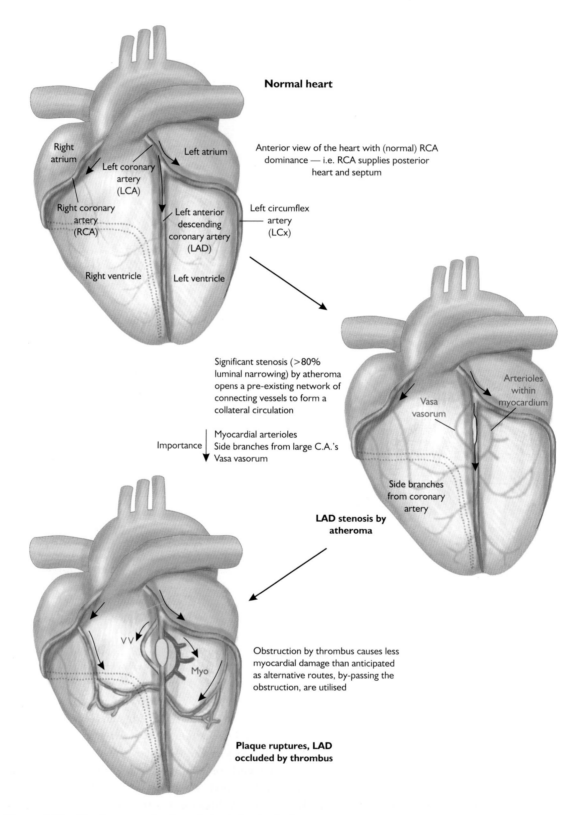

Normal heart

Right
atrium

Left coronary
artery
(LCA)

Left atrium

Right coronary
artery
(RCA)

Left anterior
descending
coronary artery
(LAD)

Left circumflex
artery
(LCx)

Right ventricle

Left ventricle

Anterior view of the heart with (normal) RCA
dominance — i.e. RCA supplies posterior
heart and septum

Significant stenosis (>80%
luminal narrowing) by atheroma
opens a pre-existing network of
connecting vessels to form a
collateral circulation

Importance

Myocardial arterioles
Side branches from large C.A.'s
Vasa vasorum

Vasa
vasorum

Arterioles
within
myocardium

Side branches
from coronary
artery

**LAD stenosis by
atheroma**

VV

Myo

Obstruction by thrombus causes less
myocardial damage than anticipated
as alternative routes, by-passing the
obstruction, are utilised

**Plaque ruptures, LAD
occluded by thrombus**

Figure 6.13   Development of collateral circulation in the heart

tance to flow increases in the main vessel, making the small-channel route attractive and hence visible on arteriograms.

Where are these vessels? This is an area of great interest because, theoretically, any patient with a large network of connecting vessels would have some protection from suffering a large myocardial infarction. There are three main possibilities which, in probable order of clinical importance, are:

- small arterioles within the myocardium
- side branches from the large coronary arteries
- vasa vasorum.

John Hunter carried out an elegant experiment to demonstrate collateral circulation. He tied one of the carotid arteries of a stag from Richmond Park and observed the effect on the corresponding antler. The carotid pulse on that side disappeared, and the antler went cold and stopped growing. Within a few weeks, however, the warmth returned and the antler started to grow again. Hunter demonstrated the collateral circulation by sacrificing the stag and injecting the carotid artery. Elegant as it was, such an experiment would not go down so well nowadays!

CHAPTER 7

EMBOLISM AND DISSEMINATED INTRAVASCULAR COAGULATION

- Embolism
- Disseminated intravascular coagulation
- Shock

EMBOLISM

One of the complications of thrombosis is embolism, and we will now go on to consider the different types of emboli and their effects.

An embolus is solid, liquid or gaseous material that is carried in the blood from one area of the circulatory system to another.

The majority of emboli arise from thrombi, and there is thus a tendency to use the term **thromboembolism** as being synonymous with embolism. This is not strictly true as there are many other, although admittedly rarer, causes of emboli, including:
- fragments of atheromatous plaques
- bone marrow
- fat
- air or nitrogen
- amniotic fluid
- tumour
- foreign material, e.g. an intravenous catheter.

Since most emboli come from thrombi, we shall start our discussion with this particular type.

Where emboli lodge depends on their size, their origin and the relevant cardiovascular anatomy. Those which arise in the venous system can travel through the right side of the heart to end up in the pulmonary circulation. Those which arise in the left side of the circulation will block systemic arteries, and the clinical effect will depend on the organ involved, be it brain, kidneys, spleen or the periphery of the limbs.

Emboli to the lungs from venous thrombosis represent an important preventable cause of morbidity in hospitalised patients, and we shall consider this first.

PULMONARY EMBOLISM

The lungs are very interesting organs because they have a dual blood supply. The lung receives not only deoxygenated blood via the pulmonary arteries but also oxygenated blood from bronchial arteries feeding directly from the aorta. Hence the lungs have an established collateral arterial circulation. This means that occlusion of a branch of the pulmonary artery rarely causes infarction of the lung parenchyma and, because the alveolar walls are intact, resolution is possible. The effects of a pulmonary embolus will depend on three factors:

- the size of the occluded vessel
- the number of emboli
- the adequacy of the bronchial blood supply.

Size of the occluded vessel

If a **large embolus occludes a main pulmonary artery** or even sits astride the bifurcation of the pulmonary trunk, a so-called **saddle embolus**, the patient's blood pressure will suddenly drop and there may even be instant death. If the patient survives and reaches hospital, it may be possible to lyse the embolus using medical therapy or remove it surgically (embolectomy). It is tempting to postulate that the circulatory collapse is a result of acute strain put on the right heart by sudden obstruction to the outflow tract. However, this cannot be the whole story because patients tolerate ligation of the pulmonary artery during removal of a lung at surgery. Possibly, the left ventricular outflow drops because the left atrial filling has been reduced, perhaps there may be a reflex vasoconstriction of the entire pulmonary vasculature.

Around 95 per cent of emboli originate in the ileofemoral venous system, a small number coming from the pelvic veins, calf muscle veins and superficial veins of the legs. Obviously, the diameter of these emboli will correspond with the diameter of the vessel of origin, which is less than the size of the major pulmonary arteries. So how does an embolus block a vessel larger than itself? It becomes coiled, as illustrated in Figure 7.1.

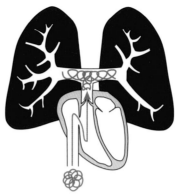

Large P.E.
Large embolus coils within major pulmonary artery. "Saddle" embolus blocks both pulmonary arteries. This produces circulatory collapse

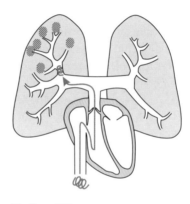

Medium P.E.
Dual blood supply protects lung from effects of pulmonary arterial obstruction

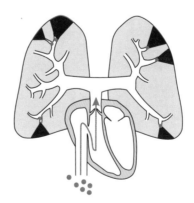

Multiple emboli combined with poor bronchial blood supply
Leads to pulmonary infarction

Bronchial artery not shown

Figure 7.1 Types of pulmonary embolism

Not infrequently, a long single embolus may fragment in the circulation to produce numerous small emboli. These may reach the small pulmonary arteries as a 'shower' to occlude several vessels at the same time, producing sudden, severe clinical effects similar to those of a single large embolus.

If a **medium-sized pulmonary artery** becomes blocked, this may produce no clinical effect because the bronchial circulation is able to supply the lung parenchyma. Generally, there will be local haemorrhage but no damage to the framework of the lung, so complete resolution can occur. If the haemorrhage is small, the patient may be asymptomatic, but if it is large, the patient may have some shortness of breath or haemoptysis.

If the **small peripheral pulmonary arteries** are involved, there may be infarction because the area is beyond the territory of the bronchial collateral supply so the pulmonary arteries are, in effect, end arteries. The area affected will generally be quite small but may produce symptoms, especially if there are multiple emboli.

Dyspnoea: sensation of shortness of breath. When associated with cardiac failure, it may be due to pulmonary oedema interfering with gaseous exchange and lung stretch reflexes. If worse on lying flat, it is called orthopnoea

Haemoptysis: coughing up blood from the respiratory tract

The number of emboli

Multiple emboli may be thrown into the lungs as a single event, or there may be successive embolic episodes. The first situation occurs when a single large embolus fragments into smaller emboli before reaching the lungs. The second scenario

happens when initially only part of the thrombus breaks off but, hours or days later, a second piece follows. If a patient survives the initial pulmonary embolus, there is a 30 per cent risk of suffering from a further embolus. This makes it extremely important that the patient receives prompt and effective anticoagulant therapy to reduce the risk. However, the anticoagulant therapy will not remove the existing embolus; that requires fibrinolytic treatment, as described earlier. Sometimes a patient will remain in 'shock' despite complete lysis of the embolus, and this is possibly a result of intense vasoconstriction of the peripheral pulmonary vessels.

The adequacy of the bronchial blood supply

If a patient suffers from heart failure or has pre-existing pulmonary disease, the bronchial blood supply will be impaired, and emboli lodging in medium-sized pulmonary arteries will result in infarction. Since the blockage is relatively proximal, the infarct will be large, extending as a cone with the apex at the blocked vessel and the base on the pleura (Figure 7.1). The area will initially be firm and purple because of the haemorrhage and congestion, but later it will be replaced by pale fibrous tissue and the area will shrink. Infarcts are most common in the lower lobes of the lungs and are multiple in 50 per cent of cases. These patients tend to get chest pain related to inflammation of the adjacent pleura and shortness of breath owing to both a reduction in lung volume and humoral and neural factors leading to vasoconstriction and bronchoconstriction (see Figure 7.5, page 117).

A typical clinical scenario is that of an elderly patient in hospital who has cardiac failure and a fractured neck of femur following a fall. The combination of recumbency, cardiac failure and postoperative dehydration combine to create an ideal situation for the formation of a deep vein thrombosis in the leg veins. A moderately-sized embolus, over a background of an inadequate collateral supply due to cardiac failure, results in significant ischaemia of the lung parenchyma and infarction.

Fate of the embolus

In some ways, this is similar to that of a thrombus. Ideally, it will be lysed by the fibrinolytic system to restore patency of the vessel. If not, organisation takes place, and the mass will be incorporated into the wall, with possible recanalisation of the vessel. Spontaneous lysis is often very good, so it is important to support the patient to allow 'nature' to do the healing.

If there are multiple emboli or repeated episodes of embolisation and organisation, the pulmonary vessel wall will thicken, resulting in a rise in pulmonary arterial pressure (pulmonary hypertension). This in turn means an increased workload for the right ventricle, which tries to compensate by becoming thicker (hypertrophy). Eventually, the right ventricle may not be able to compensate, and cardiac failure will ensue. Right ventricular enlargement due to pulmonary disease is called **cor pulmonale**.

SYSTEMIC EMBOLISM

Systemic emboli travel in the internal circulation, commonly originating in the left side of the heart from thrombi forming on areas of myocardial infarction or thrombus forming on an atheromatous aorta. Other causes include fragments of atheromatous plaques, which result from fissuring or ulceration of a plaque that releases its fibrin, lipid and cholesterol mixture into the circulation.

Arterial emboli, unless very small, nearly always cause infarction. Emboli to the lower limbs may produce gangrene of a few toes or of the entire limb. Cerebral emboli cause death or infarction unless the embolus lodges in an area that receives adequate collateral supply through the circle of Willis. Alternative sites are the upper limb and the vessels supplying the gut, kidney and spleen. A special type of systemic embolus comprises the infected material from vegetations on the heart valves in **infective endocarditis**. These produce septic infarcts and large abscesses in the affected tissues.

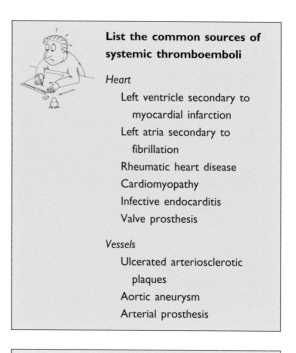

List the common sources of systemic thromboemboli

Heart
　　Left ventricle secondary to
　　　　myocardial infarction
　　Left atria secondary to
　　　　fibrillation
　　Rheumatic heart disease
　　Cardiomyopathy
　　Infective endocarditis
　　Valve prosthesis

Vessels
　　Ulcerated arteriosclerotic
　　　　plaques
　　Aortic aneurysm
　　Arterial prosthesis

Paradoxical embolus: venous thrombi that pass through a right-to-left congenital cardiac anomaly

OTHER TYPES OF EMBOLI

Other types of emboli generally enter veins rather than arteries because veins have thinner walls and a lower pressure. Therefore, most are venous emboli that lodge in the lungs.

Bone marrow emboli

Bone marrow emboli are occasionally seen in histological sections of lungs at autopsy. This is especially likely if the patient has suffered major trauma, such as a road traffic accident, but can even occur with the 'trauma' of attempted cardiac resuscitation, particularly in elderly people whose costal cartilages have ossified. Anything that fractures bone can release bone and bone marrow into the venous circulation, with resulting pulmonary emboli, but the clinical significance of this type of embolisation is unclear.

Fat emboli

Fat from the marrow cavities of long bones or from soft tissue can also enter the circulation as a result of severe trauma. However, they even form without any trauma, so alternative mechanisms must operate. Fortunately, although fat globules are found in the lungs of most victims of severe trauma, fewer than 5 per cent will suffer from the 'fat embolism syndrome', which is characterised by respiratory problems, a haemorrhagic skin rash and mental deterioration 24–72 hours after the injury. The syndrome is unlikely to result merely from the mechanical blockage of vessels but probably involves **chemical injury** to the small vessels of the lungs, producing pulmonary oedema and activation of the **coagulation pathway** to cause DIC. However, the exact mediators have not been identified. The origin of the fat in the non-trauma cases may be chylomicrons and fatty acids in the circulation coalescing to form droplets: **the emulsion instability theory**.

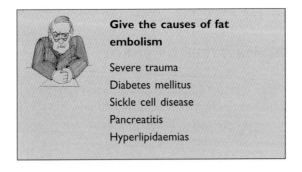

Give the causes of fat embolism

Severe trauma
Diabetes mellitus
Sickle cell disease
Pancreatitis
Hyperlipidaemias

Air and nitrogen emboli

Large quantities of air within the circulation can act as emboli by forming a frothy mass that can block vessels or become trapped in the right heart chambers to impede its pumping. Air can either enter the circulation from the atmosphere or be produced within the circulation by alteration of the pressure.

Severe trauma to the thorax may open large vessels (e.g. the internal jugular veins), allowing air to be sucked in during inspiration, or air may be

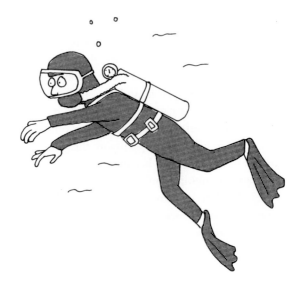

Figure 7.2

forced into the uterine vessels during badly performed abortions or deliveries. Fortunately, small quantities of air, as may be introduced during venesection, dissolve in the plasma and it probably takes about 100 ml to produce problems.

A special type of air embolism occurs in deep sea divers. Normally insoluble gases, such as nitrogen or helium, in the diver's breathing mixture will dissolve in the blood and tissues at the high pressures that occur deep beneath the sea surface. As the diver surfaces, the pressure is reduced and the gas begins to come out of solution as minute bubbles. If the reduction of pressure is rapid, these bubbles form emboli, which are particularly likely to lodge in the skeletal and cerebral circulation. The situation is slightly more complicated because platelets adhere to the nitrogen bubbles, activate the coagulation system and produce DIC (see below). The **acute form of decompression sickness**, or **'bends'**, involves pain around joints and in skeletal muscle, respiratory distress and sometimes coma and death. In the early stages, it can be treated by putting the victim in a 'decompression' chamber where the high pressure will redissolve the bubbles and allow a slow, controlled decompression. The **chronic form**, or **caisson disease**, produces multiple areas of ischaemic necrosis in the long bones. (Caissons are high-pressure underwater chambers.)

Amniotic fluid emboli

This is an uncommon but life-threatening form of embolisation. Basically, amniotic fluid is forced into the circulation as a result of tearing of the placental membranes and rupture of the uterine or cervical veins. These emboli are a mixture of fat, hair, mucus, meconium and squamous cells from the fetus and most commonly lodge in the mother's alveolar capillaries. Clinically, there is sudden onset of respiratory failure, often followed by cerebral convulsions and coma. There is also excessive bleeding as a result of DIC and the consumption of clotting factors. Over 80 per cent of the patients who develop amniotic fluid emboli will die. The exact mechanism is still unclear but it is not due simply to blockage of the pulmonary vasculature; it is postulated that some factor, such as prostaglandin F2α, in the amniotic fluid may be involved.

Tumour emboli

Embolisation of tumour is an important mechanism of tumour spread, but it is unlikely to have any immediate cardiovascular effects. The mechanisms involved in this process will be discussed in Chapter 19.

DISSEMINATED INTRAVASCULAR COAGULATION

This is a convenient moment to discuss DIC. We have just mentioned amniotic fluid embolism and are about to move on to 'shock', both conditions that can produce DIC. Furthermore, DIC results from a loss of control in the clotting and

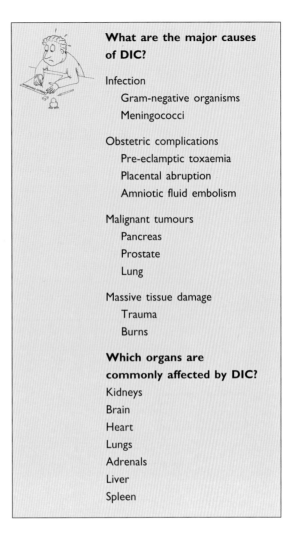

What are the major causes of DIC?

Infection
    Gram-negative organisms
    Meningococci

Obstetric complications
    Pre-eclamptic toxaemia
    Placental abruption
    Amniotic fluid embolism

Malignant tumours
    Pancreas
    Prostate
    Lung

Massive tissue damage
    Trauma
    Burns

Which organs are commonly affected by DIC?

Kidneys

Brain

Heart

Lungs

Adrenals

Liver

Spleen

fibrinolytic systems, which should still be fresh in your memory!

There is no typical clinical presentation because any organ may be affected and the major problem may be excessive clotting, which blocks numerous vessels, or inadequate clotting, resulting in haemorrhage. As a general rule, **sudden-onset DIC** presents with bleeding problems, is particularly associated with obstetric complications and may resolve once the obstetric situation improves. In contrast, **chronic DIC** is more common in patients with carcinomatosis, and thrombotic manifestations dominate.

Small thrombi form anywhere in the circulation and produce microinfarcts. In the brain, this may result in convulsions and coma, lung damage

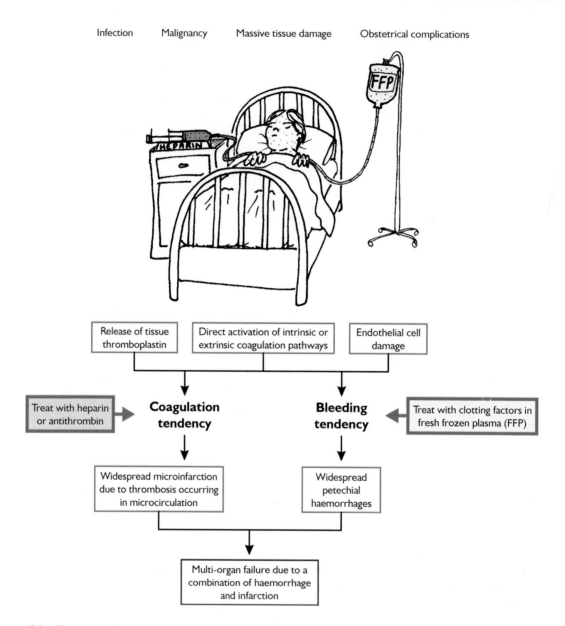

Figure 7.3 Disseminated intravascular coagulation

produces dyspnoea and cyanosis, and renal changes cause oliguria and acute renal failure. Fibrin deposition not only produces thrombi but also results in a haemolytic anaemia as the red cells fragment while squeezing through the narrowed vasculature (microangiopathic haemolytic anaemia).

The fundamental problem is that there is excessive activation of coagulation, which is ultimately complicated by consumption of the coagulation factors and overactivity of the fibrinolytic system. Clotting activation occurs through the extrinsic pathway, initiated by tissue thromboplastin, and the intrinsic pathway, commencing with activated factor XII, but it should be remembered that clotting activation will also stimulate the fibrinolytic pathways, particularly through the factor XII path, and fibrin degradation products inhibit fibrin production. These latter mechanisms will predominate in haemorrhagic DIC.

Many of the diseases mentioned produce DIC via the extrinsic pathway. For example, the placenta is believed to release tissue thromboplastin in obstetric problems, mucus from some adenocarcinomas can activate factor X, and bacterial endotoxins can prompt the release of thromboplastic substances contained in endothelial and inflammatory cells. However, nothing involving bacterial endotoxins is simple. They can also activate the intrinsic pathway directly through factor XII and indirectly by damaging endothelial cells. They even inhibit the anticoagulant activity of protein C.

Not surprisingly, the prognosis is very variable and the management extremely difficult because one is trying to balance a see-saw that is out of control. If you inhibit the clotting system too much with heparin or antithrombin III, the patient will bleed, but any bleeding tendency may require fresh frozen plasma, which may contribute to microthrombus formation.

We shall now move on to discuss 'shock', which can produce DIC and may result from many causes, including massive embolism.

SHOCK

Shock is a wonderful word. It means such different things to medical and lay people. How often we hear news reports of someone having been taken to hospital suffering from shock after witnessing some tragic event. No doubt that person is surprised and possibly emotionally disturbed, but he or she is not in a state of **circulatory collapse**, which is what a doctor regards as shock.

The 'shocked' patient is desperately ill and requires intensive treatment both to correct the condition that has produced the circulatory collapse and to cope with the widespread ischaemic damage resulting from shock. By definition, the patient will have hypoperfusion of many tissues. His blood pressure may be low but need not be, as he may either have compensated by increasing peripheral vasoconstriction to keep the pressure normal or may have had a high blood pressure that has now dropped. There may be pallor, cold extremities, sweating and a tachycardia, the first two signs from poor perfusion and the other two from the attempt to compensate, which includes the release of adrenaline.

What has happened to precipitate this disastrous state? Logically, there will be a sudden generalised poor perfusion if the pump fails or there is insufficient blood, so-called **cardiogenic** and **hypovolaemic** shock. Abrupt heart failure may result from myocardial infarction, arrhythmias and cardiac tamponade, while hypovolaemic shock follows fluid loss due to haemorrhage, severe burns, diarrhoea or vomiting. Shock following pulmonary embolism mimics cardiogenic shock, but the heart is normal and the reduced output occurs because the left atrial filling has dropped. A rather special but clinically very important form of shock is **septic shock** as a result of overwhelming infections, especially those caused by Gramnegative bacteria that have endotoxic lipopolysaccharides (see p. 61). Here pathogenesis is complicated because of the varied effects of the bacterial products on endothelial cells, platelets and leucocytes, which leads to a veritable web of interactions resulting in DIC and reduced blood volume because of vasodilatation and increased vascular permeability. Similar mechanisms probably operate in **anaphylactic shock** and **neurogenic shock**.

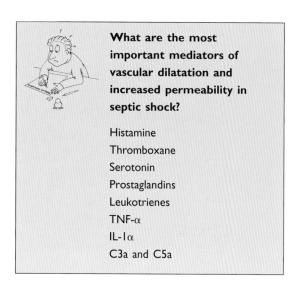

What are the most important mediators of vascular dilatation and increased permeability in septic shock?

Histamine

Thromboxane

Serotonin

Prostaglandins

Leukotrienes

TNF-α

IL-1α

C3a and C5a

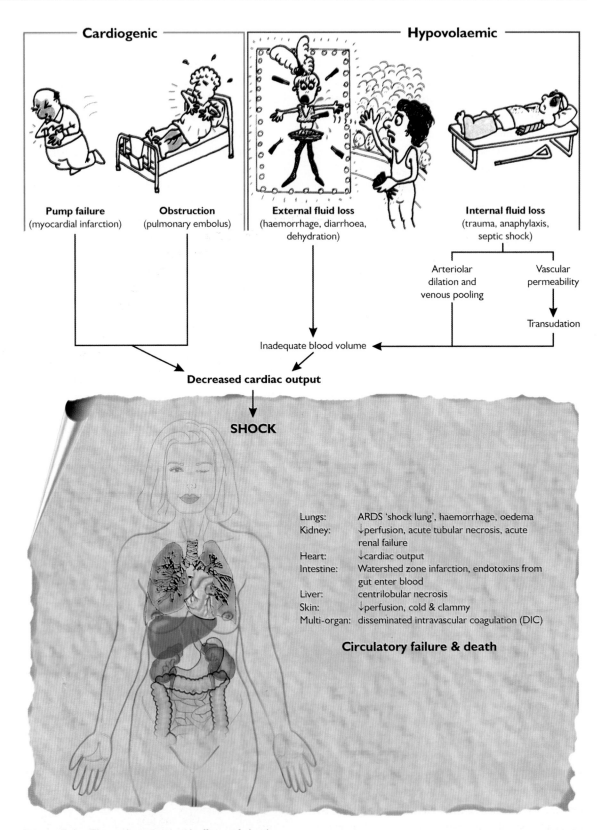

Figure 7.4 The pathogenesis and effects of shock

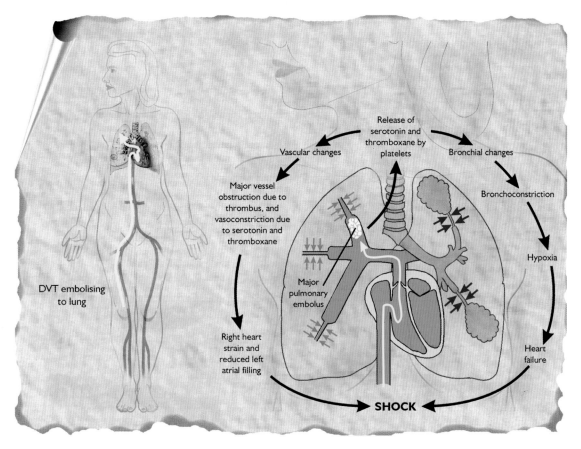

Figure 7.5 The pathogenesis of shock in pulmonary embolism

Whatever the cause, the effect at tissue level is similar, with a reduced delivery of oxygen and nutrients so that cells' normal functions are disturbed. The details of reversible and irreversible cell injury will be discussed in Part 3; here we will concentrate on the clinical effects. The most important organs for immediate survival are the heart and brain, so the body has mechanisms for shunting blood from other tissues to protect these two organs. The kidneys and lungs will frequently be underperfused and sufficiently damaged to be the immediate cause of death.

ADULT RESPIRATORY DISTRESS SYNDROME

The lungs are fairly resistant to short periods of ischaemia but, if prolonged, the patient may develop **shock lung** or **adult respiratory distress syndrome** (**ARDS**), which can be life threatening as it is difficult to maintain adequate ventilation, even with a mechanical ventilator. For oxygen to reach the alveolar blood, air must move in and out of the lungs and be able to diffuse across the alveolar septae. In 'shock lung', there is severe oedema affecting peribronchial connective tissue and alveolar septae and spaces. This both reduces the lung compliance and impairs alveolar diffusion, meaning double trouble and a mortality rate of around 50 per cent.

The probable sequence of events (Figure 7.6) is that the 'shock' causes the release of mediators, such as activated complement (C5a), leukotriene B4 and platelet activating factor, which promote leucocyte aggregation and activation in the lung. The neutrophils produce arachidonic acid metabolites, such as thromboxane, which cause

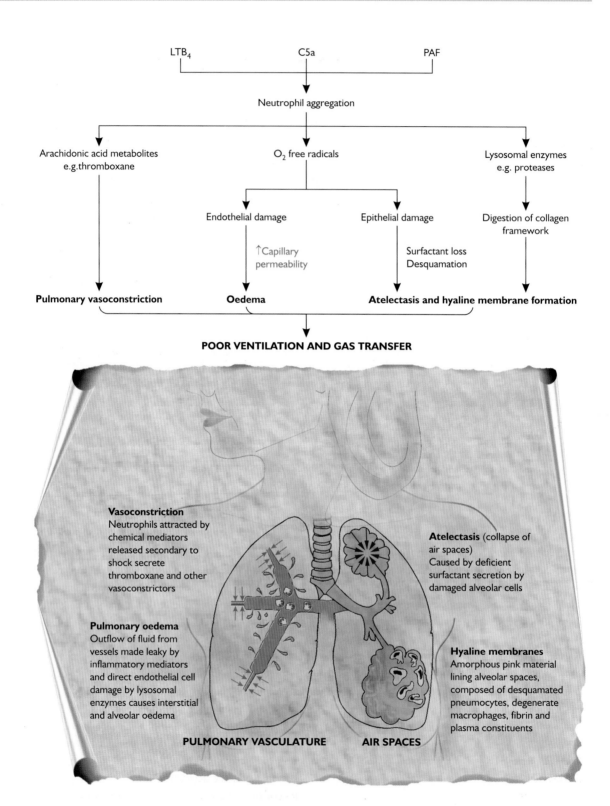

Figure 7.6   The pathogenesis of adult respiratory distress syndrome

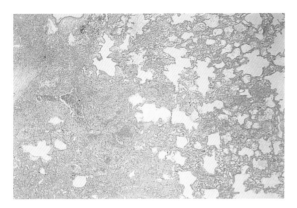

Figure 7.7 Lung photomicrograph showing adult respiratory distress syndrome. There is irregular ventilation due to the presence of hyaline membranes, exudate and cell debris within the alveolar spaces

pulmonary vasoconstriction, oxygen-derived free radicals that injure the endothelial and epithelial cells, and lysosomal enzymes that digest local structural proteins.

The damaged alveolar capillary *endothelial* cells are leaky, which leads to interstitial alveolar oedema and fibrin exudation. The damaged alveolar *epithelial* cells, particularly the type I pneumocytes, desquamate to form the characteristic **hyaline membranes** in combination with surfactant and protein-rich oedema fluid (Figure 7.7). These are the same as the hyaline membranes in neonatal hyaline membrane disease and in both situations indicate severe epithelial injury with lack of surfactant. The lack of surfactant leads to collapse of alveolar air spaces (atelectasis), so further reducing compliance and gas transfer.

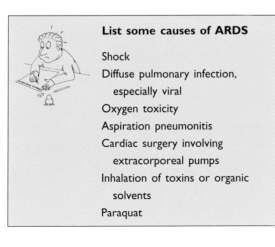

List some causes of ARDS

Shock
Diffuse pulmonary infection, especially viral
Oxygen toxicity
Aspiration pneumonitis
Cardiac surgery involving extracorporeal pumps
Inhalation of toxins or organic solvents
Paraquat

RENAL DAMAGE

Impaired renal blood flow results in **acute tubular necrosis**, a major cause of acute renal failure. This is not immediately apparent in a 'shocked' patient but will become evident once the 'shocked' state is under control and there is no circulatory reason for poor urine output. The patient will then be noted to have oliguria (a urine output of 40–400 ml/day, normal being 1500 ml/day), salt and water overload, high plasma potassium and urea levels, and a metabolic acidosis. At this stage, a renal biopsy will show numerous foci of tubular epithelial cell loss, affecting any area of the nephron, and epithelial 'casts', i.e. dead epithelial cells, present in the tubular lumens. The important clinical point is that the patient can make a complete recovery if appropriately managed, e.g. by dialysis and by rectifying the cause of the shock. After a few days, the tubular epithelium will regenerate, and the urine volume will increase, often to above normal values because the tubules are unable to concentrate the urine, and there may be excessive loss of water, sodium and potassium – the so-called diuretic phase. The tubular epithelium slowly returns to normal, and reasonable renal function is restored.

BRAIN AND CARDIAC DAMAGE

Despite the body's best efforts to protect the heart and brain, these organs may become underperfused.

Damage to the brain may be mild or devastating. The neurons, particularly the large Purkinje cells of the cerebellum and the pyramidal cells in the hippocampus, are most vulnerable to ischaemia. A short episode of hypoperfusion may not cause any irreversible neuronal damage, or the number of neurons damaged may be too few to produce any clinical effect beyond temporary confusion. However, prolonged ischaemia will result in infarction that most commonly affects the 'watershed' areas at the junctional zones between the main arterial territories (Figure 7.8). This may result in severe permanent cerebral damage or coma and death. It is important to remember that the 'watershed' effect operates in many organs if

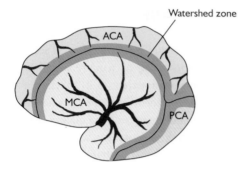

Lateral aspect of left cerebral hemisphere

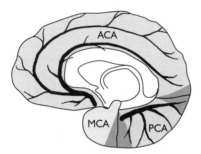

Medial aspect of right cerebral hemisphere

Key:

MCA   Middle cerebral artery
ACA   Anterior cerebral artery
PCA   Posterior cerebral artery

Figure 7.8   Watershed zones in the brain

Describe the damage that may occur in the organs of a patient with shock

Kidney	Acute tubular necrosis
Lung	ARDS
Heart	Ischaemic damage
Brain	Watershed infarcts
Liver	Fatty change/ necrosis
Adrenal	Focal haemorrhagic necrosis
Pancreas	Pancreatitis
Stomach	Erosive gastritis
Duodenum	Ulceration
Small and large bowel	Haemorrhagic gastroentero-pathy/infarction

there is poor perfusion. In the heart, this is the subendothelial zone because the endocardium is nourished by direct diffusion from the blood in the cardiac chambers and the outer myocardium is supplied by arterioles penetrating from the outside. In the gut, areas such as the splenic flexure of the colon are at the boundary between arterial supplies and thus vulnerable to poor perfusion.

CHAPTER 8

ANAEMIA

- What is anaemia?
- Iron deficiency anaemia
- Haemoglobinopathies
- Megaloblastic anaemia

We have discussed the problems related to abnormal clotting and blocked vessels, but what about abnormalities in other blood constituents? The aim of the circulatory system is to deliver nutrients to the tissues and remove waste products. This can be inadequate because of pump problems, pipe problems or the liquid itself, but the liquid is no ordinary liquid. The successful delivery of nutrients requires appropriate transport factors in the blood, the most important of which is haemoglobin. It is beyond the scope of this book to describe the whole of haematology, but we can provide a framework for thinking about blood disorders.

First it is time for a clinical scenario. A 21-year-old lady goes to see her GP for a prenatal health check as she wants to become pregnant for the first time. The doctor advises her about the risks of smoking and alcohol on the fetus and performs a physical examination, finding no abnormalities. Her blood pressure is normal, and he takes a blood sample for further analysis. The blood results and a table of normal values are produced below (Tables 8.1 and 8.2).

When the lady returns to the surgery the following week, the doctor explains that she has a minor problem because she is anaemic and probably has iron deficiency.

Table 8.1 Normal peripheral blood values

Haemoglobin (g/dl)	14–18 (male)	12–16 (female)
Erythrocytes ($\times 10^{12}$/l)	4.6–6.0 (male)	4.2–5.4 (female)
Haematocrit (PCV) (%)	42–50 (male)	37–47 (female)
MCV (fl)	80–95	
MCHC (%)	32–35	
Reticulocytes ($\times 10^9$/l)	~100 (male)	~100 (female)

PCV = packed cell volume; MCV = mean corpuscular volume; MCHC = mean corpuscular haemoglobin concentration.

WHAT IS ANAEMIA?

A few key words or parts of words will help us through the maze of blood disorders. Any word ending in 'aemia' relates to the blood (e.g.

Table 8.2 Patient's peripheral blood results

Haemoglobin (g/dl)	8.2
Erythrocytes ($\times 10^{12}$/l)	4.7
Haematocrit (PCV) (%)	0.31
MCV (fl)	69
MCHC (%)	24.5
Reticulocytes ($\times 10^9$/l)	96

PCV = packed cell volume; MCV = mean corpuscular volume; MCHC = mean corpuscular haemoglobin concentration.

Table 8.3 Glossary of haematological terms

Anaemia	Reduction in haemoglobin in blood
Pancytopenia	Reduction in all blood cell types
Neutropenia	Reduction in neutrophils
Thrombocytopenia	Reduction in platelets
Polycythaemia	Increase in red cells
Thrombocythaemia	Increase in platelets
Leucocytosis	Increase in white cells
Leukaemia	Malignant haemopoietic cells in blood
Aplastic marrow	No haemopoiesis in the marrow
Hypoplastic marrow	Reduced haemopoiesis in the marrow
Hyperplastic marrow	Increased haemopoiesis in the marrow
Leukoerythroblastic	Red and white cell precursors in the peripheral blood may indicate marrow replacement by fibrosis, tumour or abscesses

Red cell changes

Normocytic	Normal cell size
Macrocytic	↑MCV
Microcytic	↓MCV
Normochromic	Normal haemoglobin concentration
Hypochromic	↓MCHC
Poikilocytosis	Variation in shape
Anisocytosis	Variation in size
Howell–Jolly bodies	Nuclear remnants in delayed maturation

MCV = mean corpuscular volume; MCHC = mean corpuscular haemoglobin concentration.

polycythaemia or hypoalbuminaemia), just as words ending in 'uria' relate to the urine (e.g. haematuria – blood in the urine; anuria – not passing urine). A prefix of 'hypo' indicates too little, 'micro' means too small, 'hyper' is too much and 'macro' is too big. *Leuk*aemia literally means white blood but has become synonymous with a malignancy of blood cells. *An*aemia strictly means a lack of blood, which is not really correct because there is a reduction in the number of red blood cells rather than an absence of them. The term is now used to indicate a reduction in haemoglobin concentration in the blood, as in our patient's blood test. So what are the possible causes?

The red blood cells contain haemoglobin, which is important in the transport of oxygen. The haemoglobin level may drop because the number of red cells is low (reduced red cell mass) or the content of haemoglobin reduced. Red cell numbers may be reduced because of impaired production, acute or chronic blood loss through bleeding or a reduced life span for a variety of reasons.

Anaemia can be classified according to its cause (Table 8.4) or according to the appearance of the blood (Table 8.5). It is important to know both because the first investigation of a pale patient is to perform a full blood count, which will detail the haemoglobin level in the blood, the number of red blood cells, the size of the red cells (mean corpuscular volume) and the average concentration of haemoglobin in a red cell (mean corpuscular haemoglobin concentration). If the haemoglobin level indicates that the patient is anaemic, the MCV and MCHC can be used to classify the anaemia according to cell size and haemoglobin concentration, and possible causes can be looked

Table 8.4 Causes of anaemia

1. Decreased red cell production

Defective haemoglobin production

    Iron deficiency

    Anaemia of chronic disease

    Sideroblastic anaemia

Defective DNA synthesis (megaloblastic anaemia)

    Vitamin B12 deficiency

    Folic acid deficiency

Stem cell failure; e.g. aplastic anaemia

Bone marrow replacement, e.g. infiltration by
malignant disease

Inadequate erythropoietin stimulation, e.g. chronic
renal failure

Other nutritional and toxic factors

    Scurvy

    Protein malnutrition

    Chronic liver disease

    Hypothyroidism

2. Increased red cell destruction, i.e. haemolytic anaemias

Intrinsic defect of erythrocytes

    Congenital

    • Haemoglobinopathies

      – Sickle cell anaemia

      – Thalassaemias

    • Membrane defects, e.g. hereditary
spherocytosis

    • Enzyme. deficiency, e.g. glucose-6-phosphate
dehydrogenase (G6PD) deficiency

    Acquired, e.g. paroxysmal nocturnal
haemoglobinuria

Extrinsic cause for haemolysis

    Immune mediated

    • Autoimmune haemolytic anaemia

    • Haemolytic disease of the newborn

    • Blood transfusion-related haemolysis

    • Drug-induced immune haemolytic anaemia

    Direct acting

    • Infections, e.g. malaria

    • Snake venom

    • Physical trauma, e.g. microangiopathy

    • Hypersplenism

3. Blood loss

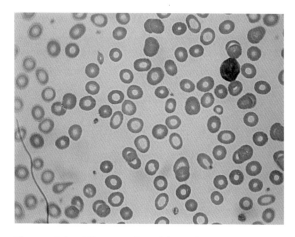

Figure 8.1 Microcytosis and hypochromia in a case of iron deficiency anaemia

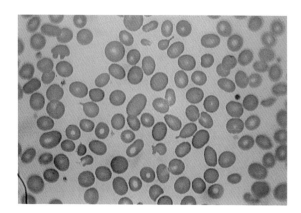

Figure 8.2 Oval macrocytes in a case of pernicious anaemia

up in Table 8.6. Try this for our patient whose results appear on page 122. Remember that 'cytic' refers to the cell and 'chromic' refers to the haemoglobin concentration.

Hopefully, you have concluded that our lady has small red cells with a reduced haemoglobin concentration, i.e. a microcytic hypochromic anaemia. To search further for a cause, you need more information. The most common causes of anaemia can be identified through a combination of:

• reticulocyte count
• the morphological appearance of the cells in the peripheral blood
• haemoglobin electrophoresis

Table 8.5 Morphological classification of anaemia

Type	MCV	MCHC	Common causes
Normocytic/normochromic	Normal	Normal	Anaemia of chronic disease Chronic renal failure
Microcytic/hypochromic	↓	↓	Iron deficiency Beta thalassaemia trait Anaemia of chronic disease (severe)
Macrocytic (megaloblastic)	↑	Normal	Folid acid deficiency Vitamin B12 deficiency
Macrocytic (non-megaloblastic)	↑	Normal	Liver disease, alcohol ingestion Hypothyroidism
Leucoerythroblastic anaemia	Normal	Normal	Replacement or infiltration of marrow

Megaloblastic refers to abnormal maturation of erythroid cells detectable on examination of the marrow.

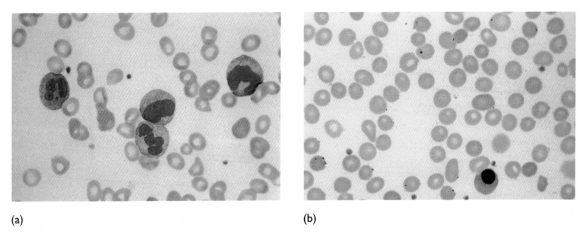

(a) (b)

Figure 8.3 Two areas from the peripheral blood from a patient with leucoerythroblastic anaemia. Photograph (a) shows myelocytes, while (b) shows an erythroblast (nucleated red cell)

- serum iron level
- bone marrow examination
- serum ferritin level (serum iron and iron binding capacity originally being used)
- serum B12 and folate levels
- the Schilling test
- antibody screens (e.g. parietal cell and intrinsic factor antibodies).

Reticulocytes are newly released red cells that are slightly larger than mature red cells and have a more basophilic (blue) cytoplasm on routine Giemsa staining. Approximately 1 per cent is the normal level, an increased value indicating an increased red cell turnover. The reticulocytes normally become mature red cells in the marrow, and it is only when the demand for red blood cells exceeds supply that these immature forms are released in significant numbers. Our lady has a normal reticulocyte count, so the most likely diagnosis is iron deficiency anaemia, which is a common finding in premenopausal and pregnant women and easily treated with iron tablets. The doctor is not likely to investigate any further unless the pregnant lady has other problems, but we shall digress to discuss the causes of iron deficiency.

Table 8.6 Investigation of anaemia

PB red cells	Macrocytic/normochromic		Microcytic/hypochromic			Normocytic/normochromic			Dimorphic
Reticulocytes	N↓	N↓	N	↑	↑	N/↓	N/↓	↑	↓
PB film				Target or sickle cells	Spherocytes			Nucleated red cells	Iron stain may show granules
PB other lines	Hypersegmented neutrophils		↑ Platelets				↓ Platelets ↓ White cells	Left-shifted white cells	
Serum iron	N	N	↓	N/↑	N/↑	N/↓	N	N	↑
Haemoglobin electrophoresis	N	N	N	Abnormal	N	N	N	N	N
Bone marrow erythropoiesis	↑ + Megaloblasts	Variable	N/↑	↑↑	↑↑	Variable	Aplasia	↓ + Fibrosis tumour cells	↑ + Sideroblasts
Bone marrow iron stores	N	N	↓	↑	N	↑	N	N	N
Vitamin B12 level	↓ or N	N	N	N	N	N	N	N	N
Folate level	↓ or N	N	N	N	N	N	N	N	N
Diagnoses	Megaloblastic anaemia, e.g. pernicious anaemia	Simple macrocytic anaemia, e.g. alcoholic liver disease, hypothyroidism, cytotoxic drugs	Iron deficiency anaemia	Haemolytic anaemia: haemoglobino-pathies	Haemolytic anaemia: immune	Anaemia of chronic disease	Aplastic anaemia	Leucoerythro-blastic anaemia	Sideroblastic anaemia

PB = peripheral blood.

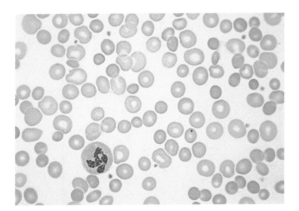

Figure 8.4 Peripheral blood in a patient with spherocytosis

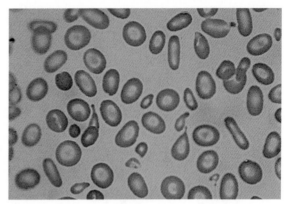

Figure 8.6 HbH disease showing marked anisopoikilocytosis

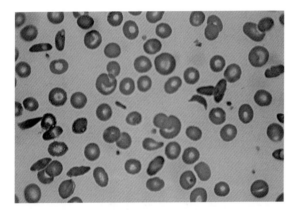

Figure 8.5 Sickle cell disease

IRON DEFICIENCY ANAEMIA

Iron is absorbed in the upper small intestine and transported in the blood bound to the glycoprotein transferrin; details of this process can be found on pages 208–211. There is no control over the excretion of iron, and iron loss from the body is through loss in secretions, exfoliated cells and menstrual blood. There is some control over the absorption of iron, between 10 and 20 per cent of dietary iron being absorbed. This does not leave much of a safety margin, so iron deficiency is the most common cause of anaemia, occurring because of an imbalance between absorption and loss. In developed countries, an average diet contains

Table 8.7 Causes of iron deficiency anaemia

Inadequate intake
Deficient diet
Malabsorption
    Generalised malabsorption, e.g. coeliac disease
    Post-gastrectomy (rapid gastrojejunal transit)

Increased iron loss
Reproductive tract
    Heavy menstruation
    Pregnancies and miscarriages
Gastrointestinal tract
    Oesophageal varices
    Peptic ulcer disease
    Chronic aspirin ingestion
    Hookworm infestation
    Haemorrhoids
    Tumours
Miscellaneous
    Epistaxis
    Haematuria
    Haemoptysis

Increased demand for iron
Early childhood
Pregnancy and lactation

about 15 mg iron, the daily requirement for *absorbed* iron being 0.5–1.0 mg for men and 0.7–2.0 mg for women. This means that any reduction in dietary iron, problem with absorption or increased requirement for iron will lead to deficiency (Table 8.7). Iron balance is particularly precarious in premenopausal women because of menstrual blood loss. Fifty millilitres of whole blood contains about 25 mg iron, which would require an extra 250 mg iron in the diet to be back in balance.

There are no immediate problems for the person developing iron deficiency because red cell production continues, but the iron stores in the marrow become depleted. Once the iron stores are inadequate, red cells are still produced but are small (microcytic) with too little haemoglobin (hypochromic); the patient will become tired and lethargic, be breathless on exertion and appear pale. Patients may also have problems owing to the effects of iron deficiency on epithelial cells if they do not receive treatment but remain chronically iron deficient. This complication, however, is rare in most countries. The mucous membranes of the mouth, tongue, pharynx, oesophagus and stomach become thin (atrophic), which may cause difficulty in swallowing (dysphagia) and produce mucosal webs in the upper oesophagus. Fingernails become spoon shaped (koilonychia) and split easily, and the thinned stomach wall does not produce a normal amount of acid. This combination of problems in severe iron deficiency is called the Plummer–Vinson syndrome and is cured by giving iron.

Paterson–Kelly–Plummer–Vinson syndrome

This syndrome was first described in 1909 by Donald R. Patterson (an ENT surgeon in Cardiff) and Adam B. Kelly (an ENT surgeon in Glasgow). It was also described by Henry S. Plummer (a physician at the Mayo Clinic, USA) and Porter P. Vinson (a physician in Virginia, USA). In medical textbooks, you may come across a variety of combinations of these names

How can we confirm that a patient's anaemia is due to iron deficiency and how can we assess the severity?

The doctor in the clinic will be taking a good history to ask about diet and blood loss in menstruation, urine and faeces, and checking whether the patient is taking any medicines, such as aspirin, that can cause repeated small inconspicuous gastric bleeds. The laboratory can look at the patient's serum iron and total iron binding capacity (TIBC). TIBC relates to transferrin, which carries the iron in the blood and is normally about 30 per cent saturated. In the early stages of iron deficiency, the body tries to increase the absorption of iron, which is reflected in an increased TIBC. The absolute level of serum iron will be normal until the iron stores are depleted, then drop. The percentage saturation decreases because of a combination of increased iron binding capacity and decreased iron.

Modern laboratories often prefer to measure serum ferritin because it is technically easier. If the serum ferritin is low, it confirms iron deficiency anaemia. If it is normal or slightly raised, it is unhelpful because serum ferritin increases nonspecifically in acute phase reactions. A very high reading suggests haemochromatosis.

If necessary, a piece of bone marrow can be examined. There will be a reduction in iron stored in the macrophages, and red cell production will be increased (erythroid hyperplasia) to try to compensate for the anaemia. However, this is not normally necessary in suspected iron deficiency anaemia.

Let us return to the doctor's surgery, where the prenatal clinic is progressing, and consider the next lady's blood results (Table 8.8). She has anaemia, but in this case the reticulocyte count is raised. You will remember that this indicates increased red cell production to compensate for red cell destruction. Why should she have red cells with a reduced life span? The answer is seen in the peripheral blood film where there are sickle cells. Sickle cells and some other abnormalities such as target cells are most common when the red cells contain an abnormal haemoglobin, so the next

Table 8.8   Table of blood results

Haemoglobin (g/dl)	8.5
Erythrocytes ($\times 10^{12}$/l)	3.2
Haematocrit (PCV) (%)	28
MCV (fl)	92
MCHC (%)	31
Reticulocytes ($\times 10^9$/l)	250

step is to perform haemoglobin electrophoresis. (You may be wondering why the MCV and MCHC are not typical of a microcytic, hypochromic anaemia: the situation is complicated when the reticulocyte count is high because reticulocytes are large and influence the MCV reading.)

HAEMOGLOBINOPATHIES

Electrophoresis is a technique for identifying molecules based on the distance that they travel along a track. There is a voltage difference on this track so that the molecule is driven by its charge and held back by its size. Haemoglobin is composed of two pairs of (i.e. four) polypeptide chains, each of which is linked to a haem group. The haem group is a protoporphorin molecule chelated with iron and able to carry oxygen. For the moment, we shall concentrate on the polypeptide chains. The normal chains are called alpha (α), beta (β), gamma (γ) and delta (δ). All normal haemoglobin has one pair of alpha chains combined with a pair of another type of chain. Hence there is haemoglobin A (α2β2), haemoglobin A2 (α2δ2) and haemoglobin F (α2γ2). HbF predominates in the fetus and HbA in the adult.

When our lady's haemoglobin is run on an electrophoretic strip, it has a band that does not correspond with the normal polypeptide chains, indicating that she has an abnormal chain. By running control specimens with known abnormal-

ities, this can be identified as sickle cell haemoglobin (HbS) in which an otherwise normal beta chain has a single amino acid altered at position 6, glutamate being replaced by valine. Unfortunately, she does not have a band corresponding with normal haemoglobin A, so we can conclude that she is homozygous for the gene (see p. 288 and Figure 23.5), i.e. she has two abnormal genes. This is called sickle cell *disease*, whereas heterozygous individuals have some normal beta chains and much less severe symptoms, the condition being called sickle cell *trait*.

Sickle cell disease is so called because the red blood cells become sickle shaped when the oxygen tension is reduced, as can occur in the tissues as oxygen is removed from the blood. The sickled cells are less flexible than normal red cells and have difficulty squeezing through small capillaries; this leads to occlusion of the small vessels. The person complains of abdominal pain, joint pains and cerebral problems because of a mixture of ischaemic and thrombotic damage. The patient is anaemic because the altered red cells are removed from the circulation by the spleen (so-called extravascular haemolysis), and the anaemia is an example of a haemolytic anaemia.

The altered amino acid in HbS acts to reduce the solubility of haemoglobin in low oxygen tensions so that it polymerises as crystalline structures called tactoids. These interact with the red cell's spectrin–actin cytoskeleton to produce the change in cell shape. In people with sickle cell trait, each cell has about 30 per cent HbS and 70 per cent HbA, while people with sickle cell disease have around 80 per cent HbS, the rest being HbF and HbA2.

Sickle cell disease is not the only haemoglobinopathy, although it is one of the most common. Haemoglobinopathies can result from an abnormal chain being present or one type of chain not being produced. In thalassaemias, the chains are normal in structure, but not enough are produced. This condition is common in people originating from the Mediterranean, Africa and Asia, and results from a wide variety of underlying genetic changes. The severity of the person's symptoms depends on the chain involved and whether he or

Normal haemoglobin types

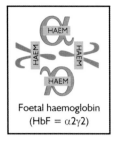

Foetal haemoglobin
(HbF = α2γ2)

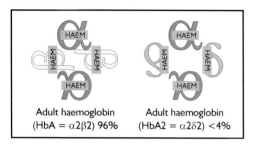

Adult haemoglobin
(HbA = α2β2) 96%

Adult haemoglobin
(HbA2 = α2δ2) <4%

Abnormal haemoglobin types

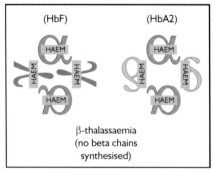

(HbF)   (HbA2)

β-thalassaemia
(no beta chains
synthesised)

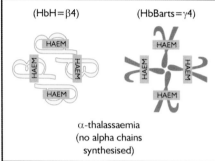

(HbH=β4)   (HbBarts=γ4)

α-thalassaemia
(no alpha chains
synthesised)

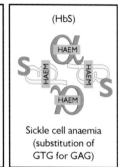

(HbS)

Sickle cell anaemia
(substitution of
GTG for GAG)

Figure 8.7 Normal and abnormal haemoglobin types

she is homozygous or heterozygous for the abnormality. All normal haemoglobin has alpha chains, so the complete absence of alpha chains is incompatible with life and an affected fetus will be oedematous (hydropic). In the absence of any alpha chains, the other chains do their best to produce a haemoglobin molecule by combining together as HbBarts (γ4) and HbH(β4). This is the position with deletion of all four genes, and, predictably, the severity decreases with the addition of each alpha chain (see written examination box, page 130). This group of conditions is called alpha-thalassaemia.

Around 95 per cent of adult haemoglobin is HbA composed of alpha and beta chains, so the other important disease is beta-thalassaemia, with absent or reduced beta chains and attempts to compensate by producing HbA2 and HbF, using the gamma and delta chains respectively.

The main clinical problems in thalassaemia result from the haemolysis of red cells with the abnormal haemoglobin. These cells have a reduced life span and are removed in the reticuloendothelial system, particularly the spleen and marrow. Here the red cell components are broken down for reuse or excretion. The iron is stored in the tissues as ferritin and haemosiderin and, if excessive, can cause tissue damage as described on pages 208–211). The protoporphyrins are degraded to produce bile pigments, any excess giving the patient a yellow tinge to the skin and sclerae, i.e. jaundice.

In intrinsic red cell problems, the haemolysis is usually extravascular, i.e. occurring in the reticuloendothelial system, and can lead to splenomegaly. There is also a group of conditions in which the haemolysis is intravascular so that the red cells rupture within the blood vessels, releasing free haemoglobin, some of which becomes bound to haptoglobin, some bound to albumin (methaemalbumin) and some excreted by the kidneys, giving rise to haemoglobinuria. These patients are also anaemic and jaundiced. Intravascular haemolysis is generally due to

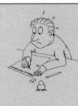

Describe the normal and abnormal forms of haemoglobin

Normal

HbA   α2β2   96% in adult

HbA2   α2δ2   3% in adult

HbF   α2γ2   1% in adult

large amounts in fetus/neonate

Abnormal

HbS sickle cell disease

> beta-chain position 6 has
> valine substituted for
> glutamate

Thalassaemias

> *Alpha*
>
> Genotype
>
> −α/αα   silent carrier
>
> −α/−α   α trait
>
> −−/αα
>
> −−/−α   HbH β4
>
> −−/−−   Hydrops fetalis with
>   HbBarts γ4
>
> generally due to gene
> deletion
>
> *Beta*
>
> β°   complete absence
>   of beta-chains
>
> β⁺   reduction in beta
>   chains
>
> Thalassaemia major =
> homozygous
>
> Thalassaemia minor =
> heterozygous
>
> generally due to defects in
> transcription, processing or
> translation of the genes

antibodies binding to the red cells, fixing complement and causing lysis. Antibodies can also promote extravascular haemolysis as the spleen will remove antibody-coated cells (see p. 37).

MEGALOBLASTIC ANAEMIA

The final lady in our prenatal clinic has Crohn's disease, which is an inflammatory disease that can affect any area of the gastrointestinal tract. The terminal ileum is commonly involved, and this can result in anaemia due to vitamin B12 deficiency. Her blood results are shown below. You have had enough practice to know the normal values without referring to page 121.

Table 8.9 Patient's blood results

Haemoglobin (g/dl)	5.0
Erythrocytes ($\times 10^{12}$/l)	1.7
Haematocrit (PCV) (%)	0.21
MCV (fl)	128
MCHC (%)	35
Reticulocytes ($\times 10^9$/l)	40

The MCV is increased and the MCHC is normal consistent with a macrocytic anaemia. We are going to concentrate on the subset of macrocytic anaemias that have abnormal erythroid maturation in the bone marrow resulting in large precursors and called 'megaloblastic'. Megaloblastic anaemia is most commonly due to vitamin B12 or folate deficiency (Table 8.10). Both are co-factors for the conversion of deoxyuridine to deoxythymidine, an essential step in the synthesis of DNA.

Working down our list of investigations, we first ask for a reticulocyte count and a peripheral blood film. The laboratory tells us that there are few or no reticulocytes but that the red cells contain Howell–Jolly bodies (nuclear remnants resulting from delayed maturation), the red cells are large (macrocytic) and of variable shape (poikilocytosis) and the neutrophils are hypersegmented (most normal neutrophils have three or four lobes, whereas hypersegmented cells have more). These are all features of megaloblastic anaemia.

Haemolytic anaemia

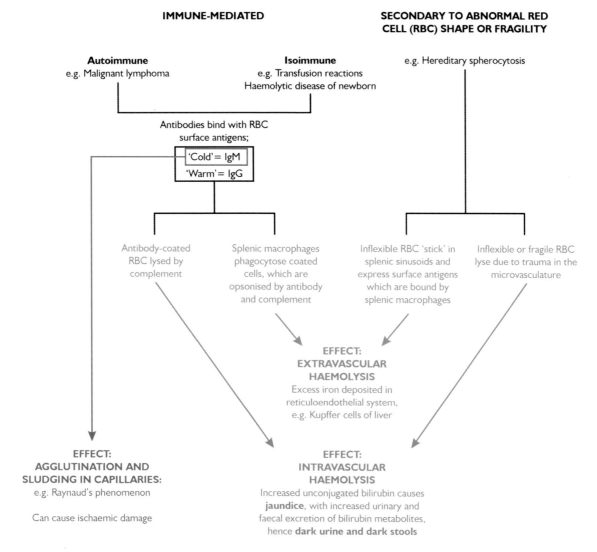

Figure 8.8 Haemolytic anaemia

The next step is to measure the serum vitamin B12 level and serum and red cell folate levels. If the folate level is low, we have a diagnosis of folate deficiency, whose cause should be identified by taking a good history. If the vitamin B12 level is low, we can investigate further and need to understand a little more about B12 absorption. Vitamin B12 is absorbed in the terminal ileum as a complex bound to intrinsic factor. Intrinsic factor (IF) is produced by the parietal cells in the stomach. This means that you need an adequate

diet and a normal stomach and terminal ileum to avoid B12 deficiency.

We assume that our lady with Crohn's disease will fail to absorb the B12/intrinsic factor complex because she has a diseased terminal ileum, but how can we prove this? We could demonstrate that her bone marrow is vitamin B12 deficient by *injecting* some vitamin B12 and observing an almost immediate increase in reticulocytes. In people with a normal terminal ileum but a damaged stomach, the parietal cells are unable to produce intrinsic

Table 8.10   Causes of megaloblastic anaemia

Vitamin B12 deficiency

Inadequate diet
  Strict vegans excluding milk, eggs and cheese
Absorption problem
  Intrinsic factor deficiency
  • Pernicious anaemia
  • Total and subtotal gastrectomy
  Terminal ileal disease
  • Crohn's disease
  • Surgical removal
Competition by microorganisms
  Bacterial overgrowth in blind loops
  Fish tapeworm infection

Folic acid deficiency

Inadequate diet
  Malnutrition
  Chronic alcoholism
Absorption problem
  Generalised malabsorption
  Tropical sprue
  Gluten-induced enteropathy (coeliac disease)
Increased demand
  Early childhood
  Pregnancy
  Erythroid hyperplasia in severe haemolytic
    anaemias
Use of folic acid antagonists
  Anticonvulsants, e.g. phenytoin
  Anticancer drugs, e.g. methotrexate

factor, so no absorption occurs. This can be detected by performing a Schilling test, in which radiolabelled vitamin B12 is given *orally* and the amount of radioactivity absorbed into the blood and excreted in the urine is measured. If lack of intrinsic factor is a problem, absorption will be low unless intrinsic factor is also given *orally*. If absorption is low when vitamin B12 and intrinsic factor are given together, the terminal ileum is likely to be damaged or there is something else blocking absorption of the B12/IF complex.

The most common cause of B12 deficiency in Britain is pernicious anaemia. This is aptly named

because patients with megaloblastic anaemia can have a very severe anaemia and may even die without treatment. Pernicious anaemia, or Addison's anaemia, occurs when the vitamin B12 deficiency is due to autoimmune damage to the stomach, resulting in chronic atrophic gastritis in which an inflamed and thinned stomach mucosa fails to produce adequate amounts of intrinsic factor or acid. This disease occurs predominantly after the age of 50 years and is more common in females. As well as severe anaemia, the sufferers may have neurological problems such as subacute combined degeneration of the spinal cord and segmental demyelination of the peripheral nerves. These are due to the lack of vitamin B12 and do not occur in folate deficiency. Patients are also at an increased risk of stomach carcinoma.

We chose an antenatal clinic as the setting for our anaemic women, so we should briefly mention the importance of folate in pregnancy. It is now clear that folate has a role in helping to prevent neural tube defects (spina bifida and anencephaly), and women should increase their daily folate intake from conception by 400 μg/day. This can be achieved by taking dietary supplements.

It is not possible for us to cover all of the causes of anaemia listed in Table 8.5, but we have discussed examples illustrating the key mechanisms, i.e. defective haemoglobin production in iron deficiency, defective DNA synthesis in vitamin B12 and folate deficiency, haemolytic anaemia due to an intrinsic cause, in this case a haemoglobinopathy, and (in Chapter 2) haemolytic anaemia due to extrinsic causes in transfusion-related haemolytic anaemia and Rhesus disease of the newborn. Abnormalities of platelets and clotting have been discussed in Chapter 6 and some of the malignancies of white cells will be covered in Chapter 16.

What would have happened to our ladies if their anaemia had not been discovered at prenatal testing? Let us first discuss the effects of anaemia. The anaemic patient has too little haemoglobin and hence a potential problem with the transport of oxygen to the tissues. The demand from the tissues will depend on the person's level of activity, so an anaemic person may be asymptomatic

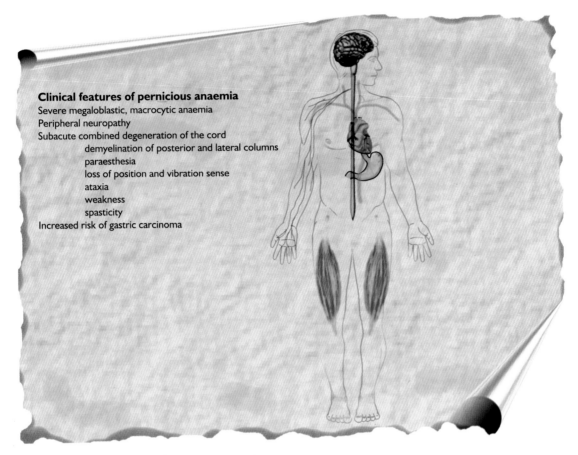

Clinical features of pernicious anaemia
Severe megaloblastic, macrocytic anaemia
Peripheral neuropathy
Subacute combined degeneration of the cord
        demyelination of posterior and lateral columns
        paraesthesia
        loss of position and vibration sense
        ataxia
        weakness
        spasticity
Increased risk of gastric carcinoma

Figure 8.9 Clinical features of pernicious anaemia

when sitting at a desk but will have problems running a marathon – and pregnancy can be regarded as a 9-month marathon (with a sprint finish!). An anaemic person can often compensate for the reduced amount of haemoglobin in the blood by pushing the blood round faster, i.e. increasing the cardiac output. The pregnant lady has the problem that in a normal pregnancy cardiac output needs to increase by around 30 per cent so compensation for anaemia may not be possible. So what will suffer? The mother will suffer with breathlessness, tiredness, weakness and possibly dizziness or fainting. The baby will suffer because nutrition through the placenta may be inadequate, leading to a 'small for dates' baby lacking the normal stores of nutrients transferred between mother and baby in the last trimester.

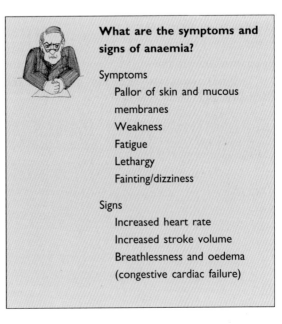

What are the symptoms and signs of anaemia?

Symptoms
    Pallor of skin and mucous
    membranes
    Weakness
    Fatigue
    Lethargy
    Fainting/dizziness

Signs
    Increased heart rate
    Increased stroke volume
    Breathlessness and oedema
    (congestive cardiac failure)

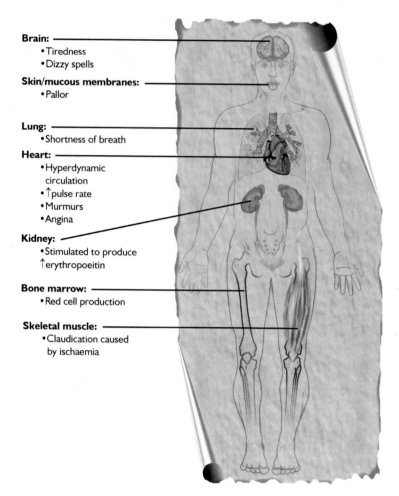

Brain:
- Tiredness
- Dizzy spells

Skin/mucous membranes:
- Pallor

Lung:
- Shortness of breath

Heart:
- Hyperdynamic circulation
- ↑pulse rate
- Murmurs
- Angina

Kidney:
- Stimulated to produce ↑erythropoeitin

Bone marrow:
- Red cell production

Skeletal muscle:
- Claudication caused by ischaemia

Figure 8.10 Systemic effects of anaemia

ACKNOWLEDGEMENT

Special thanks are due to Dr Grant Robinson for his helpful comments and for providing the haematological photographs.

CLINICOPATHOLOGICAL CASE STUDY

Clinical summary

A lady of 80 was admitted to hospital in a confused state. Relatives commented that she had been depressed for 4 years since the death of her husband, had been losing weight for 6 months and had seen her GP about shortness of breath (SOB) and swelling of the ankles (SOA), which had improved on diuretics.

Her past history included 20 years of rheumatoid arthritis treated by anti-inflammatory drugs but not requiring treatment for 2 years.

She had been a lifelong smoker but did not drink alcohol.

Physical examination:

Pulse rate 106, regular

Blood pressure 200/80

Respiratory rate 28/min

Lips and conjunctivae pale.

Heart apex beat displaced out

Soft mid-systolic murmur at apex

Swelling of ankles

Weight loss

Investigations:

Hb (g/dl) 8.2

MCHC (%) 32

MCV (fl) 80

i.e. a normochromic, normocytic anaemia with normal blood film

Chest X-ray revealed a hilar mass, and CT scanning showed lesions in the brain.

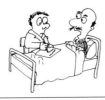

Pathological aspects

The SOB and SOA are related to cardiac failure, which would have been exacerbated by anaemia. If blood contains less haemoglobin, a larger volume of blood must be pumped through the tissues to deliver an equivalent amount of oxygen. This increases the heart's workload.

Confusion in the elderly has many causes but could be due to poor oxygen supply to the brain because of a mixture of heart failure, anaemia and narrowing of the cerebral vessels by atheroma.

Chronic disease, such as rheumatoid arthritis, produces a normochromic, normocytic anaemia by a poorly understood mechanism.

Anti-inflammatory drugs can produce gastrointestinal bleeding, leading to iron deficiency anaemia.

The increased pulse reflects the increased cardiac workload to compensate for the anaemia. Respiration rate is raised because of tissue hypoxia and reduced gas exchange in alveoli, resulting from alveolar oedema related to cardiac failure.

Red haemoglobin contributes to skin and mucosal colour in non-pigmented areas.

The murmur is produced by increased blood flow. The apex is displaced because the heart is dilated as it fails. This could be caused by malnutrition and suggests that the anaemia is due to folate or iron deficiency. Alternatively, it could result from malignancy.

These investigations exclude a macrocytic anaemia resulting from B12 or folate deficiency or a hypochromic, microcytic anaemia due to iron deficiency. Her rheumatoid arthritis is inactive and unlikely to be the cause of the anaemia, so she should be investigated for malignancy.

Features fit with a primary lung tumour metastasising to the brain. The cerebral metastases could have produced her confusion. The lung tumour is likely to be induced by smoking. Her anaemia is most probably anaemia of chronic disease secondary to malignancy.

ARTERIOSCLEROSIS

- The arteriopath
- Hyaline and hyperplastic arteriolosclerosis
- Risk factors for atherosclerosis
- How is the atheromatous plaque produced?
- What diet will prevent atheroma?
- Complications of atheroma

So far, we have concentrated on thrombosis, embolism and shock, all conditions that may suddenly affect healthy people of any age. Now we will move on to the major cardiovascular problems of later life, namely arteriosclerosis, hypertension, myocardial infarction and aneurysms. These are overwhelming causes of morbidity and mortality in developed countries but are not an inevitable consequence of aging, so it is of great importance to try to identify the causative and risk agents.

THE ARTERIOPATH

Let us briefly consider a possible clinical picture in a patient debilitated by vascular problems. A 48-year-old man complains of blurring of his vision. He is known to suffer from diabetes, which is a complex metabolic disorder characterised by hyperglycaemia (raised blood glucose). At the age of 14 years, he presented with the typical diabetic symptoms of tiredness, weight loss, polyuria

(increased urine production) and polydypsia (increased thirst). The blood glucose was raised, glucose was found in his urine, and he has been on insulin therapy since that time.

His present complaint of blurred vision started 3 months ago. On questioning, he also complains of shortness of breath, especially on exertion, and cramps in his calf muscles on exercise. On examination, he is found to have a raised blood pressure, a mild degree of cardiac failure with pulmonary oedema, small haemorrhages and small blood vessel proliferation in his retina and systolic bruits in his neck (abnormal sounds, heard through the stethoscope, caused by turbulent blood flow). His blood tests show a small rise in urea and creatinine levels, indicating a degree of renal impairment.

This unfortunate man is an 'arteriopath', i.e. he has widespread disease related to arterial pathology. The arterial pathology comes under the general heading of **arteriosclerosis**, commonly referred to as 'hardening of the arteries', although this does not relate to a specific pathologically

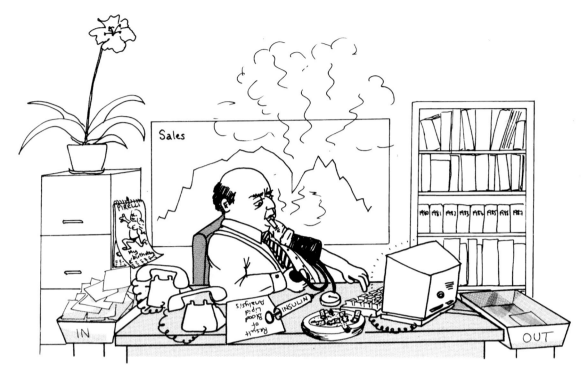

Figure 9.1 The arteriopath

Risk factors

- age
- sex (male)
- obesity
- smoking
- diabetes
- lack of exercise
- hypertension
- hyperlipidaemia
- Type 'A' personality (impatient workaholic)

recognised entity. His large and medium-sized arteries are likely to be narrowed by fibrolipid **atherosclerotic** lesions (see below), and his small arteries and arterioles will show the proliferative or hyaline changes of **arteriolosclerosis**. Atherosclerosis is principally a disease of the intima and may result in narrowing of the vessel, obstruction or thrombosis. Arteriosclerosis, on the other hand, affects the media, with a resultant increase in wall thickness and decreased elasticity, which may lead to hypertension.

Let's look at this man's symptoms to see whether we can suggest a cause for each problem:

- His longstanding diabetes makes him much more likely to develop atherosclerosis than non-diabetic people of the same age.
- Fibrolipid atheromatous plaques in his coronary arteries will reduce the perfusion of the cardiac muscle, resulting in chronic ischaemia, which damages the heart muscle so that it pumps less

efficiently. Because the left side of the heart generally fails first, this will result in pulmonary oedema.

- Atheroma in the carotid arteries produces the bruit heard on auscultation and may lead to cerebral infarction.
- The combination of poor cardiac function and atheromatous plaques in the abdominal aorta and femoral vessels will explain the pain and cramp in his calf muscle, which is secondary to poor perfusion.
- Hyaline arteriolosclerosis will affect small renal vessels, leading to glomerular damage, which will induce hypertension through a complicated mechanism involving the hormones renin and angiotensin. This exacerbates the atheroma and worsens the cardiac failure.
- The cause of his blurred vision may be of vascular origin as the retina is frequently damaged by small haemorrhages, microaneurysms and new

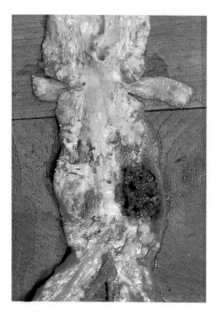

Figure 9.2 Descending aorta with atheroma and thrombus in an aneurysm

vessel formation, although diabetes can also produce a host of other ocular changes.

The next stage in understanding this man's disease is to consider the actual appearance of his vessels.

WHAT DOES THE VESSEL LOOK LIKE?

The lesion of atherosclerosis is not one specific entity but a spectrum of arterial changes including:

- atheromatous fibrolipid plaques
- fatty streaks
- intimal cushion lesions.

There is inevitably controversy over whether the different lesions are stages in the evolution of an atheromatous plaque, and we shall review the evidence when describing each lesion. From the clinical point of view, it is the atheromatous fibrolipid plaque that is to blame for producing occlusive vascular disease.

Atheromatous plaque

The **atheromatous plaque**, which is also referred to as a fibrous or fibrolipid plaque, is raised above the

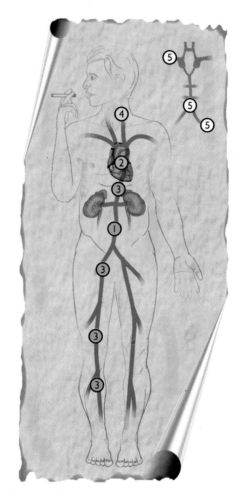

Sites in order of frequency
1. Abdominal aorta
2. Proximal coronary arteries
3. Descending thoracic aorta, femoral and popliteal arteries
4. Internal carotid artery
5. Vertebral/basilar/middle cerebral arteries

Figure 9.3 Distribution of atheroma

surrounding intima and protrudes into the lumen. It is whitish-yellow in colour, varies in size from 0.5 to 1.5 cm and may even become bigger if adjacent plaques coalesce. On slicing, the plaque is composed of a **fibrous cap** covering a soft, yellow, lipid centre, which reminded the early pathologists of porridge or gruel, so was termed **atheroma**. The intima is greatly thickened by the fibrofatty deposition, and the media may be thinned owing to a loss of smooth muscle cells, resulting in both a loss of

The atheromatous plaque

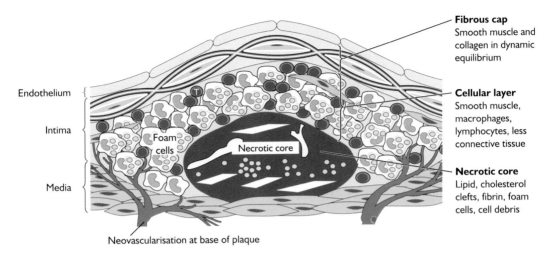

Fibrous cap
Smooth muscle and collagen in dynamic equilibrium

Cellular layer
Smooth muscle, macrophages, lymphocytes, less connective tissue

Necrotic core
Lipid, cholesterol clefts, fibrin, foam cells, cell debris

Endothelium

Intima

Media

Foam cells

Necrotic core

Neovascularisation at base of plaque

The dynamics of atheromatous plaque stability

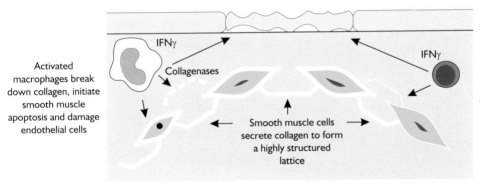

Activated macrophages break down collagen, initiate smooth muscle apoptosis and damage endothelial cells

IFNγ

Collagenases

Smooth muscle cells secrete collagen to form a highly structured lattice

IFNγ

T-lymphocytes secrete IFNγ, which inhibits collagen synthesis and damages endothelial cells

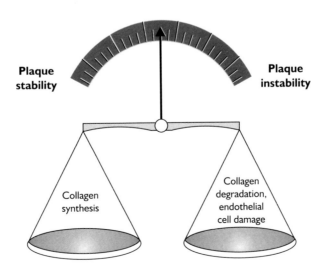

Plaque stability

Plaque instability

Collagen synthesis

Collagen degradation, endothelial cell damage

Figure 9.4 The atheromatous plaque

elasticity and a weakening of the wall. The fibrous cap is generally composed of smooth muscle cells, collagen, elastin and proteoglycans. Beneath this, there is a more cellular region of macrophages, T lymphocytes and smooth muscle cells covering the soft gruel-like mass of lipid, cellular debris, cholesterol clefts, plasma proteins and lipid-laden (foam) cells derived from macrophages and smooth muscle cells. At the edges of the lesion, there may be new vessel formation.

These plaques are more common in the aorta, femoral, carotid and coronary arteries, where they may produce clinical problems by causing partial or complete occlusion, thrombosis, embolism or aneurysm formation (see Fig. 9.13). Areas of turbulent flow are worst affected so that lesions often occur around the ostia of vessels. Interestingly, the abdominal aorta is more liable to atheroma than the thoracic aorta, but the explanation for this is unknown.

Fatty streak

Fatty streaks, like atheromatous plaques, occur in large muscular and elastic arteries but differ in that they are most common in the region of the aortic ring and the thoracic aorta. They do not affect blood flow but could represent a precursor lesion for atheromatous plaques. They first appear as tiny, round or oval flat yellow dots that become arranged in rows and finally coalesce to form a streak. The earliest streak is composed of just lipid-laden macrophages and T cells without any smooth muscle proliferation or extracellular lipid. Later, extracellular lipid and smooth muscle cells are found, together with collagen, elastin and proteoglycans. Thus the components are similar to those of an atheromatous plaque, but there is far less fat and no necrotic centre. However, some people would only use the term 'fatty streak' for the earliest stage, the other forms representing a progression towards a fibrolipid plaque.

The aortic surface area covered by streaks increases up to the third decade but then declines as atheromatous plaques occupy the intima. Interestingly, they occur proximal to branch points

and ostia in areas of low haemodynamic stress, so are not correctly sited to be the forerunners of fibrolipid plaques. The population distribution is also very different, fibrolipid plaques being more common in males in developed countries, whereas fatty streaks are found from a very early age and are independent of sex, race or geography.

Intimal cushion lesions

An **intimal cushion** is a white thickening at a branching point or ostium due to an increase in extracellular matrix and smooth muscle cells. There is almost no lipid, and the suggestion that this is a precursor lesion for fibrolipid plaques is based on the similarity in their distribution and the presence of smooth muscle proliferation. Even in early infancy, smooth muscle cells have entered the intima, raising the possibility that man is predestined to atheroma if suitable additional factors are present later.

HYALINE AND HYPERPLASTIC ARTERIOLOSCLEROSIS

Hyaline and hyperplastic arteriolosclerotic changes are very different from atheromatous damage. They only affect small vessels, do not have any increase in lipid and primarily affect the media, whereas atheroma is initially an **intimal** problem. Both are very important because of their strong association with hypertension.

Hyaline arteriolosclerosis generally occurs in elderly or diabetic patients and involves the deposition of homogenous, pink material that thickens the media, resulting in a narrowed vessel. This material is probably a combination of increased extracellular matrix, produced by smooth muscle cells, and plasma components that have leaked through a damaged endothelium.

Hyperplastic arteriolosclerosis is found in patients who have a rather sudden or severe

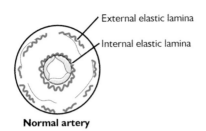

Normal artery

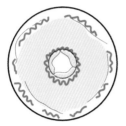

Hyaline arteriolosclerosis

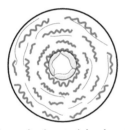

Hyperplastic arteriolosclerosis

Figure 9.5 Hyaline and hyperplastic arteriolosclerosis

prolonged increase in blood pressure. The media of the vessel wall is thickened by a concentric proliferation of smooth muscle cells and an increase in basement membrane material. In the worst cases (malignant hypertension), there may be fibrinoid necrosis of the vessel walls.

MONCKEBERG'S MEDIAL CALCIFIC STENOSIS

Another, but less important, form of arteriosclerosis is Monckeberg's medial calcific stenosis. This involves calcification of the media of muscular arteries and frequently occurs in the lower limb arteries of elderly people in association with atherosclerosis, although it can occur in any organ. It

is not thought to have much clinical significance, but it delights, and sometimes confuses, radiologists. The cause is unknown but is probably a degenerative change complicated by dystrophic calcification.

RISK FACTORS FOR ATHEROSCLEROSIS

Now that we have a mental image of the appearance and distribution of atherosclerosis, we shall consider the risk factors that are believed to be important.

AGE

Deaths from ischaemic heart disease increase with advancing age. Interestingly, the initial involvement by atheroma affects different vessels at different ages. Thus small aortic lesions appear in the first decade, coronary artery lesions in the second decade and cerebral arterial lesions in the third.

GENDER

The death rate from ischaemic heart disease is higher in males than in females up to the age of 75 years, after which the incidence is similar. Myocardial infarction is extremely rare in premenopausal women, suggesting that endocrine differences may be important and that the effect of oestrogens on lipid metabolism is a possible mechanism.

SMOKING

Smoking one packet of cigarettes a day increases the likelihood of having a myocardial infarction by 300%. Traditionally, more men than women have smoked, but as women have taken up the habit, their risk has risen. Fortunately, giving up smoking reduces the risk, which means that it is likely that smoking not only promotes atheroma but may also cause occlusion of vessels. This could result from an increased local clotting tendency because of altered platelet function. Stopping smoking for 1–2 years reduces the risk of myocardial infarction to 'only' twice that of non-smokers. So-called 'safer' cigarettes, which have a lower tar and nicotine content, reduce the risk of bronchial carcinoma but do not appear to reduce the risk of coronary heart disease. How smoking damages vessels is not known, but suggestions include increased free radical activity, raised carbon monoxide levels or a direct effect of nicotine.

HYPERTENSION

Hypertension significantly increases the risk of ischaemic heart disease and 'strokes'. The diastolic blood pressure level is considered to be more important than the systolic level, and a diastolic pressure consistently greater than 95 mmHg is deemed harmful. Drug treatment to reduce the blood pressure decreases the risk in patients with moderate-to-severe hypertension, but it is unclear whether it benefits patients with mild hypertension.

Most of the evidence suggesting the role of hypertension as a risk factor involves the complex multifactorial analysis of large studies, which, although the proper method for assessing the evidence, is not as easy to grasp as are some simpler observations. Evidence of the direct role of hypertension in producing atheroma comes from two examples of congenital abnormalities of the cardiovascular system. Patients with congenital narrowing of part of the aorta (**coarctation**) develop atheroma in the proximal hypertensive segment but not in the distal region, where the pressure is lower. The other example is the rare abnormality of having one coronary artery originating from the low-pressure pulmonary artery. The coronary artery linked to the aorta develops atheromatous changes with age, but the artery linked to the pulmonary supply remains atheroma-free.

HYPERLIPIDAEMIA

Evidence for the role of fats in atheroma comes from a variety of sources, and as the literature on the role of lipids in atherosclerosis would fill a library, we shall just highlight some of the more important points:
- Atheromatous lesions contain far more lipid than does the adjacent intima.
- Atheromatous plaques are rich in cholesterol and cholesterol esters (65–80 per cent), derived from blood lipoproteins.
- Intimal lesions can be produced in some animals by increasing the plasma concentration of certain lipids through drug or diet manipulation.
- Macrophages accumulate cholesterol from low-density lipoprotein (LDL), and this is increased if there is endothelial damage.
- In populations with a high incidence of atherosclerosis, there are high plasma concentrations of certain lipids; LDL rich in cholesterol appears most harmful, very low-density lipoprotein (VLDL) does some harm, but high-density lipoprotein (HDL) appears to be cardioprotective.
- In families with genetic disorders causing hypercholesterolaemia or in groups with acquired hypercholesterolaemia (e.g. hypothyroidism and nephrotic syndrome), atherosclerosis is increased.
- Cardiovascular mortality can be reduced by lowering the plasma cholesterol with diet or drugs (e.g. cholestyramine).

DIABETES

The risk of a myocardial infarction in a diabetic patient is twice that of a non-diabetic patient, and, as our clinical case above illustrated, their arterial disease is widespread.

OTHER POSSIBLE RISK FACTORS

These include:
- lack of regular exercise

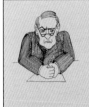

List some risk factors for atherosclerosis
Age
Gender
Smoking
Hypertension
Hyperlipidaemia
Diabetes

- obesity
- high carbohydrate intake
- 'type A' personality/stress
- hyperuricaemia and gout.

HOW IS THE ATHEROMATOUS PLAQUE PRODUCED?

Now that we know who is most likely to suffer from atherosclerosis, we need to look at the theory of how atheroma is produced. The 'reaction to injury' theory has its origin deep within the history books, while the key role of LDL is emphasised in Figure 9.6.

REACTION TO INJURY THEORY

Virchow believed that leakage of plasma proteins and lipid from the blood to the subendothelial tissue stimulated intimal cell proliferation. He regarded the cell proliferation as a form of low-grade inflammation and termed this the 'imbibition hypothesis', later often called the 'insudation' or 'infiltration' hypothesis. Rokitansky is credited with the 'encrustation' theory, which suggested that thrombi forming on damaged endothelium could become organised to form a plaque. The modern 'reaction to injury' theory was proposed by Ross and Glomset in 1976. Essentially, they suggest that some change or damage to the vascular endothelium causes increased permeability to proteins and lipid, and also leads to the aggregation of platelets and monocytes. These leucocytes release various enzymes and growth factors, which promote smooth muscle cell proliferation. Monocytes migrate from the blood into the subendothelial layers, where they become macrophages and ingest the lipid. A short, sharp injury can be completely repaired, but chronic, repeated injury leads to the formation of an atheromatous plaque.

Stable atheromatous plaques may not produce any clinical effect, but problems occur if a lipid lesion covered by a thin fibrous capsule is disrupted, releasing material that promotes local thrombosis. The thrombosis may cause an acute occlusion of the vessel, with potentially devastating effects, or cause only a partial occlusion. Partially occlusive thrombus undergoes organisation and becomes incorporated into the plaque to increase its size. The factors involved can be thought of as atherogenic factors important in producing the early plaque, and thrombotic factors important in its progression.

Endothelial cell damage is known to be produced by a variety of factors, such as haemodynamic forces, hyperlipidaemia, cigarette smoke, immune mechanisms, certain viral antigens, irradiation and various mutagens. This damage plays an atherogenic and thrombogenic role. The next stage required in the response to injury theory is that the aggregated platelets and monocytes release substances to promote smooth muscle proliferation and the influx of more leucocytes.

Platelet-derived growth factor (PDGF) is believed to be important because smooth muscle proliferation is observed *in vivo* in zones where platelets adhere to damaged endothelium, and PDGF can *in vitro* promote both the proliferation and migration of smooth muscle cells. Interestingly, there are two animal models that provide supporting evidence. In one, the platelets lack alpha granules, which contain PDGF, and the animals do not develop atheroma. In the other, pigs lacking vWF, which is necessary for platelet adherence and aggregation, are resistant to both thrombosis and spontaneous atherosclerosis. Other growth factors, such as FGF and endothelial cell growth factor are probably involved, as is

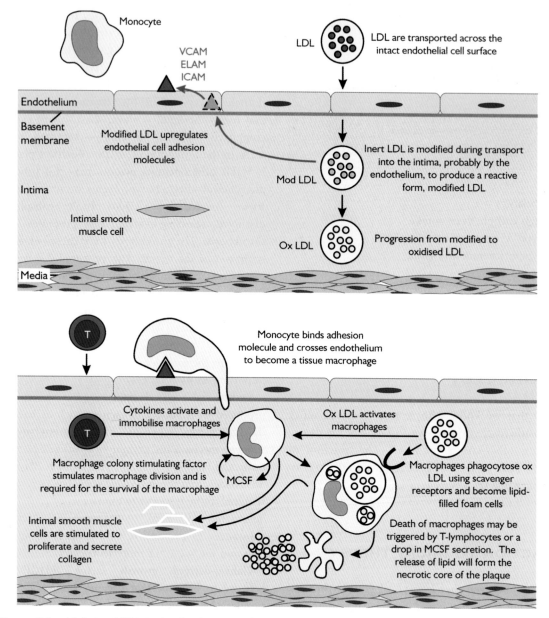

Figure 9.6 (a) Role of LDL in the development of the atheromatous plaque.

a reduction in the growth inhibitors (TGF-β and endothelial-derived relaxing factor, EDRF) produced by macrophages and endothelial cells. The end result is that smooth muscle cells migrate from the media to the intima, proliferate, accumulate cholesterol and cholesterol esters to become one of the types of **foam** cells (the other is macrophage derived) and also manufacture extracellular matrix.

The **influx of leucocytes** is apparent from simple observation, i.e. by counting the number of macrophages and lymphocytes in the atheromatous lesions and comparing the answer with the very small number present in non-atheromatous intima. Once lymphocytes and macrophages are involved, the whole complex army of cytokines can be called into action to promote chemotaxis, cell proliferation, altered permeability, etc.

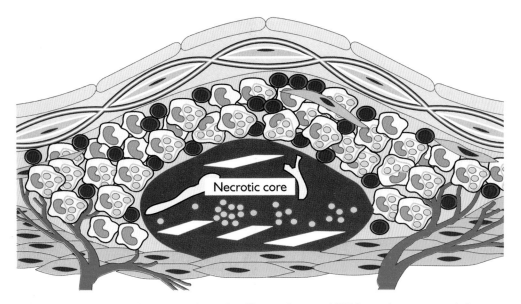

New blood vessels enter the plaque via the media. The vessels express VCAM, providing a new portal of entry for macrophages and lymphocytes

Smooth muscle cells secrete a highly structured lattice-like collagen framework, forming a fibrous cap over the cells and necrotic core. The cap requires constant renewal and there is a high turnover of smooth muscle cells

Figure 9.6 (b) Established atheromatous plaque

Oxidised lipoproteins (OLP) deserve a mention because of the clear association between LDL blood levels and coronary artery disease. It appears that OLPs may be produced by reactive oxygen species altering the lipoprotein present in plaques. The altered LDL is then recognised by the 'scavenger' receptor on macrophages and phagocytosed so that the macrophage becomes a foam cell. The OLP may ultimately contribute to the death of the macrophage.

OLP are thought to be able to cause:
• endothelial cell damage
• smooth muscle cell injury, leading to central necrosis of the plaque
• foam cell formation as the OLPs are taken up by the receptor for modified LDL
• the recruitment and retention of macrophages.

What about the role of thrombosis in plaque expansion and acute events? Figure 9.8 shows a plaque that has fissured and in which thrombus has formed over the surface, so it is possible to see the evidence for this with your own eyes. It appears that some plaques are eccentric and lipid rich, with a high

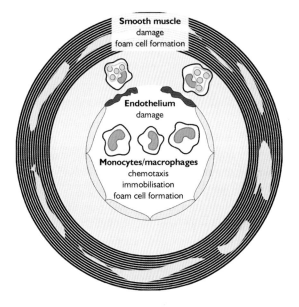

Figure 9.7 Effects of oxidised lipoproteins

tendency to rupture and promote thrombosis, while other plaques are more fibrotic, do not fissure and are thus stable (Fig. 9.4). One of the difficulties in

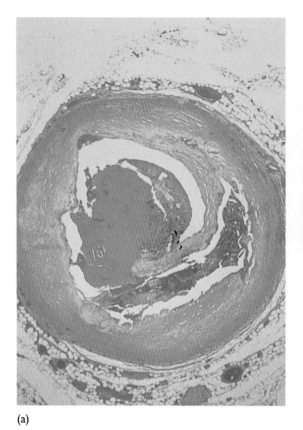

(a)

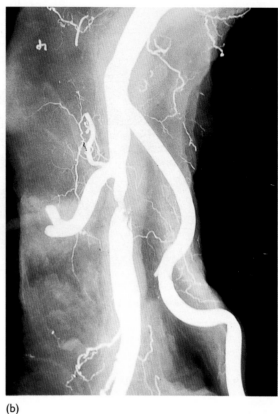

(b)

Figure 9.8 (a) Atheromatous plaque with fissuring and thrombus formation. (b) Angiogram showing narrowing of the coronary artery corresponding to (a)

predicting an individual's risk of acute coronary artery occlusion is that the likelihood of plaque rupture does not depend on the degree of vessel stenosis. Thus lowering blood LDL levels reduces the risk of coronary artery thrombosis but does not make a significant difference to coronary artery stenosis as assessed by arteriography.

Not surprisingly, there is evidence that factors promoting thrombosis are linked to coronary artery disease. Cigarette smoking is known to enhance platelet reactivity, and plasma fibrinogen levels increase with age, obesity, smoking, diabetes, stress and hyperlipidaemia. This means that the risk of acute coronary events can be reduced by reducing platelet activity with drugs such as low-dose aspirin.

Thus there is a large bank of literature supporting the 'response to injury' theory, although many questions remain unanswered.

WHAT DIET WILL PREVENT ATHEROMA?

The popular press are fond of reporting the latest diet to prevent atheroma and are then even more delighted to report the contradictions that follow, so what do we really know and what is speculation? Most of the historical evidence comes from comparing populations with distinctly different diets, for example the fish-eating Eskimos with meat-eating Danes, or the butter lovers of Belgium with the olive oil fans of the Mediterranean.

Let us digress for a minute to consider how we should define a successful diet. Ideally, we would like to prevent the formation of atheromatous plaques, but as we cannot assess the size, number and distribution of plaques in millions of living people in different populations, most researchers opt to

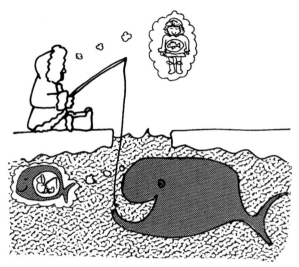

Fish-loving eskimos
low risk

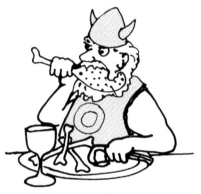

Meat-eating Danes
high risk

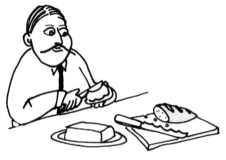

Butter-loving Belgians
high risk

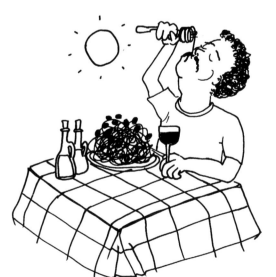

Mediterranean olive oil fans
low risk

Figure 9.9 Atheroma risk and dietary habits

monitor the major life-threatening complication of plaques, namely occlusive coronary heart disease (CHD). However, by doing that, they are really measuring the outcome of two different pathological mechanisms. The patient must not only suffer from atheroma in the coronary vessels but also undergo an occlusive event such as thrombosis or vasoconstriction; there may therefore be different dietary factors affecting the processes, i.e. 'atherogenic' and 'thrombogenic' dietary factors. Obviously, it is probable that any atherogenic factors operate over decades and that starting on a low-fat diet as you retire will cause little change to your plaques. However, the likelihood of thrombosis could be affected by an alteration of diet in later life.

LIPIDS AND CORONARY HEART DISEASE

The first stage in our discussion needs to establish which dietary-derived blood levels correlate with CHD. Then we need to review the biochemical pathways involved so that we can try to understand the complex interplay between the dietary intake of a substance and the blood levels. Finally, we can consider the observed effects of altering diets.

Risk of coronary heart disease increases with:
- raised serum total cholesterol concentration
- raised LDL cholesterol concentration
- reduced HDL cholesterol concentration.

Of course, it is good to observe the factors that increase the risk, but it is even more important to discover whether manipulating the factor can reduce the risk. We now know that in people with no other specific risk factors (primary prevention studies), the risk of CHD reduces by 10 per cent and the risk of non-fatal myocardial infarction by about 20 per cent if a 10 per cent fall in serum total cholesterol is achieved. Similar figures are available for secondary prevention studies (i.e. patients who already have CHD) to support altering the levels of LDL and HDL cholesterol.

LIPID METABOLISM

There are two important pathways for lipid metabolism: the exogenous and the endogenous.

Cholesterol enters the gut in the diet or in bile. Cholesterol and triglycerides are absorbed from the gut to be transported in the blood as chylomicrons. Triglycerides are delivered to a variety of tissues. The cholesterol is delivered to the liver when the chylomicron remnant is endocytosed via a receptor which recognises apoprotein E on its surface. Some cholesterol may be secreted in bile; the rest enters the endogenous cholesterol pathway

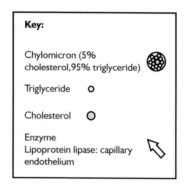

Key:

Chylomicron (5% cholesterol, 95% triglyceride)

Triglyceride   o

Cholesterol   O

Enzyme
Lipoprotein lipase: capillary endothelium

Figure 9.10 Exogenous cholesterol pathway

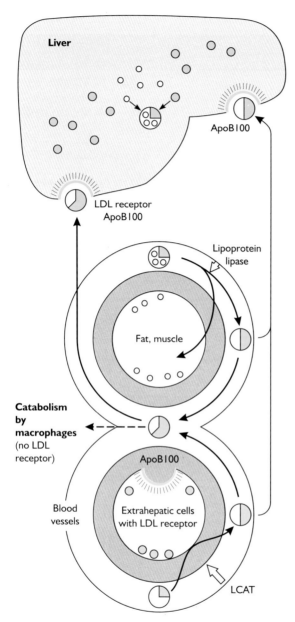

Cholesterol is secreted in very low density lipoproteins (VLDL), which are broken down by lipoprotein lipase in the endothelium of the capillaries in fat and muscle to release triglycerides and form intermediate density lipoproteins (IDL). Some IDL are absorbed by the liver via the LDL receptor, which recognises apoprotein B100; the remainder are metabolised to low density lipoproteins (LDL). LDL are taken up by the numerous extrahepatic tissues which bear the LDL receptor, and the remainder is either taken up by the liver or catabolised by macrophages. High density lipoproteins (HDL), also secreted by the liver, remove cholesterol from the tissues. This is catalysed by plasma lecithin-cholesterol acyltransferase (LCAT). IDL and LDL are formed by a series of metabolic steps

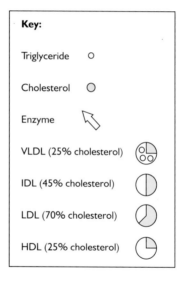

Figure 9.11   Endogenous cholesterol pathway

Exogenous (i.e. dietary) lipids are digested to release triglycerides (TGs) and cholesterol esters. These combine with phospholipids and specific apoproteins to make them water soluble, and are then called chylomicrons. The TG component of the chylomicron can move from the circulation into cells by lipoprotein lipase activity on the endothelial surface of cells. Once inside the cell, it may be converted to glycerol and non-esterified

fatty acids, which are a major energy source. Once the chylomicron has lost its TG, it is called a chylomicron remnant particle (CMR) and is rich in cholesterol. This particle attaches to liver receptors via apo-B48 and apo-E and enters the hepatocyte.

Endogenous lipid refers to the various lipids produced by the liver. The building blocks are gycerol and fatty acids, reaching the liver from fat

Table 9.1   Classification of lipoproteins

Lipoprotein	Site of production	Major lipid	Major apoprotein	Role/fate
Chylomicron	Intestinal mucosal cell	TG	B48	Transport of dietary TG
CMR	Removal of TG from chylomicron	Cholesterol	B48	Transport dietary cholesterol to liver
VLDL	Liver	TG	B100, CII, E	Transport endogenous TG
IDL	Partial removal of TG from VLDL	TG and cholesterol	B100, E	Taken up by liver or converted to LDL
LDL	Further removal of TG from IDL	Cholesterol	B100	Transport endogenous cholesterol to liver and tissues
HDL	Liver and intestinal mucosal cell	Phospholipid	A, D	Complex

CMR = chylomicron remnant particle; IDL = intermediate density lipoprotein; LDL = low-density lipoprotein; TG = triglyceride; VLDL = very low density lipoprotein.

stores or synthesised from glucose, and cholesterol derived from lipoproteins (such as the CMR) or synthesised locally from acetate and mevalonic acid using the enzyme HMG CoA (hydroxy methyl glutaryl coenzyme A). Glycerol and fatty acids combine to produce TG. The liver releases VLDL, rich in TG and containing about 25 per cent cholesterol. Loss of some TG produces intermediate-density lipoproteins (IDLs), and a further loss of TG results in cholesterol-rich LDL. This LDL is removed from the circulation by attachment to high-affinity LDL receptors via apoprotein B100 on the liver and peripheral cells, and the LDL is broken down to amino acids and cholesterol. The alternative route is through low-affinity LDL receptors, and it is these receptors which are thought to be important in atherosclerosis. If there are high levels of LDL, the liver and peripheral cells accumulate some intracellular cholesterol, which inhibits the endogenous synthesis of cholesterol and suppresses the production of their LDL receptors, thus reducing LDL uptake from the blood and probably diverting more LDL to cells with low-affinity receptors.

When we were listing the risk factors for atherosclerosis above, we had a group labelled 'other

List some causes of secondary hyperlipidaemia
Nutritional
   Obesity
   Alcohol abuse
Hormonal
   Diabetes
   Hypothyroidism
Drugs
   Beta-blockers
   High-dose steroids
Miscellaneous
   Stress
   Bile duct obstruction and primary biliary cirrhosis
   Nephrotic syndrome and chronic renal failure

possible risk factors'. Now that we know something about the relationship of serum lipid levels and CHD, it is educational to compare that list with a list of secondary hyperlipidaemias (see written examination box).

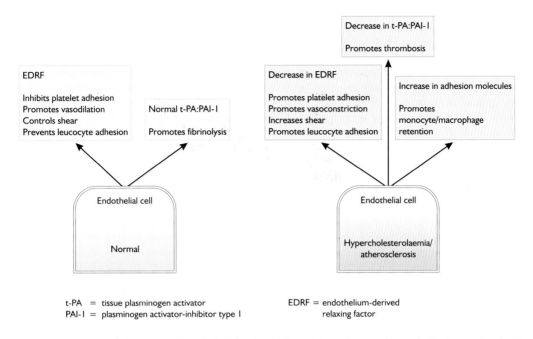

MANAGING LIPID LEVELS

So what is the ideal diet? First, you should be a reasonable weight because, in patients who are very overweight, a weight reduction of about 10 kg reduces LDL cholesterol by 7 per cent and raises HDL cholesterol by 13 per cent. Regular exercise appears to enhance this effect. The standard teaching is that diets should restrict total fat intake to less than 30 per cent of all calories, no more than 10 per cent of this fat being from saturated fat, cholesterol intake should be limited to less than 300 mg/day and fibre intake should be increased. Unfortunately, this produces a drop in total cholesterol of only about 2 per cent, and although greater reduction can be achieved with more stringent diets, they are generally too unpalatable.

The alternative is to use drugs such as statins and anion exchange resins. Statins inhibit the enzyme HMG CoA reductase and so reduce the endogenous production of cholesterol. Anion exchange resins bind to bile acids, preventing their reabsorption and thus enhancing cholesterol excretion. Both approaches reduce LDL cholesterol. The statins also produce some lowering of TG and a rise in HDL levels, whereas the resins cause an undesirable rise in TG and generally no effect on HDL.

HOW DO RAISED CHOLESTEROL LEVELS CAUSE CORONARY HEART DISEASE?

So how does this work? How might lowering LDL cholesterol prevent CHD? You must appreciate that we are now into speculation rather than experimentally proven fact. You will remember that acute events in coronary arteries often relate to plaque rupture and that plaque rupture is more likely in cholesterol-rich plaques. It is possible, therefore, that there may be a process of 'reverse cholesterol transport' from the plaque to the serum, possibly involving HDL.

Coronary symptoms occur with changes less than full plaque rupture and can relate to small local thrombi or vasospasm of coronary arteries. The link between these is in the multifunctional endothelial cell that is involved in regulating

1. Luminal narrowing causing ischaemia

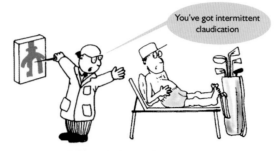

Ischaemia (luminal narrowing)
* e.g. intermittent claudication

2. Thrombosis

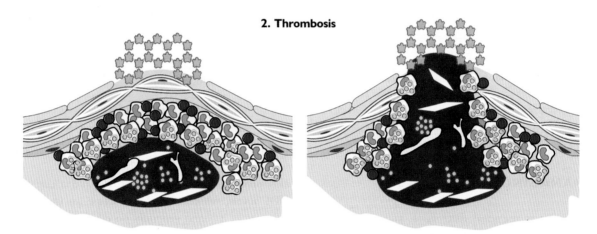

Level 1 thrombus: endothelial cell damage only.
Exposure of the basement membrane initiates thrombosis

Level 2 thrombus: plaque rupture, tear involves intima.
Basement membrane and plaque contents initiate thrombus

3. Weakening of arterial wall, with aneurysm formation

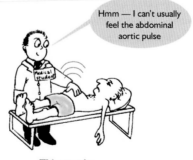

This may be complicated by:
* thrombosis
* thromboembolism
* rupture

Figure 9.13 Complications of atheroma

vasomotor tone, inhibiting platelet activity, maintaining a balance between thrombosis and fibrinolysis, and regulating the recruitment of inflammatory cells. A crucial mediator of these functions is EDRF (nitrous oxide), and the intra-coronary perfusion of acetylcholine (an EDRF agonist) produces vasodilatation of normal coronary arteries but constricts areas affected by atheromatous plaques. This is assumed to be due to acetylcholine's direct constrictor effect on the underlying smooth muscle in the absence of normal tone regulation by the endothelium, i.e. the endothelial cells are dysfunctional atheromatous plaques.

The really amazing observation is that the vasoconstriction produced by acetylcholine challenge can be reduced or even converted into slight vasodilatation by a 6-month period of lipid-lowering drugs. It is not known quite how the LDL cholesterol causes endothelial dysfunction, but there is a suggestion that it is because of increased oxidative stress, some early work raising the possibility that antioxidant drugs may have a beneficial effect.

COMPLICATIONS OF ATHEROMA

The plaques in themselves do not cause any symptoms but produce an effect by reducing the size of the lumen of the blood vessel and hence causing ischaemia or infarction of the tissues supplied by the atheromatous vessel. The atheroma can act as a base for the formation of **thrombus** and **embolus** and, by weakening the wall, can cause local dilatation: an **aneurysm**. The luminal surface of the plaque may **ulcerate**, which commonly precipitates thrombus formation. **Haemorrhage** may also occur within plaques, and the resulting haematoma may distend the plaque to cause ulceration. In almost all advanced atheromatous plaques, there is some degree of dystrophic **calcification**, which, if extensive, will turn the artery into a stiff pipe.

The two most common clinical manifestations of atherosclerosis are myocardial infarction and cerebral infarction.

MYOCARDIAL INFARCTION, ANEURYSMS AND HYPERTENSION

- Myocardial infarction
- Aneurysms
- Hypertension

MYOCARDIAL INFARCTION

Let us first consider the clinical aspects of myocardial infarction. A typical scenario may be as follows. A 63-year-old gentleman presented to the accident and emergency department complaining of chest pain. He had had central chest pain for 6–8 hours, and the pain radiated down the left arm and into his neck. He was feeling nauseated and also complained of shortness of breath. He had a history of hypertension for the past 5 years and had been receiving treatment. He also smoked 25 cigarettes per day and was obese. He had a family history of hypertension, and his father had died at the age of 55 from a 'heart attack'. His brother was also hypertensive.

On examination, he was found to have a pulse rate of 40 beats per minute and a blood pressure of 110/80, and he was in cardiac failure. An electrocardiogram (ECG) confirmed an inferior

myocardial infarction, and he was found to be in complete heart block. He received treatment for his pain, a temporary pacing wire was inserted, and he was transferred to the intensive care unit for observation.

As house physicians and residents, you will encounter this sort of situation with alarming regularity. So what is the pathological sequence of events that leads to a myocardial infarction, and what are the complications that may arise as a consequence?

WHAT MECHANISMS LEAD TO MYOCARDIAL INFARCTION?

Myocardial infarction means that cardiac muscle cells die because of a lack of nutrients, most importantly oxygen. This generally results from poor blood flow to the myocardium because of narrowing or total occlusion of one or more

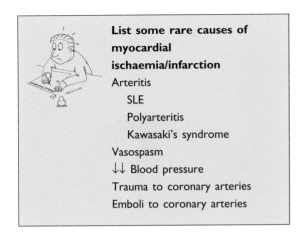

List some rare causes of
myocardial
ischaemia/infarction
Arteritis
    SLE
    Polyarteritis
    Kawasaki's syndrome
Vasospasm
↓↓ Blood pressure
Trauma to coronary arteries
Emboli to coronary arteries

coronary arteries. The extent of the infarction will depend on the amount of collateral flow, the metabolic requirements of the cells and the duration of the insult. Atheroma of the coronary vessels accounts for the majority of cases, rarer causes including vascular spasm, emboli, arteritis and anaemia (see the written examination box).

We learnt in the previous chapter that plaques can be stable or unstable. The stable plaques narrow the coronary arteries so that blood flow is insufficient for even a moderate increase in cardiac work, such as walking upstairs, and the patient will complain of chest pain on exercise, that is relieved on resting. This is called **angina** and occurs because, although the myocardial cells become ischaemic, the damage is reversible.

Unstable plaques may not produce any clinical problems until an 'acute' event occurs when the fibrous cap of the plaque splits so that blood can reach the soft, necrotic centre. This can distort and enlarge the plaque, but, most significantly, the plaque contents activate the thrombotic cascade. Platelets and fibrin will aggregate to block the lumen and the platelet constituents (TXA2, histamine and serotonin) may worsen the situation by promoting spasm in the vessel wall. It is not known why the plaque fissures, but this may be influenced by macrophage activity in the soft atheromatous centre, by vasospasm in the wall, by bending and twisting of the vessel as the heart contracts or by altered distribution of stresses on the wall. It is often stated that coronary artery stenosis is not likely to produce clinical symptoms

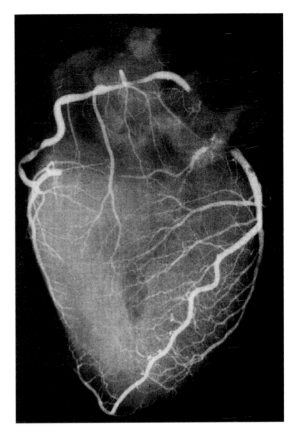

Figure 10.1 Coronary arteriogram showing main coronary arteries and numerous collateral vessels

unless the cross-sectional area is reduced by 75 per cent. This is true for longstanding fibrosed areas of atheroma, but the majority of plaques that fissure to produce occlusion are fairly small and have an abundance of soft lipid. Soft plaques are more likely to fissure than hard, fibrous plaques.

Vasospasm is an elusive mechanism for a pathologist to identify because there will be nothing to see at autopsy. However, it may be seen on angiography in some patients with angina or infarction and principally occurs in areas damaged by atheroma. It is potentially of great therapeutic importance because it may be influenced by drugs.

Patterns of infarction

Occlusion of a single vessel, as described above, will produce a **regional infarct**, occupying the

Distribution of regional myocardial infarction

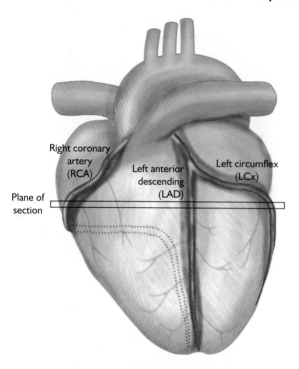

Right coronary artery (RCA)

Left anterior descending (LAD)

Left circumflex (LCx)

Plane of section

This is a normal, right CA-dominant heart

Posterior infarct: involves LV, RV (slightly) & posterior third of IV septum

RCA Occlusion

RV   LV

LCx

LAD

Anterior infarct: anterior LV, part of anterior RV and anterior two-thirds of IV septum

RCA

RV   LV

LCx

LAD   Occlusion

Subendocardial infarction

Triple vessel atheroma compromises supply to all areas of the myocardium, except the endocardial and epicardial zones.

A sudden drop in blood pressure, triggered by, for instance, the shock of hypothermia, can decrease CA flow sufficiently to cause circumferential infarction

RCA Occlusion

RV   LV

LCx

LAD

Lateral infarct: lateral wall of LV

RCA

RV   LV

LCx Occlusion

LAD

Figure 10.2 Patterns of myocardial infarction

segment of myocardium that is normally supplied by a particular coronary artery. The infarct may involve a variable thickness of the myocardial wall, but when it involves the full thickness of the wall, it is referred to as a transmural infarction. Ninety per cent of **transmural infarctions** result from thrombosis complicating atheroma. Myocardial infarction is much more common in the left ventricle and interventricular septum, but approximately 25 per cent of posterior infarctions will extend into the adjacent right ventricle or even into the atria. Occasionally, the infarcted region does not correlate with the thrombosed vessel; this is termed 'infarction at a distance'. It occurs because the patient has had previous coronary artery problems and has developed a collateral circulation so that, for example, longstanding poor flow through the left anterior descending coronary artery may make the anterior wall of the left ventricle dependent on collateral flow from the right coronary artery. Thus sudden occlusion of the right coronary artery may result in infarction of the region normally associated with the left anterior descending artery.

The other important pattern of myocardial damage is the **subendocardial infarction**. The pathogenesis of this type of infarction is different from that of regional infarction as there is generally widespread atherosclerosis in all coronary vessels but no specific occlusion. The subendocardial region is the most vulnerable part of the myocardium for two reasons: first, any collateral supply that is developed tends to supply the subepicardial part of the myocardium, and second, the subendocardium is under the greatest tension from the compressive forces of the myocardium and hence most likely to be ischaemic. Normally, blood will flow into the myocardium when the aortic root pressure exceeds the left ventricular cavity pressure, as occurs during diastole. A generalised reduction in myocardial perfusion results from any combination of coronary stenosis, reduction in aortic root pressure, increase in left ventricular cavity pressure, myocardial thickening and shortening of diastole.

Subendocardial infarction is much less common than transmural infarction. It is confined to the inner half of the myocardium and may be **regional** or **circumferential**. A very thin layer of subendocardial muscle remains viable because it receives nutrients and oxygen from the ventricular luminal blood. It should be noted, however, that even a transmural, regional infarct probably begins in the subendocardial region and then spreads to the rest of the wall.

Is myocardial infarction preventable?

You will hopefully realise from the preceding sections that any dietary or therapeutic factors that influence atherogenesis or thrombosis will alter the risk of myocardial infarction. If patients have *widespread* severe atherosclerotic coronary heart disease, they may have their diseased vessels bypassed by a graft from their leg veins or by synthetic vessels. Alternatively, the internal mammary artery can be 'plumbed' into the coronary arteries to bypass the stenotic areas. If they have only a *localised* lesion, they may have this 'stretched' by inflating an intravenous balloon catheter in the affected area, and the vessel may be stented to try to avoid restenosis. Low-dose aspirin may be used to reduce any thrombotic tendency by acting on the platelets. Once a coronary artery has become occluded, urgent action is required in the first 2 hours, while ischaemic damage is in the reversible phase. An intravenous catheter may be used to attempt to dislodge the clot, lytic agents may help to dissolve it, and the use of antithrombotic drugs will aim to prevent any extension of the thrombus. Early studies on hormone replacement therapy after the menopause suggest that this may help to prevent heart attacks and strokes.

WHAT ARE THE APPEARANCES OF INFARCTION?

Let us consider the clinical example described earlier in which the patient's ECG showed him to have had an inferior infarction. If he had died within a few hours, autopsy would have revealed a thrombus within the right coronary artery. This artery supplies the posterior wall of the left ventricle and the posterior third of the interventricular septum. Ischaemia of the septum would explain his complete heart block as this would damage the conduction pathway. No macroscopical abnormality would be seen in the myocardium, as the infarction would be only **6 hours old**, but the area of infarction could be highlighted using **histochemical techniques**.

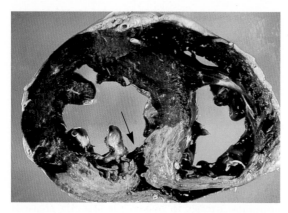

Figure 10.3 Heart slice through the right and left ventricles stained with NBTZ to demonstrate infarction in the area supplied by the left anterior descending artery. The left ventricular wall has ruptured (arrow), allowing blood into the pericardial space. (Slice viewed from below; right ventricle at the right of photograph)

Normal heart muscle contains dehydrogenases, which leak out of fibres that have been damaged by ischaemia. If a 1 cm slice of myocardium is dipped into a solution of the yellow dye nitroblue tetrazolium (NBTZ), the normal myocardium will appear blue owing to the reduction of the dye by the dehydrogenase enzymes, while the ischaemic myocardium will be pale and unstained. Had the patient died at **24 hours**, the infarcted area would either appear pale or be red-blue as a result of the trapped blood. Later, the dead myocardium becomes pale yellow, softened and better defined, with a rim of hyperaemic tissue at the periphery. Over the next few weeks, the necrotic muscle is replaced by fibrous scar tissue. This is usually complete by 6 weeks, the exact time course depending on the size of the infarct and any complications that may occur.

Under the light or electron microscope, the cardiac muscle will show the typical changes of reversible and irreversible ischaemic damage, which will be described in Figure 11.1.

WHAT COMPLICATIONS MAY OCCUR?

Our 63-year-old gentleman was in cardiac failure and complete heart block, two of the most common complications of myocardial infarction.

First, we will consider **arrhythmia**. This may be a type of heart block, ventricular tachycardia or bradycardia, ventricular fibrillation or asystole. Arrhythmias are responsible for many cases of sudden death following myocardial infarction, and their prompt diagnosis is of crucial importance in the management of these patients. Arrhythmias occur either because of ischaemia or death of the specialised conducting tissue of the heart, or because of interruption of the conduction of impulses within the damaged myocardium. A damaged atrioventricular node, for example, may lead to complete heart block, while damage to the conducting fibres within the ventricles will produce left or right bundle branch block. Damaged myocardial fibres may also be 'arrhythmogenic' and thus initiate abnormal impulses, which may terminate in ventricular fibrillation. It is interesting that many of the drugs used to treat arrhythmias, which act by altering the action potential, are also capable of inducing them.

The second complication mentioned is **cardiac failure**. This gentleman's cardiac failure could be due to complete heart block, so restoring normal sinus rhythm will be important in his treatment. Cardiac failure may also occur because of the extensive death of muscle cells in the left ventricular wall or because they have been 'stunned' by a short period of ischaemia and are temporarily unable to contract, although they may recover over a few days.

If a **papillary muscle** is damaged, mitral valve incompetence will produce cardiac failure. The papillary muscle is initially likely to be intact but incapable of contraction. After 4–5 days, the infarction has softened and the muscle may rupture, allowing the valve leaflet to prolapse, i.e. to float upwards into the left atrium.

Similar softening occurs in infarcted tissue in the left ventricular wall so that it may rupture. This occurs in transmural (i.e. full thickness) infarction but not in subendocardial infarction. Within 24–48 hours of transmural infarction, the damaged ventricular muscle stretches, i.e. becomes thinner, and is liable to aneurysm formation or rupture. This is often referred to as **infarct expan-**

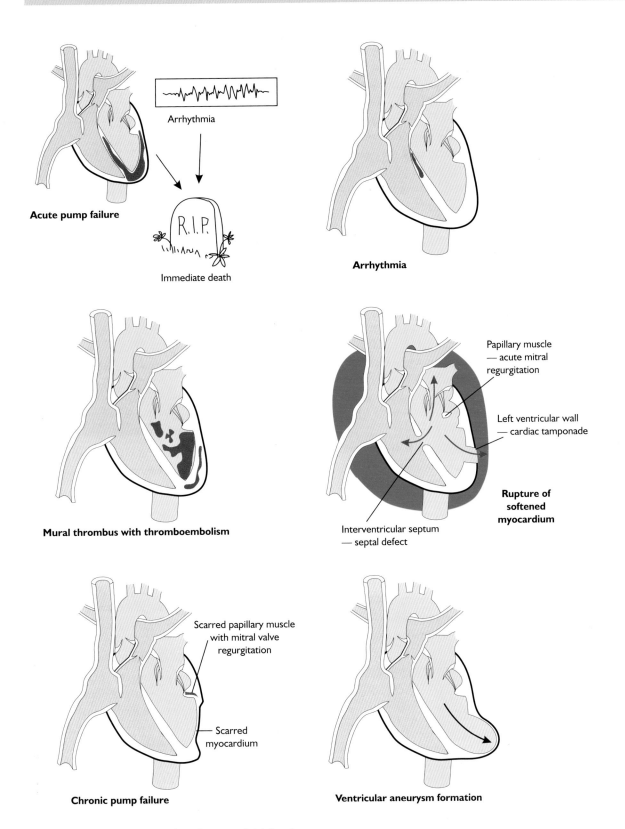

Figure 10.4 Possible sequelae of myocardial infarction

sion, but it should be appreciated that the amount of tissue damage is not increasing: it is merely a stretching of the damaged area. **Rupture** may take place in the interventricular septum, which creates a **ventricular septal defect** (**VSD**), or through the ventricular wall so that the blood leaks into the pericardial cavity, producing a **haemopericardium**, which inhibits the normal action of the heart – so-called **cardiac tamponade**. Either of these complications is generally fatal and is most likely to occur 5–7 days after a myocardial infarction.

The body's immune system responds to the infarction so that the pericardial surface overlying the infarcted area usually becomes inflamed (**pericarditis**) by the second or third day. In most cases, this is self-limiting, but the friction between the pericardial surfaces produces a **pericardial rub** that may be heard through a stethoscope. Similar changes occur on the endocardial surface of the infarct, which, in combination with stasis, predispose it to **mural thrombosis**. Whenever there is thrombosis, there is a risk of **embolism**. In this case, these would be systemic emboli affecting organs such as the brain or kidneys.

Finally, the healed and fibrotic wall may balloon out to produce a **cardiac aneurysm**, which can itself be a site of thrombus because of stasis.

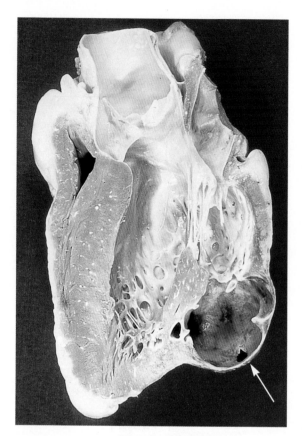

Figure 10.5 Sagittal section through the left ventricle showing cardiac aneurysms

Tachycardia: an increase in pulse rate
Bradycardia: an abnormally slow heart rate
Arrhythmia: an abnormal cardiac electrical rhythm
Asystole an absence of cardiac electrical activity
Fibrillation: uncoordinated and ineffective muscle contraction

ANEURYSMS

Cardiac aneurysms are quite rare, whereas aneurysms of large and medium-sized arteries, such as the aorta and cerebral arteries, are fairly common. An aneurysm is a localised dilatation in a blood vessel that may produce no symptoms, may cause problems through pressing on adjacent structures or may become occluded with thrombus or rupture, with potentially devastating effects.

Let us start with **berry** aneurysms. As the name suggests, these are more than just a dilatation, looking more like a cherry stuck on the side of a vessel. Berry aneurysms are usually small, less than 1.5 cm in diameter, and are globular in shape. Although referred to as congenital, they are not present at birth but develop because there is a defect in the media of the blood vessels at sites of bifurcation. They occur most commonly around the circle of Willis. Patients with berry aneurysms generally present with a sudden severe headache and some lose consciousness because the aneurysm has leaked. A patient will occasionally have ocular

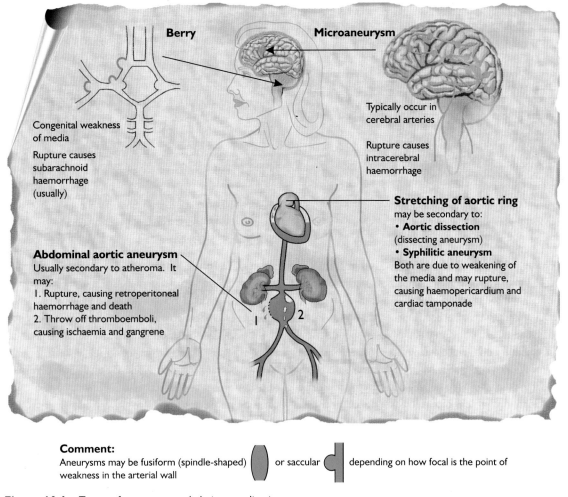

Berry

Congenital weakness of media

Rupture causes subarachnoid haemorrhage (usually)

Microaneurysm

Typically occur in cerebral arteries

Rupture causes intracerebral haemorrhage

Stretching of aortic ring
may be secondary to:
• **Aortic dissection**
(dissecting aneurysm)
• **Syphilitic aneurysm**
Both are due to weakening of the media and may rupture, causing haemopericardium and cardiac tamponade

Abdominal aortic aneurysm
Usually secondary to atheroma. It may:
1. Rupture, causing retroperitoneal haemorrhage and death
2. Throw off thromboemboli, causing ischaemia and gangrene

Comment:
Aneurysms may be fusiform (spindle-shaped) or saccular depending on how focal is the point of weakness in the arterial wall

Figure 10.6   Types of aneurysm and their complications

problems or facial pain because of pressure on the cranial nerves by an unruptured aneurysm. Frequently, these patients are young or middle-aged and are not normally hypertensive but are assumed to have raised their blood pressure by acute exertion.

The other important type of aneurysm affecting cerebral vessels is the **microaneurysm** or Charcot–Bouchard aneurysm. These are generally multiple small aneurysms, only a few millimetres in diameter, present on small arteries within the cerebral hemispheres. They occur in older, hypertensive individuals and are a common cause of intracerebral haemorrhage, a form of 'stroke'.

Atherosclerotic aneurysms are most common in the abdominal portion of the aorta and may present with massive haemorrhage or as a pulsatile mass in the abdomen, which may compress structures such as the ureters. They often become complicated by thrombosis, with the risk of shedding emboli into lower limb vessels. These aneurysms occur in individuals with risk factors for atheroma and develop as a result of thinning of the media, exacerbated by hypertension. It is not known how atheroma, an intimal disease, produces medial damage. The aneurysms are generally fusiform in shape and often extend for several centimetres along the aorta. Aneurysms greater than 6 cm in diameter are likely to rupture, so it is recommended that these are replaced by prosthetic grafts as replacement after rupture carries a high mortality.

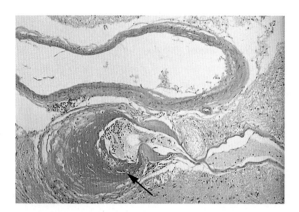

Figure 10.7 Photomicrograph showing a microaneurysm with a thrombus

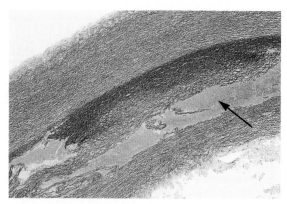

Figure 10.8 Elastin stain of aorta showing dissection of the wall by blood (stained yellow) (Courtesy of Dr S. Edwards, SGHMS)

Cystic medial necrosis is a descriptive term for necrosis of the media associated with the formation of mucoid cystic lakes. The cause of cystic medial necrosis is unknown, but it is associated with hypertension and may involve the production of abnormal collagen, elastin and proteoglycans in the media, as occurs in Marfan's syndrome. It is important as a possible aetiological factor in aortic dissection, in which blood tracks down through the media. Unfortunately, aortic dissection is often referred to as an aortic dissecting aneurysm despite the vessel not being dilated.

Aortic dissection usually occurs in the 40–60-year-old group and affects men more commonly than women, although it does occur in pregnant women, possibly because of generalised hormonal actions that soften connective tissue. Patients complain of sudden severe pain in the centre of the chest, similar to that felt in myocardial infarction, but this often radiates to the back and moves as the dissection progresses. The first event in aortic dissection is a tear in the intima so that blood enters the media and tracks down between the middle and outer thirds of the media. The tear often occurs in the ascending aorta and is thought to be due to shearing forces on the intima because of turbulent blood flow. Any hypertension will exacerbate both the turbulence and the forces splitting the media. Once the blood begins to track along the media, it can travel in either direction, can rupture back into the aorta or can rupture out into the peritoneal cavity, pericardial sac or pleural

cavity. Rupture outwards is catastrophic and common, whereas rupture into the aorta is rare but has a good prognosis and will produce a **double-barrelled aorta**. Extension of the dissection will occlude the mouths of any tributaries that become involved, this commonly affects the coronary, renal, mesenteric, iliac and carotid vessels.

Aneurysms secondary to inflammation will include those resulting from syphilis, arteritis and infection. **Syphilitic aneurysms** tend to occur in the ascending aorta and arch of the aorta, where they are ideally situated to cause mischief. Those which arise close to the aortic valve ring lead to dilatation of the ring and hence to **aortic incompetence**, the result of which is overload of the left ventricle and cardiac failure. Aneurysms may rupture into the trachea or oesophagus to produce haemoptysis (coughing up blood), haematemesis (vomiting blood) or death. Any cause of aortic expansion within the chest can produce difficulty in breathing or swallowing as a result of compression, persistent cough due to irritation of the recurrent laryngeal nerves or problems of bone erosion. Fortunately, syphilis is now an uncommon disease in the Western world, and these complications are rare.

Aneurysms secondary to **vasculitis**, such as polyarteritis nodosa, tend to occur in the renal and mesenteric vessels, where they lead to local ischaemia. Patients may therefore present with renal failure or with intestinal infarction and peritonitis, all of which have a significant mortality.

Aneurysms secondary to infection are called **mycotic aneurysms**. Such aneurysms tend to be 'saccular', i.e. the wall is weakened in a particular focus, which 'blows out' to form a sac. Most of the other conditions we have mentioned cause more diffuse weakening of the arterial wall, which dilates to form a 'fusiform' or spindle-shaped aneurysm.

HYPERTENSION

Many of the circulatory diseases we have discussed are related to hypertension. Atheroma, arteriolosclerosis, myocardial infarction and aneurysms are linked by their association with hypertension, so we cannot finish the section without discussing the aetiology and pathogenesis of hypertension.

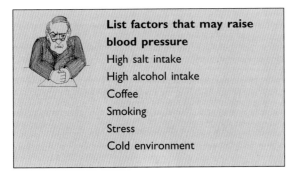

List factors that may raise blood pressure

High salt intake

High alcohol intake

Coffee

Smoking

Stress

Cold environment

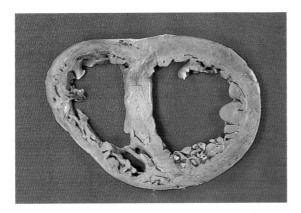

Figure 10.9 Dilated cardiomyopathy as a result of untreated hypertension. This leads to congestive cardiac failure

Hypertension is extremely common, affecting around 25 per cent of adults if a blood pressure of greater than 140/90 mmHg is regarded as abnormal. Unfortunately, organ damage may be irreversible by the time a patient presents with symptoms, so it is important to screen the people who are most susceptible. You will thus need to know about the factors influencing blood pressure. Hypertension is predominantly a condition of middle and later life that may be classified as 'benign' or 'malignant'. Fortunately, 'benign' hypertension is much more common, is relatively stable and is treatable with long term antihypertensive drugs. 'Malignant' hypertension only affects 5 per cent of hypertensive patients but is more severe and is liable to affect men under 50 years of age. It is defined as a diastolic pressure of more than 120 mmHg. The major dangers of hypertension are coronary heart disease, cerebrovascular accidents, congestive heart failure and chronic renal failure.

In 95 per cent of cases, there is no obvious cause; this is termed primary or idiopathic hypertension. Most of the remainder are due to renal disease, a small number resulting from endocrine abnormalities (secondary hypertension).

WHAT MECHANISMS MAY OPERATE IN HYPERTENSION?

We will have to be content with describing some of the theories concerning hypertension, as nobody knows the answers. First, it is useful to review the factors influencing the control of blood pressure.

In simple terms, arterial pressure will depend on the **cardiac output** and the **total peripheral resistance**. The resistance is determined by the arteriolar lumen, which may expand or contract depending on the state of the smooth muscle cells in the vessel wall. This is called **local vascular tone** and is influenced by a variety of mediators (see box on p. 165), which may act throughout the body or be produced and have their action locally, i.e. **autoregulation**. The cardiac output depends on the heart rate, its contractility and the blood volume.

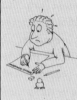

List the causes of secondary hypertension

Renal disease

Acute or chronic glomerulonephritis

Vasculitis, e.g. systemic lupus erythematosus

Renal artery stenosis

Chronic pyelonephritis

Diabetic nephropathy

Cardiovascular disease

Coarctation of the aorta (hypertension in the upper half of the body)

High cardiac output states

Hormonal

Phaeochromocytoma – excess catecholamines from tumour

Cushing's syndrome – excess corticosteroids

• Primary – adrenal cortical adenoma/hyperplasia

• Secondary – pituitary basophil adenoma, corticosteroid therapy, paraneoplastic, e.g. oat cell tumour

Conn's syndrome – excess aldosterone

• Adrenal cortical adenoma/hyperplasia

• Adrenogenital syndrome

Acromegaly – excess growth hormone

• Pituitary acidophil adenoma

Neurological

Raised intracranial pressure

• Haemorrhage

• Tumour

• Abscess

Hypothalamic or brainstem lesion

Pre-eclampsia in pregnancy

It is suggested that **essential hypertension** may result from a primary defect in renal sodium excretion, possibly combined with abnormalities in sodium or calcium transport in other cells. Many believe that the salt intake in Western countries contributes to hypertension and that salt intake should be reduced from a daily average of 9 g to 6 g. The normal kidney will increase the excretion of salt and water if the blood pressure rises, so that blood volume and hence blood pressure are reduced. It is not known what 'sets' the level at which this occurs, but if it is 'set' too high, the blood pressure will be raised, although stable. Any defect in sodium or calcium transport that leads to a rise in calcium in vascular smooth muscle will increase vascular tone responses. Vascular tone is also affected by alteration in any of the mediators already listed. The endothelium-derived ones are thought to be the most important.

Secondary hypertension is most often related to renal disease and results from abnormalities in the renin–angiotensin system, abnormal salt and water balance and renal vasodepressor substances. Angiotensin II is increased in response to raised renin levels and will increase vascular resistance, by causing vascular smooth muscle contraction, and increase blood volume through aldosterone, which promotes the distal tubular reabsorption of sodium. Negative feedback is provided via a lowering of renin levels secondary to the increase in angiotensin II, the raised pressure in the glomerular afferent arteriole and decreased proximal tubule sodium reabsorption, which influences the macula densa. Increased renin secretion occurs in all of the renal causes of hypertension listed in the written examination box on page 163, except for many cases of chronic renal failure. In chronic renal failure, there is sodium and water retention, which is probably related to a reduced glomerular filtration rate influencing tubular sodium handling. Theoretically, renal disease might produce hypertension through a reduction in its secretion of vasodepressor substances such as prostaglandins or platelet activating factor.

A new group of powerful vasoconstricters, the **endothelins**, has recently been identified. Endothelin I is the most potent vasoconstrictor yet discovered.

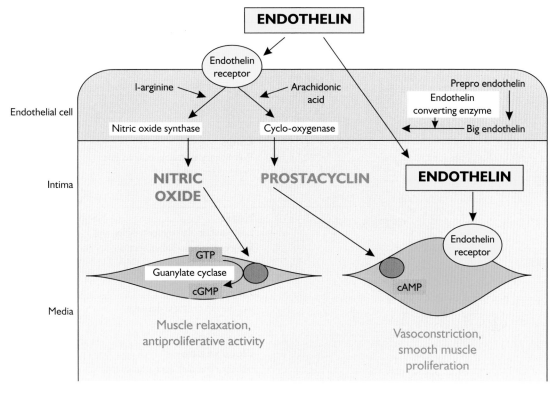

Figure 10.10 Action of endothelin on endothelial cells. (Adapted from Brown, MJ 1997: Science, medicine and the future: hypertension. *BMJ* 314. With kind permission of the BMJ Publishing Group)

Its plasma level is not raised in hypertensive individuals, but it is produced by endothelium and primarily acts locally on vascular smooth muscle. Production is increased by changes in sheer stress, hypoxia and inflammatory mediators. It may have an important role in maintaining the blood pressure following a myocardial infarction and in endotoxic shock, but may be detrimental by producing local ischaemia in heart muscle or in Raynaud's disease. Antagonists are already being tried in clinical trials. It is also mitogenic for smooth muscle cells, so may have a role in the formation of atheroma.

It is interesting to note the overlap between substances that vasoconstrict and substances that promote growth. Vasoconstrictors, such as noradrenaline and angiotensin II, promote smooth muscle growth, while growth factors, such as PDGF and epidermal growth factor, can cause vasoconstriction.

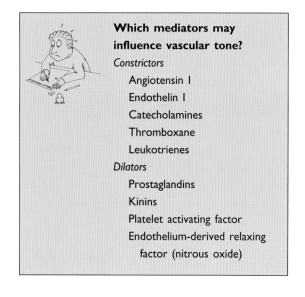

Which mediators may influence vascular tone?

Constrictors
> Angiotensin I
> Endothelin I
> Catecholamines
> Thromboxane
> Leukotrienes

Dilators
> Prostaglandins
> Kinins
> Platelet activating factor
> Endothelium-derived relaxing factor (nitrous oxide)

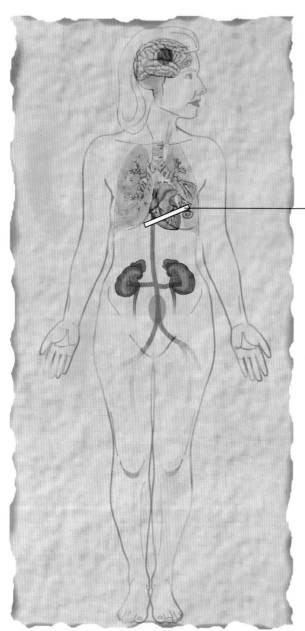

Brain
Microaneurysms and intracerebral haemorrhage

Lungs
Pulmonary oedema due to left ventricular failure

Heart
Left ventricular hypertrophy and failure; myocardial infarction

Kidneys
Ischaemic cortical damage

Blood vessels
Atherosclerosis and aneurysm formation

Figure 10.11 Complications of hypertension

We have already mentioned the morphological changes of hyperplastic arteriolosclerosis, but does wall thickness return to normal if blood pressure is lowered? This is an important question because, if vascular resistance were the result of morphological change, reversal of these changes might produce a normotensive patient who did not require continuous antihypertensive therapy. At present, it is not possible to give a complete answer, but in humans some antihypertensive drugs do produce some reduction in wall thickness, and in animals angiotensin-converting

CLINICOPATHOLOGICAL CASE STUDY

Clinical

A 65-year-old man complains of transient loss of vision in his right eye. He has had two episodes in the previous month, each lasting for approximately 7–10 minutes. Two months ago, he also had transient slurring of his speech.

Examination:
Blood pressure 180/110
Displaced apex beat and ejection systolic murmur

Carotid bruits present.

No peripheral pulses palpable below the femorals.

Chest X-ray confirm cardiomegaly but with no evidence of pulmonary oedema.
ECG shows atrial fibrillation and features of an old anterior infarction.

Echocardiogram demonstrates thrombus within the left atrium.

Carotid doppler studies indicate moderate carotid artery stenosis.
Urine analysis: no glucose detected.

Blood tests – serial cardiac enzymes: normal
Urea and creatinine: slightly raised

Management and progress:
It was decided that he should be treated with antihypertensive agents to reduce his blood pressure and anticoagulants to reduce the risk of further thrombosis/embolism. However, within 24 hours, he develops a right-sided weakness with hemiplegia and a right extensor plantar response. He dies without regaining consciousness.

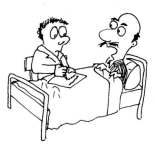

Pathology

Transient loss of vision or speech with full recovery is called a transient ischaemic attack.
It generally results from an embolus lodging in a small cerebral vessel and then being displaced or lysed. The most common sites of origin are the heart or carotid vessels.

He is hypertensive with an enlarged heart, i.e. left ventricular hypertrophy in response to increased workload.
The bruits indicate turbulent flow, which is a result of stenosis and/or irregularities of the vessel wall due to atheroma.
Absent peripheral pulses indicate widespread arteriosclerotic disease.
The presence of pulmonary oedema would have indicated cardiac failure.
In atrial fibrillation, the atria do not contract. The resultant stagnation of blood predisposes to thrombus formation.
Thrombi within the left atrium can be thrown into the systemic circulation. These can pass through the carotid arteries to lodge in the cerebral vessels.
Doppler studies detect turbulent flow. It is the electronic equivalent of the bruit.
A simple test for diabetes. Diabetics are at high risk of atheroma and may also suffer from sudden temporary loss of consciousness.
Test for myocardial infarction.
Mild renal impairment probably due to hypertension and atheroma.

The signs are of upper motor neurone damage involving the motor and sensory pathways with loss of consciousness. He has sustained a large left-sided cerebrovascular accident. The neural pathways cross; hence left-sided lesions give right-sided signs.

Post mortem findings:
Cardiovascular system – left ventricular hypertrophy. Atheroma in all three coronary arteries with an old anterior infarction. No evidence of recent infarct and no vegetations. A small amount of thrombus present in the left atrium. Extensive atheroma in aorta and carotid arteries with narrowing of the mouth of the renal arteries.
Central nervous system – a large haematoma in the region of the left internal capsule. Extensive atheroma in the cerebral vessels.
Genitourinary tract – small scarred kidneys showing ischaemic damage.
Clinically, the stroke could have been due to an embolus but, in his case, it is the result of rupture of a microaneurysm on the lenticulostriate branch of the middle cerebral artery, as a result of hypertension. These are called Charcot–Buchard aneurysms.

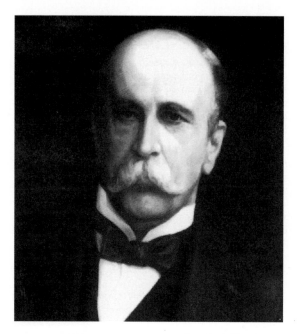

Figure 10.12 Sir William Osler (1849–1919) (Courtesy of the Wellcome Institute for the History of Medicine)

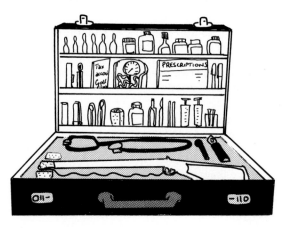

Figure 10.13 'Popgun pharmacy'

> 'A man cannot become a competent surgeon without the full knowledge of human anatomy and physiology, and the physician without physiology and chemistry flounders along in an aimless fashion, never able to gain any accurate conception of disease, practising a sort of popgun pharmacy, hitting now the malady and again the patient, he himself not knowing which'.

enzyme (ACE) inhibitors are clearly effective while thiazide and hydralazine-like vasodilators have only a minor effect. Thus, simply lowering the blood pressure is not enough, and some antihypertensives are perhaps achieving the morphological changes through other actions on smooth muscle cells.

This brings us to the end of this section on circulatory disorders. We started with the words of

William Harvey, conveying his despair at trying to understand the physiology of the motions of the heart. Physiology and pathology are of fundamental importance in clinical medicine, and the words of Sir William Osler, perhaps the greatest physician of recent times, provide an appropriate ending:

FURTHER READING

Brown, M.J. 1997: Hypertension. *British Medical Journal* **314**, 1258–1261.

Cotran, R.S., Kumar, V., Robbins, S.L. 1994: Hemodynamic factors, thrombosis and shock. In *Robbins' Pathologic Basis of Disease*, 5th edn. Philadelphia: W.B. Saunders, Ch. 4.

Fuster, V., Badimon L., Badimon, J.J., Chesebro, J.H. 1992: The pathogenesis of coronary artery disease and the acute coronary syndromes. *New England Journal of Medicine* **326**, 242–250; **326**, 310–318.

Levine, G.N., Keaney, J.F., Vita, J.A. 1995: Cholesterol reduction in cardiovascular disease. Clinical benefits and possible mechanisms. *New England Journal of Medicine* **332**, 512–519.

Lindop, G.B.M., Percy-Robb, I.W., Walker, I.D. 1992: Disturbances of body fluids, haemostasis and the flow of blood. In MacSween, R.N.M., Whaley, K. (eds) *Muir's Textbook of Pathology* 13th edn. London: Edward Arnold, Ch. 3.

Parums, D.V., Holloway, P. 1996: Cardiovascular disease. In Parums, D.V. (ed.) *Essential Clinical Pathology*. Oxford: Blackwell Science, Ch. 15.

Vane, J.R., Anggard, E.E., Botting, R.M. 1990: Regulatory functions of the vascular endothelium. *New England Journal of Medicine* **323**, 27–36.

PART 3

CELL AND TISSUE DAMAGE

INTRODUCTION TO PART 3

It would be terribly depressing if we saw dead things all around us all the time, but the fact that nature has a way of shielding us from such things also makes us view death as something abnormal and exceptional. In this section, we shall look at the pathology of cell and tissue damage, and while we will certainly examine situations in which cell damage and death occurs because of an abnormal stress or injury, we will also see that cell death has an important role in embryogenesis, growth, differentiation and immune defence mechanisms.

We will use the model of ischaemic damage to introduce the subject and then consider other forms of lethal and non-lethal cell injury. The concept of **apoptosis** or programmed cell death will be discussed, and it will be interesting to see how this type of cell death is mandatory for normal development and how it differs from **necrosis**, the cell death occurring as a result of injury. We will also consider two specific situations in which cells sustain damage: **amyloidosis** and **haemochromatosis**.

'It is a natural marvel. All of the life on earth dies, all of the time, in the same volume as the new life that dazzles us each morning, each spring. All we see of this is the odd stump, the fly struggling on the porch floor of the summer house in October, the fragment on the highway. I have lived all my life with an embarrassment of squirrels in my backyard, they are all over the place, all year long, and I have never seen, anywhere, a dead squirrel.'

Lewis Thomas

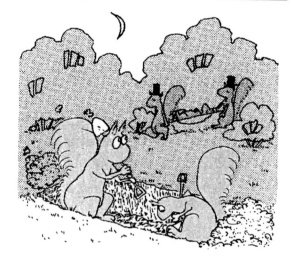

CHAPTER *11*

CELL DAMAGE AND CELL DEATH

- Clinical case – myocardial infarction
- Biochemical changes in cells
- Clinical relevance of cell changes
- Sublethal cell injury
- Necrosis
- Causes and mechanisms of cell death
- Tissue response to necrosis

Let us begin by considering myocardial ischaemia, a clinical scenario that should be familiar from Part 2.

CLINICAL CASE – MYOCARDIAL INFARCTION

A 60-year-old man complained of a sudden onset of chest pain that had started 2 hours previously. It radiated down his left arm. He was found to be in shock, with a blood pressure of 90/50 mmHg, and his ECG showed evidence of an anterior myocardial infarction. He also had bilateral pulmonary oedema. The serum cardiac enzymes, including the creatinine kinase MB isoenzyme, were elevated. Before he could be transferred to the coronary care unit, he developed ventricular fibrillation and, despite resuscitation attempts, died.

The following day, an autopsy was carried out; part of the report is illustrated overleaf.

Let us use this example to consider the changes that take place in myocardial cells following an ischaemic insult. We know that the final outcome is dependent on a number of variables. These include the **severity** and **duration** of the ischaemia and the **volume of heart muscle** affected. It will also be influenced by any **collateral circulation** and the **metabolic demands** of the myocardial cells at the time of the insult. Hence the extent of cell damage and death and whether the injury is reversible or irreversible depend on a number of factors and may be altered by medical intervention. The changes in the heart following ischaemia also vary with time.

AUTOPSY REPORT

Name: I.B. Ede   Age: 60 years

Date of admission: 24.7.97   Date of death: 24.7.97

Date of autopsy: 25.7.97

External findings:

The body was that of a Caucasian male. A central venous line in the right jugular vein and peripheral cannula in the left arm were present. There was bruising on the chest related to the resuscitation. No other abnormalities were seen

Internal examination:

Cardiovascular system – there was marked atheroma within the aorta and large vessels. The left coronary artery and the left anterior descending (LAD) artery both showed atheroma with 90% occlusion. In addition, there was an acute thrombus at the origin of the LAD. The right coronary artery showed 50% occlusion. There was no macroscopic evidence of an infarction; however, staining with NBTZ confirmed a full-thickness anterior infarct

Respiratory system – both lungs showed evidence of pulmonary oedema

Renal system – the kidneys showed evidence of ischaemic scarring

Central nervous system – there was marked atheroma in the carotids and cerebral vessels but no evidence of a cerebral infarction.

Cause of death:

	Ia	Myocardial infarction
due to	Ib	Coronary artery thrombosis
due to	Ic	Coronary artery atheroma

MACROSCOPICAL APPEARANCE

Although biochemical changes may take place very quickly, the gross appearance of the myocardium is generally entirely normal for the first 6–12 hours. As mentioned in Chapter 10, the NBTZ test can be used to highlight the area of infarction in this early period (see p. 157–158), and this is what was done in the patient described above. After about 18 hours, the myocardium generally appears slightly pale but may look reddish-blue owing to the red blood cells entrapped within the area of infarction. Each day that follows makes the area of infarction a little more defined, paler and softer. By the end of the first week, there is usually a rim of hyperaemia surrounding the pale yellowish-brown area of infarction. This is due to the ingrowth of richly vascularised connective tissue

that will be involved in the healing and repair process. As time goes by, the dead myocardial cell debris is removed and a pale firm fibrous scar laid down, a process that is complete by 6 weeks.

MICROSCOPICAL APPEARANCE

As with the gross appearance, the light microscopic changes lag behind the biochemical changes. The earliest change (4–12 hours) is mild oedema and separation of the muscle fibres. The cells adjacent to the area of infarction may also show small droplets within the cytoplasm, a phenomenon called **vacuolar degeneration**. By 24 hours, neutrophil polymorphs infiltrate the area of necrosis, and the necrotic myocytes undergo the cytoplasmic and nuclear changes typical of necrosis. The cytoplasm appears more pink (eosinophilic), and the nuclei become pyknotic. Later, the nuclei are lost and the cross-striations disappear. By day 3, the infiltrate of neutrophils is heavy, and by the end of the week, the cellular debris from dead cells is being removed by macrophages. The fibrovascular connective tissue, which gives the hyperaemia seen macroscopically, is also evident. Examination at later stages shows the varying amounts of fibrous scar tissue seen on gross inspection.

Figure 11.1 summarises the main findings on gross and microscopic examination of the myocardium at different times following the ischaemic episode.

BIOCHEMICAL CHANGES IN CELLS

There are two important questions to consider:
- What are the biochemical changes that occur in an injured cell?
- What distinguishes reversible from irreversible injury?

There are four sites within the cell that are of paramount importance in cell damage and death:
- the mitochondria
- the plasma membrane
- the ionic channels in cell membranes
- the cytoskeleton.

The first effect of ischaemia is to reduce the production of adenosine triphosphate (ATP) by the mitochondrial oxidative phosphorylation system. If the production of energy slows down or stops, the cells cannot function; in the case of heart muscle, the cell cannot contract. Obviously, if the ischaemic cells cannot partake in aerobic metabolism, they will switch over to anaerobic metabolism to derive energy from the stored glycogen. The enzyme creatinine kinase, which is present in the myocardial cells, is also utilised to produce energy from the anaerobic metabolism of creatinine phosphate. The net effect of these mechanisms is to deplete the cells of glycogen and to produce

acidosis within the cells by the production of lactic acid and inorganic phosphates. This further inhibits the normal function of the myocardial cells. The acidosis within the cells is thought to be responsible for one of the observed histological hallmarks of cell damage – the clumping of the nuclear chromatin and **pyknosis** of the nuclei.

Ischaemia also has profound effects on the plasma membranes and on the ionic channels situated within the membranes. You will recall that these are vital in maintaining the normal ionic gradients across the cell membranes, sodium and calcium concentrations being low inside the cells, and that of potassium lower in the extracellular space. These concentrations are maintained by pumps that are energy dependent; hence it is not difficult to see that the loss of the oxidative phosphorylation and any direct damage to the membranes will disrupt the function of these pumps. So what is the effect?

First, failure of the pumps will result in the leakage of sodium into the cells and potassium out of the cells. Sodium has a larger hydration shell than potassium, so more water moves in association with sodium ions than exits with the potassium. Additional water enters because the acidosis and raised intracellular concentrations of high molecular weight phosphates will increase the osmotic pressure inside the cell. The result is acute swelling of the cell from **cellular oedema**. The endoplasmic reticulum also swells, the ribosomes detach from the endoplasmic reticulum, the mitochondria become swollen, and blebs begin to appear on the cell surface. This last phenomenon is intriguing as the changes in cell shape and surface blebbing imply alterations in the cytoskeleton of the cell. The changes in the microfilaments of the cytoskeleton are believed to be due to the increased concentration of calcium, which also results from the failure of the membrane pumps. Calcium is a very important ion in cell death and we will see why in a minute.

You might find it difficult to believe, but all the changes described so far are reversible. If the oxygen supply is restored, the cells still have the capacity to return to the normal state, and the ability of the myocardial cells to contract is

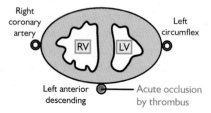
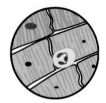

0–12 hours: *Potentially reversible*

Gross: nil, but NBTZ positive 2–8hrs
Light microscopy (LM): Nuclear pyknosis, vague
loss of striations, scanty PMN infiltrate
8–12hrs.

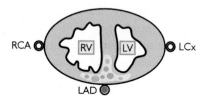
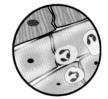

12–24 hours: *Ischaemic damage*

Gross: blotchy, pale, slightly soft
LM: Increase in PMN's, obvious loss of
striations, coagulative necrosis of
myocytes.

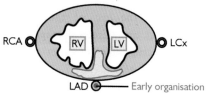
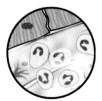

1–3 days: *Necrosis & inflammation*

Gross: Mottled pale infarct, red hyperaemic
border.
LM: as above, more marked mainly PMN
infiltrate and early capillary ingrowth,
particularly at periphery.

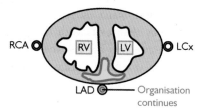
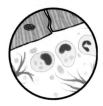

**4–7 days: *Removal of debris, early
organisation***

Gross: Depressed, soft, yellow infarct, prominent
hyperaemic edge
LM: as before, with increased macrophages
phagocytosing debris from dead myocytes,
peripheral granulation tissue formation.

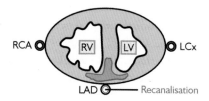
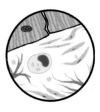

7–14 days: *Organisation*

Gross: 'bruised' look: red/purple colour,
increasingly firm as granulation tissue
forms
LM: Decreased inflammation as dead tissue is
cleared, granulation tissue replaces
damaged area.

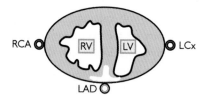
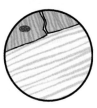

2–6 weeks: *Scar formation*

Gross: Infarct becomes firm and white and
eventually contracts, the LV wall is
thinned.
LM: Capillaries and fibroblasts are replaced by
acellular fibrous scar tissue

Figure 11.1   Myocardial infarction: changes with time

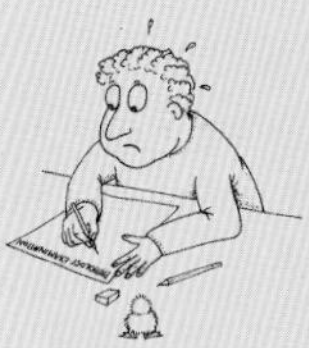

List the features of reversible and irreversible cell damage

Reversible	Irreversible
Cell swelling	Release of lysosomal enzymes
Mitochondrial swelling	Protein digestion
Endoplasmic reticulum swelling	Loss of basophilia
Detachment of ribosomes	Membrane disruption
'Myelin' figures*	Leakage of cell enzymes and proteins
Loss of microvilli	Nuclear changes: pyknosis, karyorrhexis, karyolysis
Surface blebs	
Clumping of nuclear chromatin	
Lipid deposition	

'Myelin' figures are derived from the cell surface and organelle membranes that lose lipoprotein molecules and take up extra water

restored. So what are the changes that finally tip the cell beyond the point of no return? The morphological hallmarks are a severe disruption of the mitochondrial membranes with the deposition of matrix lipoproteins, disruption of the plasma membranes and rupture of the lysosomes, with the release of enzymes. **Calcium** is thought to play a central role in this final progression to irreversible cell death.

In the normal cell, the concentration of calcium is tightly controlled by the calcium pump in the cell membrane. Inside the cell, it binds to two important proteins: troponin and calmodulin. Troponin has a role in muscle contraction, and calcium binding to calmodulin is a switch to turn on phosphorylation of important enzyme systems inside the cell. Ischaemia disrupts oxidative phosphorylation, thus affecting the energy-dependent calcium pump, leading to a rapid influx of calcium and saturation of the calcium-regulating proteins. The high levels of calcium are toxic to the cell, leading to changes in the cytoskeleton, cell surface blebbing and damage to the mitochondria, the lysosomal membranes and cell membranes. The calcium also binds to the phosphates within the cells, leading to a precipitation of hydroxyapatite crystals, which can be observed in the mitochondria. The release of enzymes from the ruptured lysosomes also contributes to the final destruction of the cellular components.

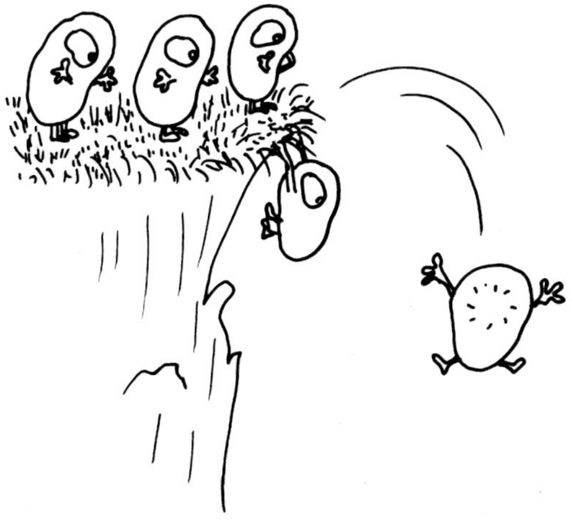

The biochemistry of cell damage and death is a complex process, with many systems interacting. In summary, ischaemia decreases the energy production by the oxidative phosphorylation system in mitochondria, which leads to loss of integrity of the plasma membrane, loss of function of the Na^+/K^+ and Ca^{++} pumps and severe injury to the mitochondria, nucleus, cytoskeleton and lysosomes. Experimental evidence suggests that calcium has a pivotal role in pushing the cell into irreversible cell damage and death.

Figure 11.2 Reversible and irreversible changes

Clinical relevance of cell changes

So much for science. Do these microscopical and biochemical changes help us to understand any of the clinical manifestations of our patient with myocardial infarction and cardiac failure? We know that ischaemia leads to a decrease in mitochondrial function and hence a decrease in ATP formation so that the cells stop contracting. What is absolutely staggering is that an ischaemic episode lasting only 1 minute can produce this change.

The cellular damage may be reversible, but the changes still profoundly affect the *function* of the organ. If the area of ischaemia is large, enough cells stop contracting to reduce the pumping power of the heart and cause **cardiac failure**. Any **arrhythmia** will exacerbate the cardiac failure. You will know that the rhythmic contraction of the heart results from the passage of electrical impulses down the specialised conduction pathways and within the myocardium. Abnormal conduction can occur if there is damage to the sinoatrial or atrioventricular node, the conduction bundles or the myocardium. Conduction of electrical impulses requires an intact cell membrane and functioning ionic channels within the membrane, so ischaemia produces abnormal conduction.

The right coronary artery supplies the atrioventricular node in 85 per cent of people; hence right coronary artery occlusion can produce complete heart block as well as inferior infarction. If the area of ischaemia involves the specialised bundles, the bundles may be selectively affected, resulting in either a right bundle branch block or a left bundle branch block. Occlusion of the left anterior descending artery produces an anterior infarction, which may be complicated by a blockage of both conduction bundles. This is frequently fatal, not purely because of the conduction problem but also because it is associated with a large area of infarction. Finally, the myocardium itself may affect the passage of impulses. An infarcted area of myocardium may not only slow down or stop the passage of electrical current but also generate an arrhythmia.

An **ECG** is a standard investigation for these patients and will detect disorders of cardiac rhythm and the approximate position and size of the infarction. The 12-lead ECG essentially produces a three-dimensional electrical picture of the heart. When part of the myocardium is damaged by ischaemia, the normal path of the electrical wave is impeded and the impulse has to travel via an alternative route. Consequently, the ECG pattern is altered and the type of change on the tracing helps to identify the area and the approximate size of the infarction.

Our patient had elevated levels of **cardiac enzymes** in his blood. Many enzymes are common to a variety of cells, but other enzymes are associated with the cell's specialist functions and will be restricted to only a few cell types. The cardiac muscle cell contains creatinine kinase (CK), aspartate aminotransferase (AST) and lactate dehydrogenase (LDH). Ischaemic damage to the myocardial cells disrupts the cell membranes, allowing leakage of these enzymes. If it is suspected that a patient has suffered a myocardial infarction, serial measurements of these 'cardiac enzymes' can be helpful in confirming the diagnosis and give a rough indication of the size of the damage. Since CK is also found in skeletal muscle, it is customary to measure CK-MB, which is an isoenzyme specific to cardiac muscle.

You can see how a knowledge of the cellular events helps us to understand the gross and histological appearances as well as the clinical measurements that are useful in diagnosis and management of the patient. Since mild reversible injury to cells is probably more common than irreversible injury, we will examine the histological patterns of reversible sublethal injury before going on to look at types of necrosis.

Sublethal cell injury

There are two patterns that we need to consider: cloudy swelling and fatty change.

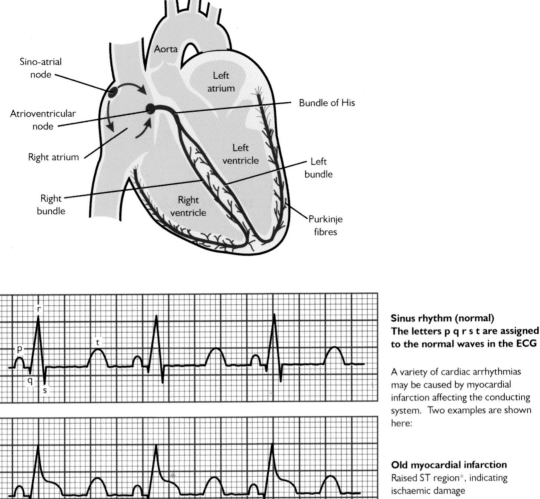

Sinus rhythm (normal)
The letters p q r s t are assigned to the normal waves in the ECG

A variety of cardiac arrhythmias may be caused by myocardial infarction affecting the conducting system. Two examples are shown here:

Old myocardial infarction
Raised ST region*, indicating ischaemic damage

Atrial fibrillation
Complexes are irregularly spaced and lack 'p' waves

Figure 11.3 Conduction system of the heart and ECG patterns in ischaemic damage

CLOUDY SWELLING

This has already been mentioned when considering myocardial ischaemia. The insult affects membrane ion exchange mechanisms to alter the ionic gradients, leading to increased intracellular sodium and water. This produces acute cellular oedema or 'cloudy swelling'. At the light microscopic level, this appears as expansion of the cell and a pale granular look to the cytoplasm. Vesicles may also appear as a result of distension of the endoplasmic reticulum. This picture of cellular oedema is also referred to as **hydropic** or **vacuolar degeneration**. Remember that cellular oedema may be precipitated by a whole range of insults and is not specific to ischaemia. Chemical toxins, infections and radiation can all induce similar changes. Remember also that cellular oedema is reversible.

FATTY CHANGE

This refers to an excess of intracellular lipid, which appears as vacuoles of varying size within the cytoplasm. Like cellular oedema, it is entirely reversible and is a non-specific reaction to a variety of insults. It is sometimes present adjacent to tissues that are more severely damaged or show frank evidence of necrosis. Fatty change can occur in any organ but is most frequent in the liver, which is not surprising since the liver is the major site of lipid metabolism. For this reason, we will use the liver as an example to discuss the pathogenesis of fatty change.

Figure 11.6 illustrates the fate of fatty acids after uptake by the liver and the possible sites at which alteration may lead to an increased accumulation of lipid within the liver cells. Very simply, adipose tissue releases fat as free fatty acids, which enter the hepatocytes, where they are converted to triglycerides and, to a smaller extent, cholesterol. Triglycerides are complexed with apoproteins to form lipoproteins, which are then secreted into the blood. Changes at any of the illustrated sites will lead to lipid accumulation within the hepatocytes. This is not just a hypothetical model derived from experimental systems but a common problem in people who abuse alcohol.

Alcohol is a hepatotoxin that has wide-ranging effects on fatty acid metabolism. It increases the peripheral tissue release of fatty acids so that more is delivered to the liver, and, within the liver, it is implicated in increasing fatty acid synthesis, decreasing the utilisation of triglyceride, decreasing fatty acid oxidation and blocking lipoprotein excretion. It is thus common for the causative agent to interfere with a variety of biochemical

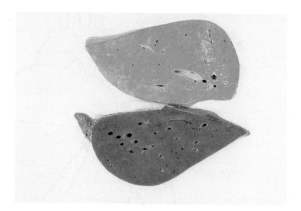

Figure 11.4 Normal and fatty (pale) liver

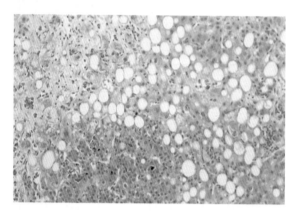

Figure 11.5 Photomicrograph of liver showing fatty (vacuoles) change

pathways. **Malnutrition** particularly affects two steps. It increases the release of fatty acids from peripheral tissue, and protein deficiency reduces the cell's ability to combine the triglyceride with apoprotein. **Carbon tetrachloride** also exerts its effect through reducing the availability of apoprotein. Disordered carbohydrate metabolism in uncontrolled **diabetes** leads to the excessive peripheral release of fatty acids.

Gross examination of the organs affected by fatty change will show that they are enlarged, yellow and tend to be greasy to the touch. Microscopically, the characteristic finding is of vacuoles within the cytoplasm. These may begin as small vacuoles, but if the fatty accumulation continues, they will coalesce to form larger vacuoles or 'fatty cysts'.

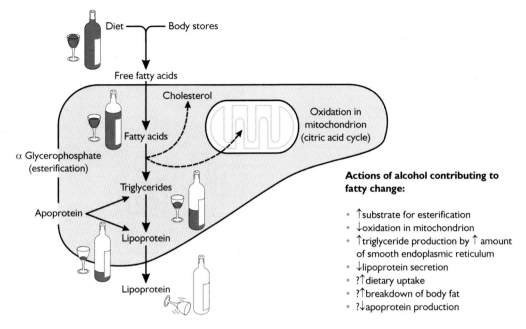

Figure 11.6 Alcohol and fatty change in the liver

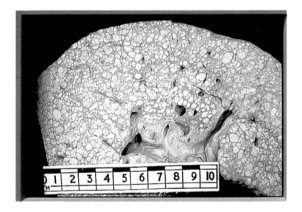

Figure 11.7 Cirrhosis of liver

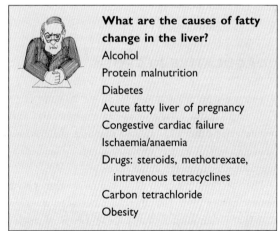

What are the causes of fatty change in the liver?

Alcohol

Protein malnutrition

Diabetes

Acute fatty liver of pregnancy

Congestive cardiac failure

Ischaemia/anaemia

Drugs: steroids, methotrexate, intravenous tetracyclines

Carbon tetrachloride

Obesity

To reiterate, this type of change is entirely reversible if the insult is withdrawn. A binge in the medical school bar on a Friday night may produce fatty change, but this will disappear if one is able to abstain for a few days afterwards! The chronic abuse of alcohol may produce sufficient fatty change to interfere with the normal function of the hepatocytes, and, in the long term, excessive alcohol consumption will lead to cell death, scarring and cirrhosis, which is *not* reversible.

NECROSIS

Necrosis is cell death due to injury.

In general terms, the microscopic changes include **eosinophilia** of the cytoplasm, **pyknosis** and disintegration of the nuclei (**karyorrhexis**), and finally complete dissolution of the nuclei (**karyolysis**). However, there are different patterns of necrosis in different circumstances. The principal types are:

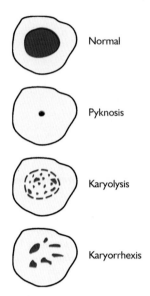

Figure 11.8 Nuclear changes in cell death

- coagulative
- colliquative or liquefactive
- caseous.

COAGULATIVE NECROSIS

If you consider Figures 11.9 and 11.10, one is of a normal kidney with normal glomeruli and tubules, the other of a kidney that has suffered an ischaemic insult and is showing coagulative necrosis. Can you spot the difference?

The second picture is essentially the ghost outline of the first. The difference between the two is that the damaged kidney shows a loss of nuclei from the cells, and the cytoplasm stains a darker pink with eosin. This pattern of necrosis is the most common type and occurs in many solid organs, such as the heart and kidney. The necrosis following a myocardial infarction is therefore of the coagulative type. Strange isn't it? Why should the basic architecture and cellular outline be preserved if the cells are dead?

Perhaps the offending injury destroys not only the vital structural proteins within the membrane, cytoplasm and nucleus but also the enzymes within the lysosomes that would otherwise degrade the cellular and extracellular components. The tissue,

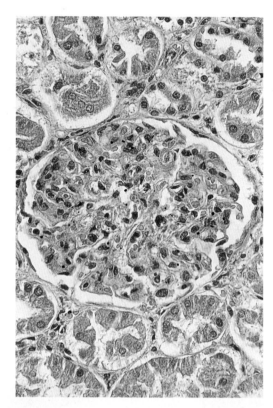

Figure 11.9 Normal kidney

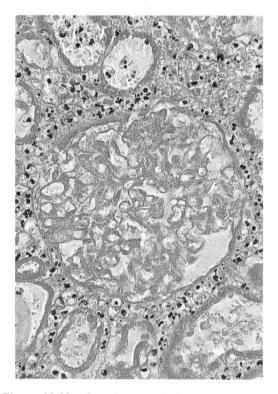

Figure 11.10 Coagulative necrosis

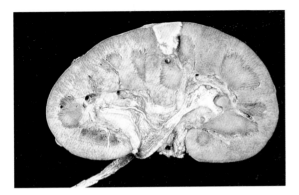

Figure 11.11 Kidney, showing wedge-shaped cortical infarct

of course, does not remain in that state for ever. If you remember the example of myocardial infarction, we stated that polymorphs move in within 24 hours of infarction. These inflammatory cells release enzymes that digest the cellular components, and the resulting debris will be removed by phagocytic cells such as the macrophages. It should be clear from this that the appearance of an area of coagulative necrosis will change with time.

COLLIQUATIVE OR LIQUEFACTIVE NECROSIS

The hallmark of this type of necrosis is the release of powerful hydrolytic enzymes that degrade cellular components and extracellular material to produce a proteinaceous soup. It characteristically

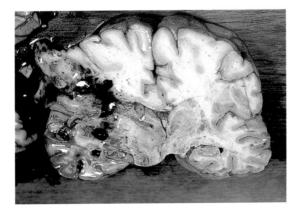

Figure 11.12 Brain with cerebral infarction

occurs in the brain, where it produces a cystic cavity containing fluid and necrotic debris.

Liquefaction may also be encountered in tissues when there is a superadded bacterial infection. Enzymes are then released from both the bacteria and the inflammatory cells that have been recruited to fight the infection.

CASEOUS NECROSIS

Caseous necrosis typically occurs in tuberculosis and is so called because of a resemblance to soft, crumbly cheese. The necrotic area is not quite liquid, but neither is the outline of the tissue retained as in coagulative necrosis. On microscopic sections stained with haematoxylin and eosin (H&E) (Figure 11.13), the necrotic area appears homogeneously pink (eosinophilic) with a surrounding inflammatory response involving multinucleate giant cells, macrophages and lymphocytes (see granulomatous inflammation, p. 70).

It is believed that lipopolysaccharides in the capsules of the Mycobacteria may be responsible for this peculiar reaction, but the mechanism is unclear.

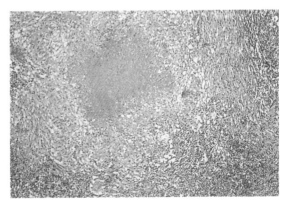

Figure 11.13 Photomicrograph of lymph node with tuberculous granuloma and caseous necrosis

OTHER TYPES OF NECROSIS

Although these are the main types of necrosis, we should, for completeness, briefly mention four

Compare and contrast coagulative and liquefactive necrosis		
Coagulative		**Liquefactive**
Severe ischaemia destroying proteolytic enzymes	*Mechanism*	Strong proteolytic enzyme action destroying tissue
Initial preservation of cell outlines and tissue architecture	*Appearance*	Loss of cell outlines. Tissue becomes cystic or fluid
Kidney, heart	*Occurrence*	Brain, bacterial infections

others: fat necrosis, gangrene, fibrinoid necrosis and autolysis.

Fat necrosis

This type of necrosis is peculiar to fatty tissue and is most commonly encountered in the breast following trauma and within the peritoneal fat as a result of pancreatitis.

Within the breast, trauma may lead to the rupture of adipocytes and the release of fatty acids. This will elicit an inflammatory response, and the area will become firm because of scarring. Clinically, the lump may be mistaken for a carcinoma, and excision and microscopic examination may be required to determine the diagnosis.

In pancreatitis, damage to the pancreatic acini results in the release of proteolytic and lipolytic enzymes, which denature fat cells in the peritoneum and lead to an inflammatory reaction. Calcium is also deposited in the tissues in combination with fatty acids to form calcium soaps. This is a form of dystrophic calcification; we will consider calcification again in the section on tissue response to necrosis, below.

Gangrene

This does not represent a distinctive type of necrosis but is a term used in clinical practice to describe black, dead tissue. It is most commonly seen in the lower limb in patients with severe atherosclerosis, which often causes irreversible ischaemic damage to the most peripheral tissues in the body. If the pattern of necrosis is mainly of the coagulative type, it is referred to as **dry gangrene**, while the presence of infection with Gram-negative bacteria converts it into a liquefactive type of necrosis, called **wet gangrene**. It will be apparent from the preceding discussion that the type of necrosis encountered depends on a number of different factors, including the type of tissue involved and the nature of the offending agent.

Fibrinoid necrosis or fibrinoid change refers to the microscopic appearance seen when an area loses its normal structure and resembles fibrin. It does not have any distinctive gross appearance.

Autolytic change is completely different from the other types as it refers to cell death occurring after the person has died. Obviously, the heart stops pumping, and all the tissues become irreversibly ischaemic. Enzymes leaking from the cells digest adjacent structures, but there is no inflammatory response because the inflammatory system is dead.

CAUSES AND MECHANISMS OF CELL DEATH

We have considered the biochemical and morphological changes that occur with cell injury and death, but what are the causes and what are the mechanisms?

There is a wide range of insults that can cause cell death, ranging from the obvious, such as trauma and burns, to more subtle causes arising as a result of specific metabolic abnormalities. The causes include:

- ischaemia
- physical agents, e.g. temperature, radiation and trauma
- chemical agents, e.g. corrosive agents, alcohol and carbon tetrachloride
- infections, e.g. bacterial, viral and parasitic
- nutritional disorders, e.g. obesity and malnutrition
- immunological disorders, e.g. autoimmune disease, and hypersensitivity reactions
- genetic disorders, e.g. sickle cell disease.

Let us consider the possible mechanisms involved in these varied causes of cell injury and death, bearing in mind that it is not always possible to define the exact site of action of the initial insult. Since the cell membrane, oxidative phosphorylation and DNA are vital to the cell, it is very likely that these will be involved. You will also recall that the final outcome is dependent on the severity and duration of the insult and the metabolic demands of the tissues at the time of the insult.

Physical and chemical agents are well known for causing cell death. We are all aware of the devastating effects of dropping an atomic bomb and the mass destruction caused by chemical warfare. Radiation and chemicals produce cell death by the production of oxygen free radicals, the details of which have been illustrated in Part 1. Temperature is another important factor. Heat applied to the skin in low doses may induce a coagulative type of necrosis, but with intense heat, the tissue may simply vaporise. Those interested in Arctic exploration will be aware of the gangrene induced by extreme cold, which is due to a combination of thrombosis in small vessels and ice crystal formation in the tissues (frostbite).

The role of infections in tissue death was discussed earlier. Briefly, microorganisms may injure tissues by producing toxins, by competing for essential nutrients, by a direct cytopathic effect as a result of cell invasion or by provoking an attack by the immune system. In the course of fighting infection, there is usually some damage to

the normal tissue through the release of degradative enzymes and the chemical mediators of inflammation. Similar indirect mechanisms operate in the autoimmune diseases as well as immunologically mediated injury, as discussed under hypersensitivity reactions (see p. 36).

Sickle cell disease is caused by a genetic change in DNA that results in the production of an abnormal haemoglobin molecule. This molecule is susceptible to changes in oxygen concentration, and hypoxia leads to a configurational change that results in the 'sickling' of red blood cells. These cells are unable to pass through the capillaries, thus blocking the local circulation to produce local tissue ischaemia. The abnormal red cells are also prone to removal from the circulation by the reticuloendothelial system. Sickle cell disease is therefore a good example of a genetic abnormality that results in cell injury and death. It is dealt with in more detail in Part 5.

So the tissue receives an insult in the form of infection, alcohol or ischaemia, and the result is cell death and some type of necrosis. What then? What are the possible tissue responses to and sequels of necrosis?

TISSUE RESPONSE TO NECROSIS

HAEMORRHAGE

Haemorrhage is not really a reaction to necrosis but is the consequence of endothelial cells being damaged. This may be due to the same agent as is causing the necrosis of the parenchymal cells or may be a secondary effect related to the inflammatory response. Severe endothelial cell damage may result in leakage of blood from the vessels, so areas of haemorrhage are common in necrotic tissues. The blood will eventually be removed by the phagocytic mechanisms involved in repairing the area of necrosis.

Tumours also often show macroscopically evident haemorrhage. This is thought to be due to

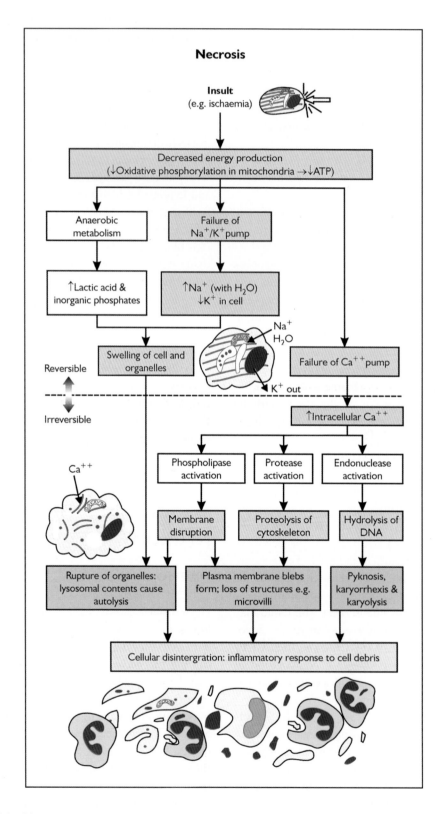

Figure 11.14   Necrosis

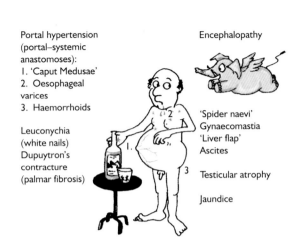

Portal hypertension (portal–systemic anastomoses):
1. 'Caput Medusae'
2. Oesophageal varices
3. Haemorrhoids

Leuconychia (white nails)
Dupuytron's contracture (palmar fibrosis)

Encephalopathy

'Spider naevi'
Gynaecomastia
'Liver flap'
Ascites

Testicular atrophy

Jaundice

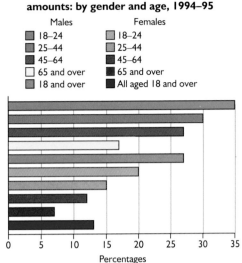

Adults consuming alcohol above sensible amounts: by gender and age, 1994–95

Males
■ 18–24
■ 25–44
■ 45–64
□ 65 and over
■ 18 and over

Females
□ 18–24
□ 25–44
■ 45–64
■ 65 and over
■ All aged 18 and over

Percentages

Figure 11.15 Stigmata of liver disease (data from Social Trends 1994–1995 (Alcohol), General Household Survey. Office for National Statistics, Crown copyright 1997)

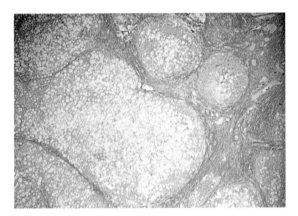

Figure 11.16 Photomicrograph of liver with cirrhosis

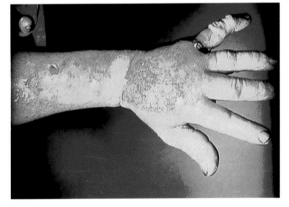

Figure 11.17 Severe burn resulting in scarring and contractures

the action of cytokines such as TNF, which damage endothelial cells and induce thrombosis in small vessels, resulting in haemorrhage and necrosis in the tumours.

REPAIR AND ITS COMPLICATIONS

In the first part of the book, we looked at the processes of inflammation and repair. The healing and repair associated with necrosis follow identical pathways, which is not surprising because

inflammation is one of the causes of necrosis. The inflammatory process is responsible for clearing cell debris from areas of necrosis, the final result being dependent on the site of injury and the extent of the damage. In the liver, for example, minor degrees of injury may not be noticeable after the liver cells have regenerated. More severe damage with loss of the supporting tissue will produce scarring and fibrosis, and may lead to cirrhosis.

Cirrhosis is an example of a problem caused by the healing and repair process. What happens is that

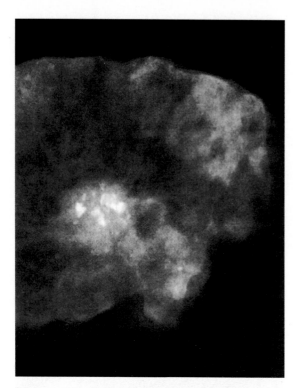

Figure 11.18 X-ray of breast tissue (mammogram) showing a circumscribed abnormality, which is radio-opaque because of dystrophic calcification

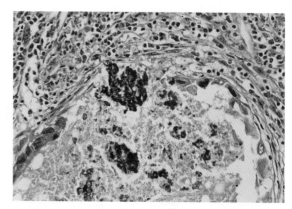

Figure 11.19 Dystrophic calcification in necrotic tumour

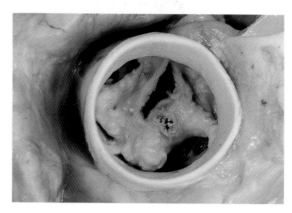

Figure 11.20 Dystrophic calcification in damaged aortic valve, producing stenosis

the hepatocytes regenerate as parenchymal nodules without central veins or portal tracts, which ruins the normal blood flow through the liver. This means that the liver vasculature cannot cope with the blood coming through the portal vein, so the pressure rises to produce **portal hypertension**. The blood takes alternative routes through anastomoses that link the portal and systemic circulations, but this can produce more problems as the dilated anastomotic vessels, termed **varices**, are liable to rupture and cause life-threatening haemorrhage.

Almost every organ has a set of complications related to the repair following necrosis. In the heart, a myocardial infarction may be followed by rupture or aneurysm formation. Lung fibrosis may impair both ventilation and gas transfer. Scarring of the skin may be disfiguring and induce contractures. All of these problems involve the formation of fibrous tissue, and we will now turn to a complication that may affect the fibrosis itself, namely calcification.

CALCIFICATION

Calcification in tissues is divided into two types:
• dystrophic calcification
• metastatic calcification.
The written examination box on page 189 illustrates the salient features of these two types of calcification. In this discussion, it is the first type that is important. **Dystrophic calcification** occurs in tissues that are dying or are non-viable following some type of injury, involution or alteration. The patient has a normal serum calcium level, which contrasts with the situation in **metastatic calcification**, in which patients with high serum calcium levels calcify their previously normal tissues.

<table>
<tr><th colspan="3">Compare and contrast dystrophic and metastatic calcification</th></tr>
<tr><th></th><th>Dystrophic</th><th>Metastatic</th></tr>
<tr><td>Serum calcium</td><td>Normal</td><td>Raised</td></tr>
<tr><td>Tissues affected</td><td>Dead or damaged</td><td>Previously normal</td></tr>
<tr><td>Examples</td><td>Scars, atheroma, damaged heart valves, tuberculous lymph nodes, neoplasms, dead parasites</td><td>Renal failure, bone metastases, sarcoidosis, myeloma, primary and tertiary hyperparathyroidism</td></tr>
</table>

In this section, we have already mentioned the calcification that occurs in fat necrosis following an episode of pancreatitis, and, in the previous section, we described the calcification that commonly complicates atheroma. Dystrophic calcification can sometimes be an aid in detecting lesions by X-ray examination, as occurs in breast screening programmes that use mammography. Dystrophic calcification can be intracellular and/or extracellular and may progress to bone formation (osseous metaplasia). The mechanism of dystrophic calcification involves two stages – **initiation** followed by **propagation** – which results in the formation of hydroxyapatite crystals. When the cell undergoes necrosis, large amounts of calcium enter the cell as the membrane ionic pumps fail. This calcium combines with the phosphates within the mitochondria to produce the hydroxyapatite crystals. The mechanism for extracellular calcification is similar, crystals forming in membrane-bound vesicles derived from degenerating cells. After this initiation, the propagation of crystal formation depends on the local concentration of calcium and phosphate, whether there are inhibitors and the amount of collagen, since collagen enhances crystal production. Dystrophic calcification generally acts only as a sign of previous injury, but at certain sites, such as the heart valves, it may affect function.

Metastatic calcification arises from an abnormality of calcium metabolism resulting in high levels of serum calcium. There are many causes of hypercalcaemia, which include primary and tertiary hyperparathyroidism, hyperthyroidism, sarcoidosis, metastatic cancer in bone and excess vitamin D ingestion. This form of calcification occurs in normal tissues, the favoured sites being soft tissues, blood vessels, lungs and kidneys. Extensive calcification in the kidney may impair renal function, while soft tissue calcification may be nothing more than a minor nuisance. The mechanism of metastatic calcification is thought to be similar to the dystrophic variety, with the formation of hydroxyapatite crystals commencing in mitochondria.

Having considered necrosis and its complications, we will now move on to apoptosis, the paradox of cell death.

APOPTOSIS

- Can cell death be useful?
- Structural changes in apoptosis
- Biochemical changes in apoptosis
- Genetic events in apoptosis
- Apoptosis and disease
- Apoptosis versus necrosis
- Apoptosis and therapeutic implications

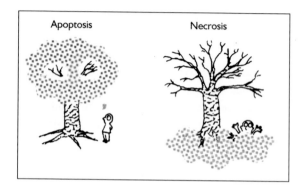

The word apoptosis is derived from Greek and was originally used to describe the falling of individual leaves from a tree. In pathology, it is a specific type of cell death that involves single cells or small groups of cells in a tissue where the other cells are functioning normally. A similar pattern of cell death is also encountered in plants and invertebrates and is called programmed cell deletion. The term **programmed cell death** may be more appropriate than apoptosis as it emphasises that programmed cell death appears to be under physiological and, possibly, genetic control, whereas cell necrosis is the result of injury. The genetic control of death – that is quite a statement to make for it implies that our own genes, selected by the pressures for survival, are also involved in causing cell death. Can death be a necessary part of life? The philosophers and gardeners among you will have no difficulty with this concept; after all, a good rose garden requires a certain amount of pruning.

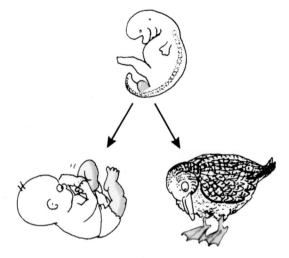

Figure 12.1 Apoptosis at the embryonic stage

CAN CELL DEATH BE USEFUL?

The importance of programmed cell death is evident from the earliest stages of the embryo through to the involutional changes of the menopause.

Let us consider the production of a limb with its five digits. To achieve this, tissue growth has to occur by cell division, but it is also necessary to produce interdigital cell death. It is either that or ending up as a duck! This type of cell death is genetically controlled.

Similarly, there are the stages of metamorphosis that take place to turn a tadpole into a frog. Metamorphosis requires not only mitotic activity and tissue growth but also a large amount of programmed cell death. When a tadpole turns into a frog, the most obvious change is that limbs are formed and the tail is resorbed. During the process of resorption, there is an increase in thyroxine, which appears to lead to the activation of collagenases and hence destruction of the tail. Here, we have an example of how programmed cell death may depend on the production of a hormone, with activation of protein enzyme systems to assist the process.

A hormonal effect on cell death is also important in the maturation of the human reproductive system. The reproductive system has an early indifferent phase when it is neither male nor female. The wolffian duct will differentiate into the epidydimis and vas deferens in the male, while the müllerian duct forms the uterus and fallopian tubes in the female. We know from experimental observations that the administration of oestrogens at a critical time will feminise the male, whereas the administration of testosterone will masculinise the female. In order for that to happen, there has to be regression of the primitive wolffian or müllerian structures, and this occurs via programmed, controlled cell death.

The development of the nervous system is also dependent on programmed cell death. There is an excess of neurons, and only those which produce the correct synaptic connections with their target

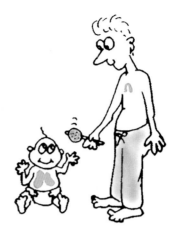

Figure 12.2 Thymic atrophy due to apoptosis

cells survive. The rest, up to 50 per cent, die as a result of apoptosis.

The thymus is large in the fetus and infant but atrophies before adulthood. This involution occurs via cell death that is thought to be steroid sensitive. The steroid hormones are produced in the adrenal gland, so that, in this case, one organ is responsible for the involution of another via its secreted product. This observation is useful in perinatal autopsies for deciding whether the death of a newborn baby is a sudden event or whether it has followed several days of problems *in utero*. If the baby has been stressed *in utero*, adrenal steroids will cause premature involution of the thymus so that it is less than half its normal size. If the baby has been normal *in utero* but has suffered a problem during delivery (e.g. birth asphyxia), the thymus will be its normal size. There is some recent evidence that this steroid sensitivity is under the control of a single gene, and the same gene may be involved in apoptosis caused by cytotoxic T lymphocytes (see below).

The endometrium is a hormone-dependent tissue that undergoes cyclical changes during the reproductive period as well as involutional changes after the menopause. The oestrogens secreted by the ovary in the early part of the menstrual cycle induce endometrial proliferation, and if pregnancy does not occur, there is programmed cell destruction that results in **menstrual shedding**. If pregnancy occurs, there is hyperplasia of the breast

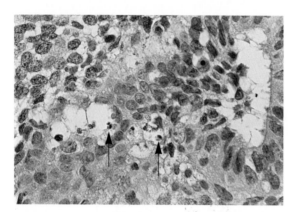

Figure 12.3 Photomicrograph showing apoptosis in the endometrial glands

in preparation for lactation, which will be followed by **physiological atrophy** involving apoptosis after weaning. This atrophy is not only due to cell loss but also results from a reduction in cell size and a loss of extracellular material. Following the menopause, the withdrawal of the hormonal influence results in **involution of the uterus and ovaries**.

Apoptosis plays an important role in the immune system. It is necessary for the selection of specific subpopulations of both T and B lymphocytes and is also important in the destruction of target cells by cytotoxic T cells. Now we will discuss apoptosis initiated by immune cells, which differs in that individual target cells die after a local stimulus from an immune cell. For example, in a liver infected by hepatitis B virus, a liver biopsy will reveal many individual apoptotic cells; this is due to the immune cells attacking hepatocytes bearing the antigens of hepatitis B. It appears that cytotoxic T cells and natural killer cells are capable of directing a target cell to commence apoptosis, i.e. to commit suicide.

STRUCTURAL CHANGES IN APOPTOSIS

The original term for apoptosis was 'shrinkage necrosis', apoptotic cells tending to shrink while necrotic cells initially swell. Apoptotic cells lose their contact with neighbouring cells early on. After 1–2 hours, the nuclear chromatin condenses on the nuclear membrane, and the membrane then 'packages' these small aggregates of nuclear material to give membrane-bound nuclear fragments. The cytoplasm shrinks and the cell's organelles also become parcelled into membrane-bound vesicles. These are called **apoptotic bodies** and contain morphologically intact mitochondria, lysosomes, ribosomes, etc. Finally, these apoptotic bodies are phagocytosed by neighbouring cells or by macrophages. Experimental evidence suggests that an apoptotic cell acquires molecules on its surface that allow neighbouring cells and macrophages to identify it as having committed suicide, hence leading to clearing of the fragments.

A crucial feature of apoptosis is that the cell's contents are not allowed to leak into the extracellular space, where enzymes may digest adjacent structures or proteins may stimulate an immune response. Instead, the cell packages itself into small membrane-bound vesicles that contain functioning mitochondria and other cell organelles. These survive long enough to be phagocytosed by macrophages, which can degrade the components in secondary lysosomes. This mechanism is essential for allowing cell death without secondary inflammation and scarring.

BIOCHEMICAL CHANGES IN APOPTOSIS

The biochemical processes responsible for the structural changes described above are beginning to be understood. DNA transcription leads to production of proteins – the endonucleases that result in cleavage of DNA and the production of the characteristic 'DNA ladder' seen in apoptosis. The cytoskeletal proteins undergo proteolysis. Activation of transglutaminase results in protein–protein cross-linking. The appearance of phosphatidylserine and other charged sugar molecules on the outer and inner surfaces of the cell membrane seems to be responsible for the recognition of apoptotic cells by macrophages and their neighbours. These sugars are not usually exposed on the cell membrane, and their presence during cell death is an active process by which the debris is cleared.

GENETIC EVENTS IN APOPTOSIS

The genetic events in apoptosis were elucidated by the study of the nematode *Caenorhabditis elegans*. The development of this organism is remarkably well understood, and it is known that 131 somatic cells out of 1090 are eliminated by apoptosis. The genes responsible for this programmed cell death have been identified. Two genes, *ced-3* and *ced-4*, induce apoptosis, while a third gene, *ced-9*, inhibits it. The mammalian counterparts of these genes have been identified. *Ced-3* is related to a family of cystein proteases known as the ICE (IL-1β converting enzyme) protease family. These play a key role in apoptosis and confirm that the proteolytic cleavage of critical proteins is important in the induction of apoptosis. The *ced-9* gene encodes a protein that shows homology to proteins of the *bcl-2* family, which are known inhibitors of apoptosis in humans. *bcl-2* is a member of a large family, some of which, like *bcl-2* and *bcl-xL*, inhibit apoptosis, whereas others, e.g. bax, bad and *bcl-xS*, promote cell death.

Since most cells contain members of the ICE family of proteases, the initiation of apoptosis seems to be dependent on the activation of this proteolytic cascade. The balance between the destructive signals from the ICE members and the protective signals from proteins such as the bcl-2 family will determine whether, in a given case, the cell survives or dies.

Cytokines also play a very important role in cell death. The first receptor identified as being associated with apoptosis was the CD95/apo-1/fas. It is a member of the CD40/TNF receptor family and is expressed in hepatocytes, enterocytes and some lymphocytes. The activation of this fas receptor

has been shown to be a key event in the killing of target cells by cytotoxic T cells.

Besides *bcl-2*, discussed above, there is a number of other oncogenes involved in apoptosis. c-*myc* is an oncogene with mitogenic actions and has a role in cell proliferation. Strangely, if c-*myc* is expressed in the absence of other growth stimulatory factors, it induces apoptosis. Hence c-*myc* appears to be able to produce cell replication or cell death, the outcome being dependent on the availability of other growth factors.

The tumour suppressor gene *p53* induces apoptosis and appears to be important in inducing apoptosis following DNA damage by irradiation. Mutation of the *p53* gene and hence inactivation of the protein will therefore tip the balance towards cell survival.

APOPTOSIS AND DISEASE

It will come as no surprise that cell death is important not only in normal development and normal physiology but also in disease processes.

The pathology associated with AIDS is linked to the phenomenon of apoptosis. In HIV-positive patients, the mitogenic stimulation of peripheral lymphocytes results in apoptosis. The data suggest that gp120, a protein released into the circulation in HIV-positive patients, activates the fas receptor, thus initiating apoptosis. The cells characteristically affected are the CD4+ T cells, which are the cells important for the generation of memory to intercurrent and opportunistic infections.

When viruses infect cells, they attempt to take over the cell's replication machinery in order to proliferate and spread. The apoptotic mechanism will come into play when breaks occur in DNA strands as the viral genome incorporates itself into the cell's DNA. Many viruses code for proteins that block apoptosis. Examples include the inactivation of p53 by HPV16 and EBV, which produces proteins that either simulate *bcl-2* or block molecules related to the TNF/CD40 pathway.

Since viruses play a role in carcinogenesis (see Part 4), the question arises of whether apoptosis

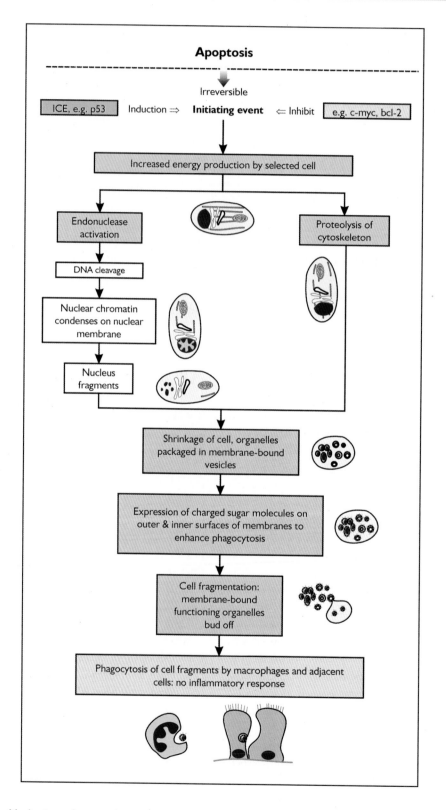

Figure 12.4 Mechanism of apoptosis

Compare cell necrosis with apoptosis: how do they differ?

Necrosis	**Apoptosis**
Group of cells affected	Single or few cells selected
Caused by injurious agent/event	Programmed death
Reversible events precede irreversible	Irreversible once initiated
Energy deprivation causes changes	Events are energy-driven
Cells swell due to influx of water	Cells shrink as cytoskeleton is disassembled
Haphazard destruction of organelles and nuclear material by enzymes from ruptured lysosomes	Orderly packaging of organelles and nuclear fragments in membrane-bound vesicles
Cellular debris stimulates inflammatory cell response	New molecules expressed on vesicle membranes stimulate phagocytosis, no inflammatory response

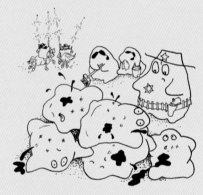

Necrosis is a messy business

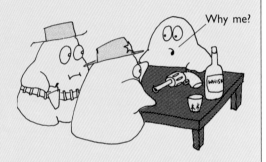

Apoptosis is an ordered event

Figure 12.5 Necrosis and apoptosis – how do they differ?

also has a role in the development of tumours. It is clear that, for tumours to arise, there must be both an increase in proliferation and a decrease in cell death. Since some genes are protective by inducing cell death when genetic damage has occurred, it is not surprising that the inactivation of such genes allows the transmission of genetic damage to daughter cells by allowing cell replication to take place and preventing death that would otherwise have occurred. The tumour suppressor gene *p53* plays a crucial role in inducing apoptosis following DNA damage resulting from radiation and carcinogens. The inactivation of *p53* (which is one of the most common genetic alterations in tumours) prevents apoptosis. In the presence of mutations in genes responsible for DNA repair and the simultaneous inactivation of apoptotic pathways, genetic damage will be transmitted to the next generation of cells, thus creating the first step in the process of oncogenesis.

APOPTOSIS VERSUS NECROSIS

Cell death is certainly useful, as we have seen, both in normal development and in abnormal conditions such as with infection or malignancy. But what are the fundamental differences between apoptosis and necrosis? The important differences are listed in the written examination box.

APOPTOSIS AND THERAPEUTIC IMPLICATIONS

The study of cell death and apoptosis has raised important therapeutic issues, none more so than in the field of oncology. It is now generally accepted that tumour growth is a result of a fine and precarious balance between cell proliferation and cell loss. Tumours that grow fast do so not only by proliferating fast but also by keeping cell death to a minimum.

The mainstay of cancer treatment has been surgery, radiation and chemotherapy. The mode of action of the latter two is to change the rate of cell proliferation, and this has proved successful with many types of cancer. The first reported cure with radiotherapy was in 1899 on a basal cell carcinoma of the skin. Therapeutic radiation damages cells, both malignant and normal, by generating ions in the tissue, the most common of which are the oxygen free radicals derived from water. These are the same as those involved in bacterial killing in inflammation (see p. 18). Indirect biochemical damage includes the peroxidation of molecules (especially lipids), interference with oxidative phosphorylation, changes in membrane permeability and the inhibition of some enzymes. All of these would produce the necrosis type of cell death. In addition, radiation damages DNA (as we shall discuss on pages 308 and 309) producing breaks in the strands. These are normally repaired promptly, but there may on occasions be errors in the repair, leading to cell death.

There are numerous chemotherapeutic agents with a variety of modes of action. **Alkylating agents** (e.g. cyclophosphamide and melphalan) form covalent links with certain molecules, the most important of which is the guanine base in DNA. This leads to breaks in the DNA and faulty transcription. **Antimetabolites** (e.g. cytarabine and

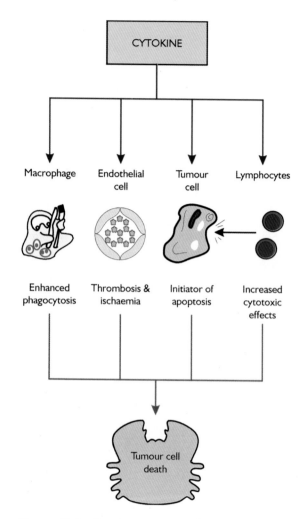

Figure 12.6 Postulated actions of cytokines on tumours

methotrexate) resemble naturally occurring substances but are subtly different so that they block an enzyme pathway or damage the macromolecular structure in which they are incorporated. Many are analogues of purine or pyrimidine bases and affect nucleic acid synthesis, while methotrexate interferes with folic acid metabolism, thus blocking DNA and RNA synthesis. **Antibiotics** useful in chemotherapy (e.g. adriamycin and daunorubicin) often produce a local distortion of the DNA helix that interferes with the function of DNA and RNA polymerases. The **vinca alkaloids** (e.g. vinblastine) act in a completely different manner and bind to tubulin in the microtubules of the mitotic spindle to block division. The hallmark of both radiotherapy and chemotherapy is that the cell's metabolism becomes irreversibly damaged and the proliferating cell is most likely to perish, i.e. undergo necrosis.

What about apoptosis? Does that have any therapeutic potential? The answer is yes. We are still at an early stage but there is considerable interest in the various cytokines that might be able to promote apoptotic tumour cell death. Cytokines are produced by lymphocytes and macrophages following stimulation and, besides modifying the immune response, may act directly to cause death of tumour cells.

Tumour necrosis factor (TNF or cachectin) is produced by activated macrophages, and its action on tumour cells takes place via various distinct mechanisms. It has a role in inflammation that alters endothelial cells, promoting thrombosis and thus causing ischaemic cell necrosis in the tumour. Although the death of cells in a tumour is rather complex, ischaemia playing a major role, there is evidence that at least some of the cells die as a result of attack by lymphocytes. In experimental models, TNF also causes an increase in apoptotic cell death, which appears to be a direct effect as there is an early rise in the synthesis of RNA in the affected cell. We have already discussed the interaction of the TNF pathway with the fas receptor. Various interleukins appear to produce tumour cell death secondary to stimulation of cytotoxic T cells and NK cells, which then act on the tumour cells to initiate apoptosis.

Interferons, on the other hand, appear to exert their effects by acting in synergy with the above factors. They have been shown to enhance the cytotoxicity of T lymphocytes and NK cells, and they also increase the phagocytic activities of macrophages on tumour cells. They are known (in combination with TNF) to reduce the rate of tumour cell multiplication.

The study of mediators and mechanisms of cell death has caused a tremendous thrill in clinical oncology. With the advent of genetic engineering, it is possible to produce the quantities of cytokines necessary for cancer treatment. The initial euphoria has been dampened a little as some cytokine treatment is rather toxic, but advances will continue to be made in both the biology and the clinical regimens.

As Lewis Thomas says, cell death is indeed a natural marvel! It seems to be such an integral part of life, yet until recently we paid little attention to it. The study of cell death is assuming an increasingly important role in the understanding of such diverse processes as embryogenesis, infections and neoplasia.

We will now go on to consider the two specific types of tissue damage caused by amyloidosis and haemochromatosis.

CHAPTER 13

AMYLOID

- Clinical case – myeloma and cardiac failure
- How do we explain the signs and symptoms?
- Microscopical features of amyloid
- What is amyloid?
- The nature of amyloid
- Systemic amyloidosis
- Localised amyloidosis
- Pathogenesis of amyloid
- Staining characteristics of amyloid

CLINICAL CASE – MYELOMA AND CARDIAC FAILURE

A 60-year-old lady complained of tiredness, weakness, loss of weight, pain in her ribs and shortness of breath that had been getting worse for 6 months. Her exercise tolerance had decreased to 100 m, and she had noticed that her urine was frothy. On examination, she was thin, appeared anaemic and had a raised jugular venous pressure and peripheral oedema. She was tachycardic with a pulse rate of 110 beats per minute and her blood pressure was 110/90 mmHg. Auscultation revealed evidence of pulmonary oedema. Dip-stick testing of the urine sample showed the presence of protein.

Investigations showed that she was anaemic with a haemoglobin of 9.0 g/l, serum albumin was low at 20 g/l, and calcium was raised at 3.5 mmol/l. Her urea was raised at 25 mmol/l and

her creatinine was 180 μmol/l, indicating impaired renal function. Urine analysis confirmed proteinuria and protein casts. A chest X-ray showed cardiomegaly with pulmonary oedema and, in addition, revealed lytic lesions in the ribs. This prompted a further skeletal survey, which showed lytic lesions in the skull and pelvic bones, and serum electrophoresis demonstrated the presence of a paraprotein band and a reduction of other immunoglobulin levels. Bence Jones protein was found in the urine.

A diagnosis of myeloma appeared likely, and it was felt that her cardiac and renal failure might be the result of amyloid deposition, so a renal biopsy was performed that confirmed the presence of amyloid.

We will follow our familiar pattern and consider the pathophysiology behind the signs and symptoms, the appearances of biopsy material that help us to make the diagnosis of amyloid and then the classification of amyloidosis.

How do we explain the signs and symptoms?

Myeloma is a disorder of plasma cells in which there is overproduction of part of one immunoglobulin. In essence, it is cancer of the plasma cells. Amyloidosis is one of the complications of myeloma, as amyloid protein can be formed from the light chains of immunoglobulin molecules. The amyloid protein is deposited at various sites in the body, including the heart and kidneys, and can interfere with normal function.

In the heart, amyloid is deposited within the extracellular space of the myocardium, so infiltrates around the myocardial fibres. Here, it restricts movement of the myocardial cells, leading to poor ventricular contraction. This results in decreased cardiac output with cardiac failure and a compensatory increase in heart rate (**tachycardia**). Failure of the left ventricle will increase the hydrostatic pressure in the pulmonary veins to produce **pulmonary oedema**, while failure of the right ventricle results in a **raised jugular venous pressure** and **peripheral oedema**. In addition, amyloid infiltration may affect the conduction system, leading to arrhythmias and hence exacerbation of the cardiac failure, which is also being worsened by the patient's anaemia.

This lady had evidence of **renal failure**, with a raised plasma urea and creatinine concentration and protein in the urine, which makes the urine frothy. Amyloid damages the kidney by being deposited within the glomerular tufts, where it both reduces the amount of fluid filtered and makes the filter more leaky so that protein can pass into the urine. The protein and immunoglobulin light chains in the tubular fluid can precipitate to cause obstruction and hence cause direct damage to the tubules, which further compromises renal function. Amyloid is also found in the blood vessel walls and around tubular basement membranes. We will consider the microscopic appearances later in the chapter.

The other symptoms and signs in this patient are related to the malignant plasma cells that proliferate in the bone marrow. These may depress

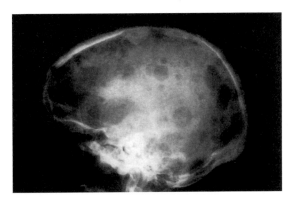

Figure 13.1   Skull X-ray with multiple 'punched-out holes' in a patient with a myeloma

haemopoiesis, leading to **anaemia**, and produce **bone pain** and **hypercalcaemia** as the tumour expands and erodes the bone to produce the lytic lesions seen on X-rays.

Now that we understand the reasons for the signs and symptoms, let us consider the microscopic features that may help us to make a diagnosis of amyloid.

Microscopical features of amyloid

In this patient, a renal biopsy was carried out to assess the degree of damage and to confirm the presence of amyloid. Where a renal biopsy is not indicated, a simpler way of looking for amyloid is to use a rectal biopsy or to obtain peritoneal fat by fine needle aspiration, which is easier and less traumatic. Figures 13.2 and 13.3 are of renal biopsies from a normal kidney and from a patient with amyloid secondary to myeloma.

Let us first consider the glomeruli. The glomerular tuft is expanded by the presence of amorphous hyaline material, which is causing distortion of the tuft and obliteration of the capillary lumina. Compare this with the normal kidney, in which the mesangium contains only a few cells and the lumina of the vessels are clearly identified. The blood vessel in the case of amyloidosis shows thickening of the wall due to the deposition of

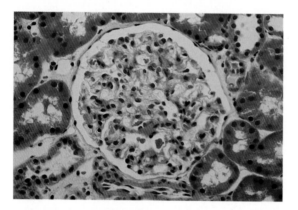

Figure 13.2   Normal kidney

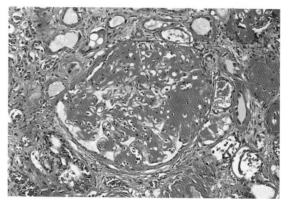

Figure 13.3   Renal amyloid

hyaline material which can be demonstrated to be amyloid. The narrowing of these arterioles leads to ischaemia of the tubules, and you can see that, compared with the normal kidney, there is evidence of tubular loss (atrophy). Some of the tubules also contain protein casts within their lumina owing to the leakage of albumin and immunoglobulin light chains. Calcification is not seen in this section but may occur. In the earlier

discussion of calcification, we mentioned that metastatic calcification occurs when there is an abnormality of calcium metabolism. Myeloma is one of the causes of hypercalcaemia, and metastatic calcification is a recognised finding that may also contribute to the renal failure. There is a mild inflammatory infiltrate within the interstitium of the myeloma kidney, and this is secondary to the tubular damage caused by ischaemia. It is not uncommon for these patients to develop ascending infections related to the tubular blockage caused by the protein casts, and severe interstitial inflammation with polymorphs in the tubular lumina is an indication of pyelonephritis.

Now that we know about the clinical aspects of amyloid, we need to ask:

- What is amyloid?
- In what circumstances is it formed?
- Which organs are affected?
- How are they damaged?
- How can we be sure that the amorphous pink material in a biopsy is amyloid?

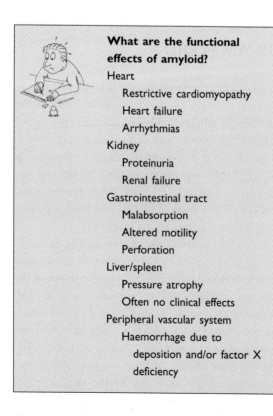

What are the functional effects of amyloid?

Heart
  Restrictive cardiomyopathy
  Heart failure
  Arrhythmias
Kidney
  Proteinuria
  Renal failure
Gastrointestinal tract
  Malabsorption
  Altered motility
  Perforation
Liver/spleen
  Pressure atrophy
  Often no clinical effects
Peripheral vascular system
  Haemorrhage due to
    deposition and/or factor X
    deficiency

WHAT IS AMYLOID?

Amyloid is an extracellular deposit of proteinaceous material.

We have known about amyloid for a very long time and, as early as 1842, Rokitansky had reported the presence of a 'waxy, eosinophilic' material in tissues. It was Rudolf Virchow,

Table 13.1   Classification of amyloidosis

Clinical disorder	Amyloid fibril	Related serum protein
Systemic amyloidosis		
Immunocyte dyscrasia with amyloidosis		
Monoclonal gammopathy, myeloma	AL	Ig light chains, mostly
Waldenström's macroglobulinaemia		λ type
Reactive systemic amyloidosis	AA	SAA
Heredofamilial systemic amyloidosis		
Neuropathic form (type I)	ATTR	Transthyretin
Non-neuropathic form (familial Mediterranean fever)	AA	SAA
Haemodialysis-associated amyloidosis	$A\beta_2m$	β_2-Microglobulin
Senile amyloidosis	Asc	Transthyretin
	Ascl	Atrial naturetic peptide
Localised amyloidosis		
Cerebral amyloid		
Alzheimer's disease, Down syndrome, hereditary cerebral angiopathy (Holland, Iceland)	$A\beta_2$	APP
Endocrine-related amyloid (AE)		
Medullary carcinoma of thyroid	ACal	Calcitonin
Islet cell tumours	AIAPP	Islet amyloid peptide
Plasmacytoma	AL	Ig light chains
Cutaneous amyloid	AD	?Keratin

SAA = serum amyloid associated; APP = amyloid precursor protein.

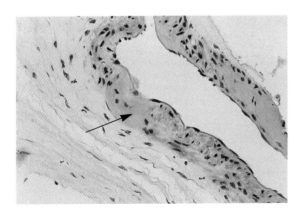

Figure 13.4   Extracellular amyloid deposition in blood vessel

however, who coined and popularised the term 'amyloid' because of the reaction of the material with iodine and sulphuric acid, an indication that the material was 'starch-like'. Organs affected by amyloid are generally enlarged and firmer than normal. The amyloid is not toxic but causes damage by producing **atrophy of parenchymal cells** through pressure or ischaemia, or by interfering with function by impairing, for example, the heart's contractions or the kidney's glomerular permeability, as already described.

Amyloid deposition may be **localised** or **systemic**. The important point is that, despite the fact that amyloid appears identical on light microscopy in different disorders, its chemical composition differs. Amyloidosis is therefore not a single entity but a group of disorders whose amyloid has a different composition but common physical properties because of the three-dimensional folding pattern of the protein.

Amyloid

Excess production
Chronic inflammation AA
Myeloma AL
etc

Decreased excretion
Renal dialysis Aβ2m

Abnormal protein
Familial ATTR

Aetiology

Amyloidogenic proteins

Mechanism

Partial degradation
in macrophage

Addition of Serum
Amyloid P (SAP) &
carbohydrate moiety

except cerebral
amyloid

SAP

+

Glycosaminoglycan

Clinical relevance

The extent of amyloid
deposition in the body
can be assessed with
radio-labelled SAP,
which localises to
amyloid deposits

Starch-like staining
property due to
carbohydrate
component

Anti-parallel β-pleated
sheet

Extracellular deposition
(except cerebral amyloid):
Systemic: e.g. AL, AA,
Aβ2m, ATTR
Localised: e.g. AE, AD

Congo red stain binds
to parallel amyloid
fibrils and can refract
polarised light, causing
apple green
birefringence when
viewed through
polarisers

Figure 13.5 Mechanisms operating in amyloid production

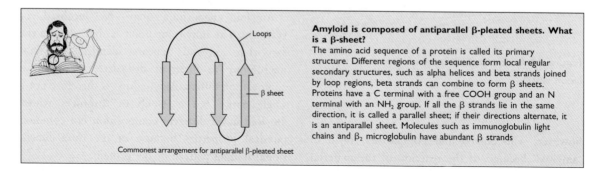

Loops

β sheet

Commonest arrangement for antiparallel β-pleated sheet

Amyloid is composed of antiparallel β-pleated sheets. What is a β-sheet?
The amino acid sequence of a protein is called its primary structure. Different regions of the sequence form local regular secondary structures, such as alpha helices and beta strands joined by loop regions, beta strands can combine to form β sheets. Proteins have a C terminal with a free COOH group and an N terminal with an NH_2 group. If all the β strands lie in the same direction, it is called a parallel sheet; if their directions alternate, it is an antiparallel sheet. Molecules such as immunoglobulin light chains and β_2 microglobulin have abundant β strands

THE NATURE OF AMYLOID

Amyloid's rather uninteresting and bland appearance on routine microscopy belies quite a complex structure. Electron microscopy reveals that it is a fibrillary protein with fibrils arranged in non-branching rods, which are orientated longitudinally. The length of the fibres is indefinite, but the diameter is between 7.5 and 10 nm. Each of the fibrils is composed of two or more filamentous subunits 2.5–3.5 nm in diameter. The feature that gives amyloid its common properties is its 'cross-β' pleated configuration, which can be visualised using X-ray diffraction crystallography. For some unknown reason, this prevents the material from being digested and removed by phagocytic cells. The chemical properties of amyloid protein are more variable but fall into distinct groups, as indicated in Table 13.1 on p. 201.

There are two protein components in amyloid: the variable component and a glycoprotein common to all amyloid except cerebral amyloid, which is called **amyloid P component**. This may be derived from serum amyloid P component, which is an identical acute phase reactant molecule found in the plasma. Component P does not contribute to the fibrils but combines as five globular subunits to form a pentagonal doughnut shape with an internal diameter of 4 nm and an external diameter of 9 nm.

Before we proceed to discuss the different types of amyloid, it is important to appreciate that only amyloid related to immune disorders (AL) and amyloid related to chronic reactive conditions (AA) are reasonably common and cause significant disease. Familial amyloid is rare, and endocrine-related and dermal amyloid are of little clinical importance. Senile amyloid is common but of uncertain significance. It may turn out to be very important because of the presence of amyloid in the brain in many dementias. Table 13.1 contains a recent classification of amyloidosis.

Looking at Table 13.1, you can see that the amyloid types are designated using two letters. The first, A, refers to amyloid. The second letter – L, AH, S or D – refers to the biochemical classification, and we will now consider these individual groups in a little more detail.

SYSTEMIC AMYLOIDOSIS

AL OR IMMUNE-ASSOCIATED AMYLOID

Although the reactive type (AA) of amyloid is most common worldwide, the AL form is the most common in most developed countries. It is the type of amyloid that is associated with plasma cell dyscrasias, such as multiple myeloma, Waldenström's macroglobulinaemia and monoclonal gammopathies. Approximately 6–15 per cent of the patients with myeloma develop amyloid, and most will die within a year of the diagnosis. Fifty per cent die from cardiac failure, since the heart is the most important organ affected by AL-type amyloid. It is important to appreciate that AL amyloid affects a somewhat different group of tissues from those in AA amyloid, which is reflected in the patient's presentation and problems (see the oral examination box below).

AL amyloid is so designated because it is derived from the *light* chains of immunoglobulin molecules, which is why it occurs in disorders of the immunoglobulin-producing cells, i.e. plasma cells. Only part of the light chain is involved in amyloid production, this part being derived from the variable region of the molecule. Interestingly, although more myelomas produce kappa than lambda light chains, it is more common to find amyloid in patients with lambda light chain myeloma. It is thought that this is because the light chains must undergo proteolysis before fibril formation, and only some light chains have suitable regions for proteolysis. Similarly, AA amyloid precursors are believed to require cleavage, and some patients' serum AA protein is not suitable for proteolysis; thus not all patients with predisposing conditions will actually develop amyloid.

AA OR REACTIVE AMYLOID

This type of amyloid is called secondary or reactive amyloid because it is associated with

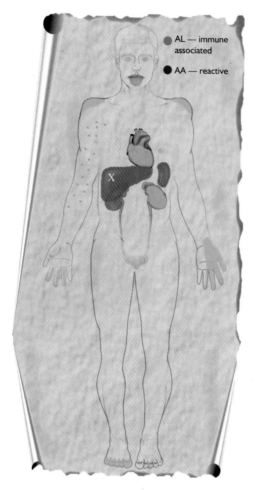

Figure 13.6 Distribution and nature of amyloid

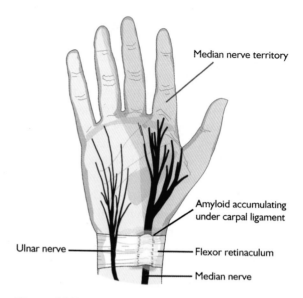

Figure 13.7 Carpal tunnel syndrome due to amyloid deposition. Intermittent compression of the median nerve in the carpal tunnel produces tingling of the fingers served by the median nerve

chronic infective or inflammatory disorders such as rheumatoid arthritis, tuberculosis, chronic inflammatory bowel disease and osteomyelitis. Approximately 10 per cent of patients with rheumatoid arthritis will develop amyloid, generally after 10–15 years of active rheumatoid disease. The kidney is most commonly affected (70 per cent), and half of the patients will die from the effects of amyloid within 5 years.

Amyloid A protein is not derived from immunoglobulins but is a 76 amino acid protein with a molecular weight of 8500 Da. It is produced by cleavage of a circulating 12 000 Da protein, termed SAA (serum amyloid A-associated) protein, which is produced by the liver and is one of the acute phase proteins.

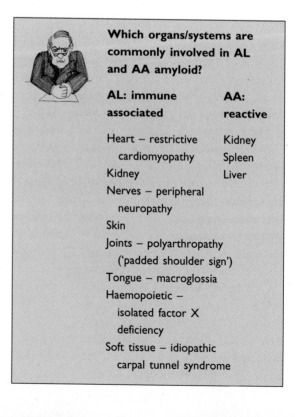

Which organs/systems are commonly involved in AL and AA amyloid?

AL: immune associated	AA: reactive
Heart – restrictive cardiomyopathy	Kidney
Kidney	Spleen
Nerves – peripheral neuropathy	Liver
Skin	
Joints – polyarthropathy ('padded shoulder sign')	
Tongue – macroglossia	
Haemopoietic – isolated factor X deficiency	
Soft tissue – idiopathic carpal tunnel syndrome	

The AA type of amyloid is also associated with familial Mediterranean fever (FMF) and some neoplasms, such as renal cell carcinoma and Hodgkin's disease. FMF is an autosomal recessive disorder in which there is inflammation affecting the pleura, peritoneum, skin and synovium. FMF is the 'odd man out' of the familial forms of amyloid because its protein component is derived from SAA, probably related to recurrent bouts of inflammation.

HEREDOFAMILIAL AMYLOID (ATTR, AA)

This is a group of inherited disorders in which the amyloid is deposited principally in nerves (familial amyloid polyneuropathy). It occurs in small clusters throughout the world and has an autosomal dominant pattern of inheritance. The genetic abnormality appears to affect the production of transthyretin (previously called prealbumin), whose normal role is the *trans*port of *thy*roxine and *retin*ol, hence its name. The abnormal transthyretin molecules can aggregate to form amyloid fibrils. In contrast to AL and AA amyloid, where the relevant light chain or precursor (SAA) serum level is elevated, serum transthyretin levels are normal, but it is the structural abnormality of the molecule that is important.

AH OR HAEMODIALYSIS-ASSOCIATED AMYLOID (Aβ_2M)

A distinct form of amyloid has been identified in patients receiving *haemodialysis* for chronic renal failure, which particularly affects the joints and tendons and may cause carpal tunnel syndrome. In patients with renal failure, there is an accumulation of β_2 microglobulin because this molecule is not-filtered during haemodialysis. β_2 Microglobulin is a normal serum protein and a component of MHC class I molecules. Here is an example of amyloid that does not result from overproduc-

tion of the precursor or an abnormality in the precursor but arises simply from a failure of normal excretion of a normal molecule.

ASc OR SENILE AMYLOID

How many people have senile amyloid? Well, it depends on how hard you look. Autopsy studies report that 25 per cent of people over 65 years old and 100 per cent of people over 80 years have some deposits. The deposits are often localised, most commonly in the heart, but 25 per cent of people have widespread deposits, especially affecting the heart, lung, pancreas and spleen. A more important question is, how many people *suffer* from senile amyloid? The answer is very few as the amyloid deposition is generally asymptomatic except for occasional cases of senile cardiac amyloid.

The amyloid protein of generalised senile amyloidosis, called ASc, is formed from an abnormal transthyretin molecule, suggesting a genetic predisposition. Senile cardiac amyloid, however, is derived from atrial naturetic peptide and is referred to as AScI. Cerebral amyloid is sometimes included under senile amyloid, but it is biochemically different and can also occur in young people, so we will discuss it separately.

LOCALISED AMYLOIDOSIS

CEREBRAL AMYLOID

Our knowledge and theories concerning cerebral amyloid are changing quite rapidly. Cerebral amyloid differs from other forms of amyloid in that it does not contain component P and can occur in intracellular (neurofibrillary tangles) as well as extracellular locations. The functional significance of cerebral amyloid is not known but it occurs in Alzheimer's dementia, Down syndrome, transmissible encephalopathies, some hereditary cerebral angiopathies and some elderly normal individuals. The amyloid may be deposited in:

- vessel walls
- neuritic plaques
- neurofibrillary tangles.

$A\beta_2$ Protein has been isolated from these lesions, and the gene coding for it is on chromosome 21. It is also interesting that this type of amyloid is believed to be synthesised locally rather than being derived from a serum precursor, as are the other types of amyloid.

ENDOCRINE-RELATED AMYLOID (AE)

Certain endocrine tumours, such as medullary carcinoma of the thyroid and islet cell tumours of the pancreas, contain amyloid derived from the hormone or prohormone produced at that site. Thus in medullary thyroid carcinoma, the amyloid is derived from calcitonin and precalcitonin, and in islet cell tumours, insulin and proinsulin are often implicated. The amyloid does not appear to have any clinical significance.

AD OR DERMAL AMYLOID

Primary cutaneous amyloid deposits have been noted, and it is thought that the amyloid is derived from keratin. The skin may also be involved in immune-associated systemic amyloid (AL) when the deposits involve degraded immunoglobulin light chains.

DYSTROPHIC AMYLOIDOSIS

This category did not feature in Table 13.1 because this entity is not yet easy to categorise. It was used originally to describe localised amyloid in damaged cardiac valves that was not associated with systemic disease or old age. Similar deposits were noted in a quarter to a half of all osteoarthritic joints, and it has also been found in damaged or abnormal tissue, such as endometriotic cyst walls, fibrotic epidermal cysts, hernial sacs and skin ulcers. The biochemical nature of the amyloid has not been identified.

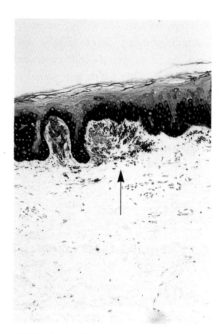

Figure 13.8 Dermal amyloid stained with cytokeratin antibody

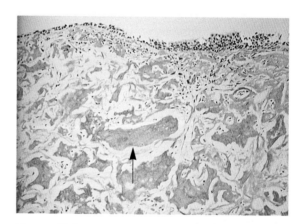

Figure 13.9 Amyloid deposition in the bladder

PATHOGENESIS

The pathogenesis of amyloid formation is far from clear, but the mechanism illustrated (p. 202) is the currently held view. It is generally believed that there is production of 'amyloidogenic' fragments through the catabolism of precursor molecules. These precursors may result from:

- an elevated production of normal proteins, e.g. light chains or SAA

- a reduced excretion of normal protein, e.g. β_2-microglobulin
- an abnormal form of protein, e.g. transthyretin.

STAINING CHARACTERISTICS OF AMYLOID

At autopsy, amyloid can be demonstrated in fresh organ slices by applying 1 per cent acetic acid followed by iodine. If amyloid is present, the tissue will stain a deep brown colour, which will turn blue-violet when 10 per cent sulphuric acid is added. In formalin-fixed, paraffin-embedded microscopic sections, amyloid may be demonstrated using Congo red, crystal violet, methyl violet or thioflavine T. Congo red is most commonly used and stains amyloid a pinkish-red colour. Collagen and elastic fibres may also stain pink, but these may be distinguished by viewing the section under polarised light, when only amyloid will give an apple green colour.

All of the forms of amyloid will stain by these techniques, and it is sometimes useful to distinguish the various types. If AA or the hereditary type of AH amyloid is treated with potassium permanganate before Congo red staining, it fails to stain, whereas the other forms of amyloid are resistant to potassium permanganate. Alternatively, specific antisera to the different forms of amyloid may be used on tissue sections by the immunoperoxidase technique.

We now know how to prove that the amorphous pink material is amyloid, but what if

Table 13.2 Examples of hyaline change

	Material
Intracellular site	
Proximal renal tubule in proteinuria	Protein
Russell bodies in plasma cells	Immunoglobulin
Viral inclusions in cells	Viral protein
Mallory's alcoholic hyaline in liver cells	Intermediate filament
Extracellular site	
Hyaline arteriosclerosis and glomerular hyalinisation	Basement membrane material and plasma proteins
Hyaline membranes in lung	Surfactant and degenerate pneumocytes

it isn't? Amyloid is not the only amorphous pink material, two common causes of a similar microscopic (but not clinical) picture being hyaline and fibrinoid change.

Hyaline change does not refer to a specific entity but is a descriptive term for a variety of intracellular and extracellular materials (Table 13.2). These have nothing in common except for their microscopic appearance. **Fibrinoid change** refers to a similar pink homogeneous material that has the histochemical staining characteristics of fibrin and may result from deposition of fibrin in the tissues. Fibrinoid necrosis classically occurs in blood vessel walls as a result of immune complex disease or malignant hypertension and also occurs in the subcutaneous nodules of rheumatoid arthritis, so called rheumatoid nodules.

CHAPTER 14

HAEMOCHROMATOSIS

- Clinical case – heart and liver failure
- How does the excess iron account for the symptoms?
- What causes haemochromatosis, and what is the pathogenesis?
- Appearance of involved organs
- Distinguishing pigments at light microscopy

Haemochromatosis is the other form of tissue damage that we should like to discuss in more detail because it allows us to look at various aspects of iron metabolism and the diseases associated with accumulation of excess iron. First, let us begin with a clinical history.

CLINICAL CASE – HEART AND LIVER FAILURE

A 40-year-old gentleman complained of tiredness, weight loss and increased frequency of micturition. The symptoms had been present for 9 months but had been worse for the past 3 months. He gave no other relevant history. The doctor noticed that the patient appeared suntanned although he had not been on a recent holiday. Examination showed a mild degree of pulmonary oedema, an enlarged liver and small testes. Dip-stick examination of the urine revealed glycosuria but no proteinuria or blood. The patient had a raised fasting blood sugar and abnormal liver function tests, with raised alanine transaminase, gamma GT and alkaline phosphatase levels. Serum ferritin and iron levels were also raised, and a chest X-ray showed a normal-sized heart with a mild degree of pulmonary oedema. Liver biopsy showed increased parenchymal iron but no evidence of cirrhosis or malignancy. The doctor concluded that his patient had 'bronzed diabetes', or haemochromatosis.

Let us consider this gentleman's symptoms and see whether they could all be due to haemochromatosis. The fundamental problem in haemochromatosis is an increase in the total body iron, and we will discuss the possible causes and mechanisms of the increased iron later. For the present, how can we explain the symptoms on the basis of the increased iron?

HOW DOES THE EXCESS IRON ACCOUNT FOR THE SYMPTOMS?

Excess iron in the body is deposited in the macrophages of the reticuloendothelial system (lymph nodes, bone marrow, spleen and Kupffer cells of the liver) and in the parenchymal cells of

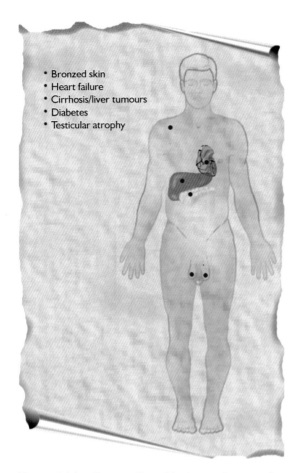

- Bronzed skin
- Heart failure
- Cirrhosis/liver tumours
- Diabetes
- Testicular atrophy

Figure 14.1 Organs affected by haemochromatosis

various organs, most commonly the pancreas, liver and heart.

Deposition of iron in the **pancreas** leads to the destruction of islet cells, resulting in deficient insulin secretion and hence **diabetes**. The symptoms of tiredness, weight loss and increased frequency of micturition are all explained by the presence of diabetes. This also accounts for the glycosuria and raised blood sugar.

Mild iron deposition in the **skin** leads to a massive increase in melanin production and thus tanned skin. Note that most of the colour results from melanin rather than iron. The combination of the above two findings is the reason for the old name of 'bronzed diabetes'.

Deposition of iron in the **liver** may have serious consequences and, in this gentleman, has produced an enlarged liver and abnormal liver function. Iron

within parenchymal cells is toxic and leads to hepatocyte cell death, with resultant scarring and fibrosis. If left untreated, the liver will eventually become cirrhotic and predispose the patient to **carcinoma of the liver (hepatocellular carcinoma)**.

His **heart failure** is explained by the deposition of iron in myocardial cells, necrosis of the myocytes and, ultimately, fibrosis. The small testes are most likely to be a result of some toxic effect of iron on the hypothalamic-pituitary axis, resulting in secondary atrophy of the testes, since iron is not found in large amounts within the testes.

WHAT CAUSES HAEMOCHROMATOSIS, AND WHAT IS THE PATHOGENESIS?

Primary haemochromatosis is a disorder of iron metabolism that is inherited in an autosomal recessive fashion. The gene for haemochromatosis has been localised to the short (p) arm of chromosome 6 (6p21.23), close to the HLA gene locus. There is an association with HLA-A3 in 70 per cent of patients; an association with B7 and B14 is also seen, although not as frequently. Recently, a candidate gene that is an MHC class I-like gene has been cloned and shown to be mutated in hereditary haemochromatosis, but its function remains elusive. Males are affected more than females, in a ratio of 7:1. This is called primary haemochromatosis to distinguish it from haemochromatosis secondary to haemolytic anaemias, liver disease or high iron ingestion (see the written examination box on page 211).

The other form of systemic iron overload is much less severe and is termed **haemosiderosis**. It results from causes similar to those of secondary haemochromatosis, but the excess iron is insufficient to swamp the reticuloendothelial cells of the bone marrow, lymph nodes, spleen and liver, so the iron remains in macrophages and does not cause toxic damage to the parenchymal cells.

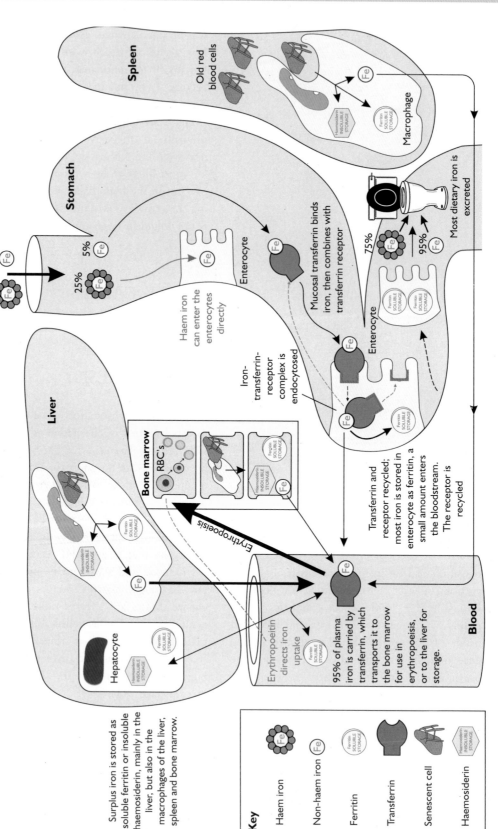

Body iron is derived predominantly from the breakdown of haemoglobin, myoglobin and cytochrome pigments by macrophages in the spleen, liver & bone marrow.

Dietary iron replaces iron lost through daily cell loss, menstruation, haemorrhage etc. Children & adult males must eat 5–10mg iron/day, whereas pregnant or menstruating females require 7–20mg/day. Haem iron can enter the enterocytes directly, whereas non-haem iron must be bound by mucosal transferrin.

Spleen

Old red blood cells

Macrophage

Fe

Stomach

5%

Fe

Fe

25%

Fe

Enterocyte

Haem iron can enter the enterocytes directly

Mucosal transferrin binds iron, then combines with transferrin receptor

Enterocyte

75%

Fe

Iron-transferrin-receptor complex is endocytosed

95%

Fe

Most dietary iron is excreted

Liver

Bone marrow

RBC's

Erythropoeisis

Transferrin and receptor recycled; most iron is stored in enterocyte as ferritin, a small amount enters the bloodstream. The receptor is recycled

Hepatocyte

Erythropoeitin directs iron uptake

95% of plasma iron is carried by transferrin, which transports it to the bone marrow for use in erythropoeisis, or to the liver for storage.

Blood

Surplus iron is stored as soluble ferritin or insoluble haemosiderin, mainly in the liver, but also in the macrophages of the liver, spleen and bone marrow.

Key

Haem iron

Non-haem iron Fe

Ferritin SOLUBLE STORAGE

Transferrin

Senescent cell

Haemosiderin INSOLUBLE STORAGE

Figure 14.2 Normal iron metabolism

These disorders result from an imbalance between the amount of iron ingested and the amount excreted, so it is a convenient moment to remind ourselves of how iron is absorbed, transported and excreted in normal circumstances.

Iron is an important element with well-known roles in haemoglobin, myoglobin, cytochromes and various enzyme systems in the cells. Approximately 80 per cent of the body's iron is in one of these functional forms while the remaining 20 per cent is stored as ferritin or haemosiderin. There is no control over the excretion of iron, and so the total iron in the body is regulated by its absorption. Some iron is lost through exfoliation of cells at the epithelial surfaces, and small amounts of blood are lost in the gastrointestinal tract. Menstruation is an important source of iron loss in premenopausal females and may account for the higher incidence of haemochromatosis in men.

Food contains iron in two forms. The more important one is **haem** iron from animal haemoglobin and myoglobin. This is first released from its apoproteins by the action of gastric acids and taken into the epithelial cell, where enzyme degradation releases the iron. This iron can be temporarily stored in the cell as the protein–iron complex **ferritin** or immediately dispatched into the plasma for transfer to other sites bound to the glycoprotein **transferrin**. Approximately 25 per cent of the haem iron in food is absorbed, whereas only 1–2 per cent of non-haem iron is. **Non-haem iron** absorption requires a different mechanism and probably involves secreting transferrin into the gut, where it binds to iron and then joins to a specific receptor on the epithelial surface. The iron–transferrin–receptor complex will undergo endocytosis so that the iron enters the epithelial cell's cytoplasm. Most iron is absorbed in the duodenum, although some enters through the stomach, ileum and colon.

The normal total adult body iron is between 2 g and 6 g, but this is increased to 50–60 grams in haemochromatosis. The hypothesis is that the basic defect in haemochromatosis resides at the level of iron absorption in the gastrointestinal tract. The exact defect is not known, but it may be an alteration in the transport proteins or

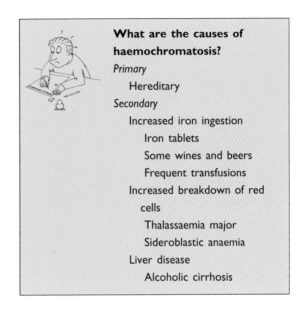

What are the causes of haemochromatosis?
Primary
   Hereditary
Secondary
   Increased iron ingestion
     Iron tablets
     Some wines and beers
     Frequent transfusions
   Increased breakdown of red cells
     Thalassaemia major
     Sideroblastic anaemia
   Liver disease
     Alcoholic cirrhosis

membrane receptors of the mucosal cells that allows excess iron to enter. Alternatively, there may be a lack of the immediate post-absorption excretion of iron or an impairment in the normal role of macrophages in controlling mucosal absorption. Once the iron has been absorbed in excess in primary haemochromatosis, it accumulates in the parenchymal cells of various organs.

What happens to the cells that have accumulated a lot of iron, and does it inevitably lead to cell death? The answers are 'don't know' and 'no'. It is possible that iron is involved in the production of free radicals that may damage the cell's membranes and organelles. Iron also tends to accumulate in the lysosomes, and any damage to the lysosomal membrane will release degradative enzymes that could damage the cellular components and lead to cell death. However, we also know that cells containing excess iron do not inevitably die, and their iron content can sometimes be reduced with iron-chelating drugs such as desferrioxamine.

APPEARANCE OF INVOLVED ORGANS

The affected organs will have a rusty-brown colour to their cut surface and can be stained for

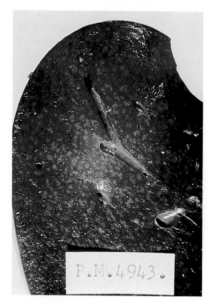

Figure 14.3 Liver stained with Prussian blue, showing iron deposition – gross anatomy

iron using Prussian blue. The texture of the organs may be altered because of the fibrosis, which makes them firmer and may cause shrinkage. Microscopic examination will show large amounts of golden-yellow pigment within the cells and often some atrophy or loss of normal cells, with varying degrees of fibrosis. The liver classically shows micronodular cirrhosis.

DISTINGUISHING PIGMENTS AT LIGHT MICROSCOPY

Iron is not the only pigment that appears brown or golden-yellow on light microscopy, the others being melanin, lipofuscin and bile. Identifying the type of pigment present may be essential in reaching a diagnosis. For example, excess brown pigment in the liver may be iron suggesting haemochromatosis, bile suggesting obstructive liver disease or lipofuscin, which is probably of no significance. Distinguishing these pigments at light microscopy depends on their appearance, their distribution and their histochemical staining pattern.

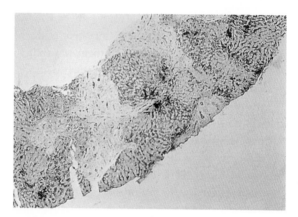

Figure 14.4 Liver stained with Prussian blue, showing iron deposition – histology

IRON

Iron stored as haemoglobin is brown or golden-yellow, tends to be granular and is found in the cells of the reticuloendothelial system as well as the parenchymal cells. The technique most commonly used for demonstrating iron is **Prussian blue** staining, which renders iron blue.

MELANIN

Melanin can vary in colour from light brown to black. It is found in normal skin and retina but can also be seen in benign naevi and malignant melanoma. While malignant melanomas often contain melanin, they may also contain iron because of haemorrhage within the tumour, and the two pigments may appear very similar on H and E sections. Thus distinguishing melanin from iron in a tumour may establish the diagnosis of melanoma. This can be achieved by the **Masson–Fontana technique**, with which melanin stains black.

LIPOFUSCIN

Lipofuscin is composed of pigments derived from the oxidation of lipids and lipoproteins and is found mainly in lysosomes, also being seen in mitochondria. They have been referred to as 'aging'

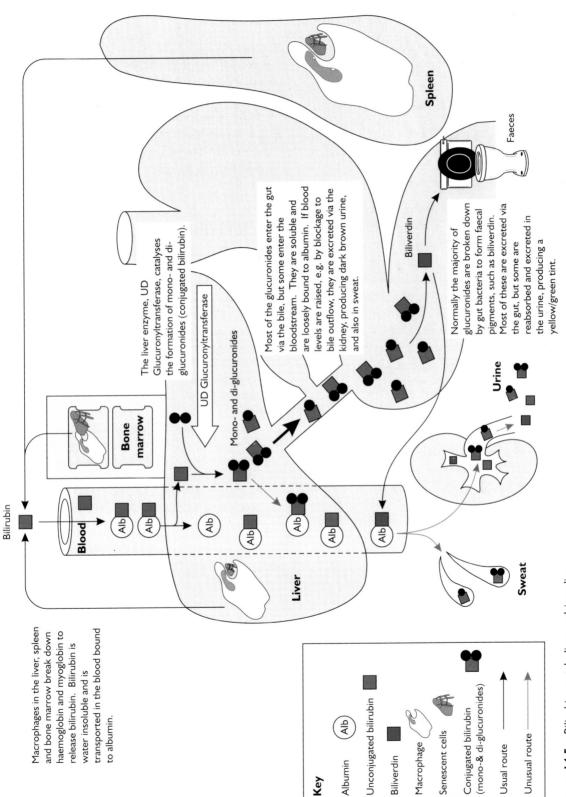

Figure 14.5 Bilirubin metabolism and jaundice

or 'wear and tear' pigments because their amount increases with the patient's age. It is thought that they represent the residue of degradation, i.e. what is left after everything else has been processed for excretion or recycling. The most common sites of deposition are the liver and heart.

The **Sudan black technique** turns lipofuscin black.

BILE

Bile pigments result from the breakdown of red cells (Figure 14.5). Following the removal of haemoglobin and iron, biliverdin is transported to the liver, where it is conjugated with glucuronic acid and excreted into the hepatic duct. These pigments can be seen in the bile canaliculi as well as in the hepatocytes and appear either as brown or greenish-yellow pigment. There is a number of methods that can be used to demonstrate this pigment, one being the **Fouchet** technique, which stains bile pigments blue-green.

That brings us to the end of this section on cell and tissue damage. A basic understanding of cell death and how tissues react to injury is vital not only for understanding clinical signs and symptoms but also for allowing us to formulate theories on embryogenesis and normal development. Paradoxically, this study of death is funda-mental to our knowledge of life, and as Lewis Thomas says:

> 'We will have to give up the notion that death is catastrophe, or detestable, or avoidable, or even strange. We will need to learn more about the cycling of life in the rest of the system, and about our connection to the process. Everything that comes alive seems to be in trade for something that dies, cell for cell.'

FURTHER READING

Alberts, B., Bray, D., Lewis, J., Raff, M., Roberts, K., Watson, J.D. 1989: *Molecular Biology of the Cell*, 2nd edn. New York: Garland Publishing.

Cooper, G.M. 1997: The cell: a molecular approach. Washington: ASM Press.

Cotran, R.S., Kumar, V., Robbins, S.L. 1994: Cellular injury and cellular death. In *Robbins' Pathologic Basis of Disease*, 5th edn. Philadelphia: W.B. Saunders, Ch.1.

Lackie, J.M., More, I.A.R. 1992: Cells and tissues in health and disease. In MacSween, R.N.M., Whaley, K. (eds) *Muir's Textbook of Pathology*, 13th edn. London: Edward Arnold, Ch. 1.

Wyllie, A.H. 1997: Apoptosis. In Anthony, P.P., MacSween, R.N.M., Lowe, D.G. (eds) *Recent Advances in Histopathology*. London: Churchill Livingstone, 1–14.

CLINICOPATHOLOGICAL CASE STUDY

Clinical

A 60-year-old man with longstanding history of alcohol abuse presented with a three-week history of general malaise, weight loss, loss of appetite and productive cough.

Examination:

He was noted to be short of breath with an increased respiratory rate, and was jaundiced. He had a fever and tachycardia of 110 beats/min. He also had supraclavicular lymphadenopathy and a mildly enlarged and tender liver. Auscultation of his chest revealed coarse crackles over both his lung fields.

Investigations:

The liver function tests were abnormal, with a raised bilirubin of 45 μmol/L and a raised γ-GT of 90 IU/L. His chest X-ray showed bilateral consolidation with a small right pleural effusion. A lymph node and liver biopsy were carried out.

The lymph node showed numerous caseating granulomas with calcification. The Ziehl–Neelson stain showed abundant acid-fast Mycobacteria. The liver biopsy showed an acute alcoholic hepatitis with marked fatty change and liver fibrosis, but without cirrhosis.

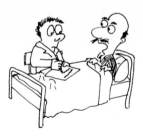

Management and progress:

He was started on antituberculous therapy and was counselled for his alcohol abuse.

While in hospital, he had a bout of abdominal pain and diarrhoea. Endoscopy showed gastritis, but sigmoidoscopy was unremarkable. The rectal biopsy revealed the presence of amyloid in the mucosa.

He was discharged on antituberculous therapy and sent for rehabilitation for his alcohol abuse, but he defaulted from his appointments and was lost to follow-up.

Pathology

He had a long history of alcohol abuse, which predisposes to many illnesses. Alcoholics tend to be malnourished as they derive most of their calories from alcohol and are therefore deficient in many vitamins, especially the B group. They damage the liver by episodes of hepatitis which heals with scarring, producing fibrosis and eventually cirrhosis. They are also predisposed to infections because of depression of the immune system caused by the alcohol, and, in this man, clinical examination revealed signs of a chest infection. Tuberculosis is a particular problem in alcoholics.

The liver function tests were in keeping with alcoholic damage with raised bilirubin and liver cell enzymes. The chest X-ray confirmed a pneumonic process involving both lungs.

Caseous necrosis with granuloma formation is a classical picture of tuberculosis, and special stains revealed the Mycobacteria. Immune suppression due to the alcohol abuse is responsible for the reactivation or secondary tuberculosis.

In areas of necrosis, calcification is common, this type being called dystrophic calcification. The serum calcium levels are normal, as opposed to those in metastatic calcification, which are raised.

His liver showed the classical fatty change common in alcohol abuse, with some hepatitis, i.e. inflammation of the hepatocytes with liver cell necrosis. The result is healing by scarring with resultant fibrosis. He did not have cirrhosis, which is irreversible, unlike fatty change, which is.

Alcoholics are predisposed to gastritis, i.e. inflammation of the gastric mucosa. They may also have gastric ulcers. Other complications include oesophageal varices if portal hypertension has developed as a result of cirrhosis.

Patients with longstanding chronic inflammatory diseases such as rheumatoid arthritis and tuberculosis are prone to reactive amyloidosis (AA). Rectal biopsy is a good way of diagnosing amyloid. The amyloid may have been responsible for the diarrhoea, but infective causes should be excluded. Lack of compliance is a common problem with alcoholics.

PART *4*

CELL GROWTH AND ITS DISORDERS

INTRODUCTION TO PART 4

Does early death come
As a punishment?
Or
Does it come too late,
For those who are tortured
By incurable pain?
Is death really cruel?
Or
Is it merciful?

Gitanjali, 1961–1977

Gitanjali, as beautiful as the poem by Rabindranath Tagore, died at the age of 16 of cancer. To many people, cancer is a disease that appears suddenly, takes a tight grip, progresses relentlessly and causes a slow and painful death.

In 1731 Lorenz Heister, a German surgeon wrote:

'The name *Scirrhus* is given to a painless tumour that occurs in all parts of the body, but especially in the glands, and is due to stagnation and drying of the blood in the hardened part. ...When a scirrhus is not reabsorbed, cannot be arrested, or is not removed by time, it either spontaneously or from maltreatment becomes malignant, that is, painful and inflamed, and then we begin to call it *cancer* or *carcinoma*; at the same time the veins swell up and distend like the feet of a crab (but this does not happen in all cases), whence the disease gets its name; it is in fact, one of the worst, most horrible, and most painful of diseases.'

Is this pessimism really justified? About 20 per cent of people will die of cancer, which is less than the number dying from cardiovascular disease (approximately 30 per cent), but heart disease does not usually generate such intense dread.

First, let us take a brief look at the history of cancer.

Johannes Müller, a German microscopist, established that tumours were made of cells (1883). This laid the foundation for his pupil, Rudolf Virchow, who divided tumours into 'homologous' and 'heterologous'. The homologous group resulted from the proliferation of cells already present and were generally benign, while the heterologous group showed a change in the character of the cell and were generally malignant. Virchow, however, failed to recognise the mechanism of metastasis, which was later described by Billroth (1856) and von Recklinghausen (1883).

Many investigators have looked for causes of cancer. One of the most famous was Percival Pott who, in 1775, identified that scrotal cancer in chimney sweeps was related to chronic contact with soot. Occupational exposure to industrial tar and paraffin was recognised by von Volkmann in 1875 as causing cancers, and many such associations have since been described. Advances in molecular and cell biology techniques have recently facilitated the investigation of these associations at the level of genetic material. We are now in a position to attempt to answer some of the fundamental questions relating to the control of normal growth and differentiation, and how these mechanisms go wrong in the process of neoplasia.

In Part 4, we shall consider the benign disorders of cell growth and the premalignant changes that are clues of early cancer and are important in screening programmes. We will go on to look at the symptoms that occur in cancer, how it is diagnosed and which features are important for its prognosis and treatment. Then we will turn to the aetiology (causes of cancer) and the pathogenesis (natural history) of tumours, and finally to how they behave and what treatments are available.

CHAPTER 15

BENIGN GROWTH DISORDERS

- Clinical case – prostatic disease
- Hyperplasia and hypertrophy
- Atrophy
- Metaplasia and dysplasia
- Benign neoplasms
- Hyperplasia and hypertrophy versus benign neoplasms

Cells have to adapt to any changes in nutrient supply or workload in order to survive and continue performing their cellular function. These adaptations take place at both the cellular and subcellular levels. We will discuss these adaptations, with an emphasis on the changes that are important in pathology, and we will consider the clinical situations in which they are encountered. The changes that we will discuss are **hyperplasia, hypertrophy, atrophy, metaplasia** and **dysplasia,** and **benign neoplasms.**

CLINICAL CASE – PROSTATIC DISEASE

A 70-year-old man visited the urology clinic complaining of difficulty with micturition. He passed urine 15–20 times per day and several times during the night (nocturia). The stream of urine was poor, and he found that on some occasions it dribbled. The urologist detected an enlarged prostate on rectal examination, and the patient had part of his prostate removed to improve the flow.

Some of you may be wondering why an enlarged prostate obstructing urine flow through the urethra should result in increased urinary frequency. The reason (as indicated in Figure 15.1) is that the enlarged median lobe protrudes into the bladder to produce a dam behind which some urine stagnates. This means that, after micturition, there is still urine in the bladder and the patient feels the urge to pass urine again. The stagnant urine is also prone to infection or stone formation. The poor urine flow is due to narrowing of the prostatic urethra and the 'ball-valve' effect of the median lobe pressing forward on the urethral orifice.

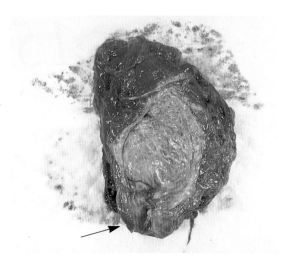

Figure 15.1 Macroscopic specimen with prostatic hyperplasia and bladder showing numerous trabeculae due to urinary obstruction

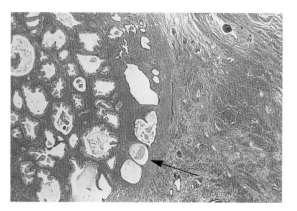

Figure 15.2 Photomicrograph showing nodular hyperplasia of the prostate

HYPERPLASIA AND HYPERTROPHY

Hyperplasia is defined as an increase in the *number* of cells in an organ or tissue, while hypertrophy is an increase in *cell size*. The two often coexist in a tissue because some cell types are incapable of division so must increase their size (hypertrophy) to cope with any extra work, while other cells can proliferate to share their additional work (hyperplasia). In Chapter 1, we noted that cardiac and skeletal muscle and nerve cells are unable to replicate, whereas epithelial cells and fibroblasts can. Smooth muscle cells can respond by a combination of hyperplasia and hypertrophy. This means that, in the prostate, the glandular epithelium and the fibroblastic stroma will show hyperplasia, and the smooth muscle is hypertrophic and hyperplastic. Why should the prostate enlarge with age, since its workload does not increase? There is presumably an overreaction to years of androgen stimulation, but nobody really knows.

When the hypertrophy or hyperplasia is useful, i.e. it allows the organ to cope with extra work, it is called **physiological**. If the enlargement does not appear to serve a purpose, it is termed **pathological**. Thus the prostatic changes are pathological.

Physiological hyperplasia and hypertrophy may be mediated through hormonal changes or growth factors. Pregnancy is an example of hormone-induced hyperplasia and hypertrophy that allows an organ the size of a pear to enlarge to accommodate a full-term baby and prepares the breasts for lactation. The smooth muscle cells of the uterus enlarge (hypertrophy and hyperplasia) ready for the work of pushing the baby into the world (aptly named 'labour'), and the number of glandular milk-producing cells in the breast increases (hyperplasia).

A fascinating example of physiological hyperplasia that occurs in the body is the regeneration of the liver following partial hepatectomy, encapsulated in the Greek myth of Prometheus. Prometheus, who was Atlas's brother, had incurred the wrath of the mighty Zeus. In anger, Zeus had Prometheus chained naked to a pillar in the Caucasian mountains, where a vulture tore at his liver all day, year in, year out, and there was no end to his pain because the liver grew back each night. It is not recommended that you try this experiment on your colleagues. The evidence suggests that the remaining liver produces a growth factor, transforming growth factor-alpha, which causes an increase in mitotic activity and hence an increase in the cell number. What is remarkable is that it knows when to stop! It is believed that a growth inhibitor, transforming growth factor-beta, is involved in this process. The ancient Greeks had remarkable insights into the body's capacity to regenerate.

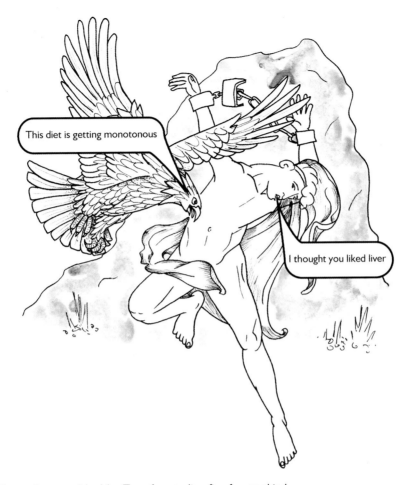

Figure 15.3 Prometheus punished by Zeus for stealing fire for mankind

1. List some examples of hyperplasia and hypertrophy and their causative factors
2. Are they physiological or pathological?

1. Hypertrophy of myocardium due to hypertension
   Skeletal muscular hypertrophy due to exercise
   Red cell hyperplasia in bone marrow secondary to low atmospheric oxygen (living at high altitude)
   Uterine hyperplasia/hypertrophy secondary to hormonal changes of pregnancy
   Hyperplasia of epidermis and connective tissue due to release of growth factors to aid wound healing
2. All these are examples of physiological hyperplasia or hypertrophy

ATROPHY

Atrophy is defined as a decrease in *cell size* and/or *cell number*. Extra cells are lost through the process of apoptosis described in Chapter 12. Strictly speak-

ing, the reduction in *cell numbers* is called **involution**. Since this is part of normal development, it is termed **physiological atrophy**, the classic example being the involution of the thymus gland during development. It is distinguished from **pathological** atrophy, which results from an abnormal state. An example of pathological atrophy is the severe muscle wasting that may follow an episode of poliomyelitis or the muscle wasting that is commonly observed in limbs immobilised in plaster following a fracture.

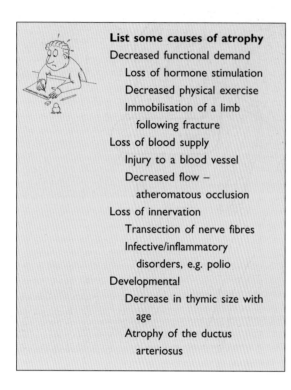

List some causes of atrophy
Decreased functional demand
  Loss of hormone stimulation
  Decreased physical exercise
  Immobilisation of a limb
    following fracture
Loss of blood supply
  Injury to a blood vessel
  Decreased flow –
    atheromatous occlusion
Loss of innervation
  Transection of nerve fibres
  Infective/inflammatory
    disorders, e.g. polio
Developmental
  Decrease in thymic size with
    age
  Atrophy of the ductus
    arteriosus

METAPLASIA AND DYSPLASIA

The uterine cervix serves as a useful model for this discussion of **metaplasia and dysplasia**. The changes in the cervix are now well documented because of the national programme designed to screen women of reproductive age to detect early changes associated with cancer. Screening involves scraping some cells from the junctional zone of the cervix using a spatula. These are spread onto a glass slide, fixed and stained by the Papanicolaou technique.

The cervix has a transitional zone between the squamous epithelium of the ectocervix and the columnar epithelium of the endocervix. If there is

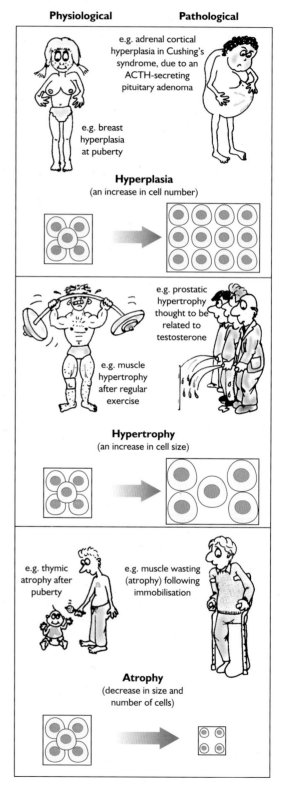

Figure 15.4 Physiological and pathological examples of hyperplasia, hypertrophy and atrophy

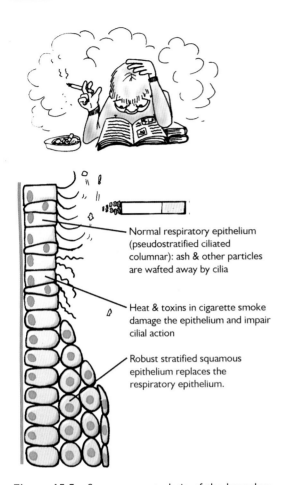

Figure 15.5 labels:
- Normal respiratory epithelium (pseudostratified ciliated columnar): ash & other particles are wafted away by cilia
- Heat & toxins in cigarette smoke damage the epithelium and impair cilial action
- Robust stratified squamous epithelium replaces the respiratory epithelium.

Figure 15.5 Squamous metaplasia of the bronchus

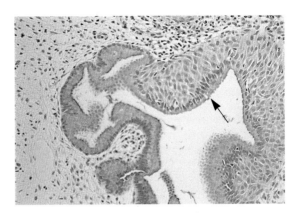

Figure 15.6 Photomicrograph showing squamous metaplasia of endocervical glands

chronic inflammation of the cervix, the columnar epithelium may be replaced by squamous epithelium – so-called squamous metaplasia. **Metaplasia** is the *conversion of one type of differentiated tissue into another type of differentiated tissue.* This is most common in epithelial tissue, although it can occur in other types of tissues such as mesenchymal tissues. It is generally a response to chronic irritation and is a form of adaptation that involves, for example, replacing a specialised glandular or respiratory epithelium with a more hardy squamous epithelium.

Metaplasia is benign and reversible, but its importance lies in the fact that the stimulants and irritants causing the metaplasia may persist and play a role in carcinogenesis.

The exfoliated cervical cells may show dysplasia, which is more worrying because it is a step on

the road to an invasive tumour. The term **dysplasia** was originally used to mean an abnormality of development. Unfortunately, it is a term that is used too loosely, and this causes confusion. In pathology reports concerning the microscopy of tissues, dysplasia refers to a combination of **abnormal cytological appearances and abnormal tissue architecture**. Its importance lies in its **precancerous** association. However, 'dysplasia' is still used to describe some gross abnormalities of development encountered in neonatal pathology, such as renal dysplasia and bronchopulmonary dysplasia, which have no precancerous association.

Dysplasia in the cervical squamous epithelium involves an increased cell size, nuclear pleomorphism, hyperchromatism, loss of orientation of the cells so that they are arranged rather haphazardly and abnormally sited mitotic activity (Figure 15.8). These appearances are, of course, the same as those described in malignant change, but they differ in extent. When the full thickness of the epithelium is involved, it can be called 'carcinoma *in situ*', while involvement of only the lower third is 'mild dysplasia'.

Many pathologists and clinicians felt that it was inappropriate to have different names for various stages of the same process, so the term 'cervical intraepithelial neoplasia' (CIN) was introduced. CIN I is the equivalent of mild dysplasia and describes abnormalities affecting the lower third of the epithelium, CIN II (replacing moderate dysplasia) is used for changes reaching the middle third,

Lung cancer: by region

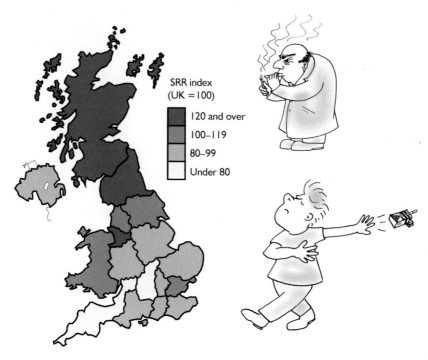

SRR index
(UK = 100)

- 120 and over
- 100–119
- 80–99
- Under 80

SRR = Standardised registration rate

This is calculated by dividing the observed incidence of lung
cancer in a population by the incidence that would normally be
expected. The product of this ratio is multiplied by 100

Figure 15.7 Social trends in smoking over the UK (1996) (Data from the General Households Survey, Office for National Statistics, Crown copyright 1997)

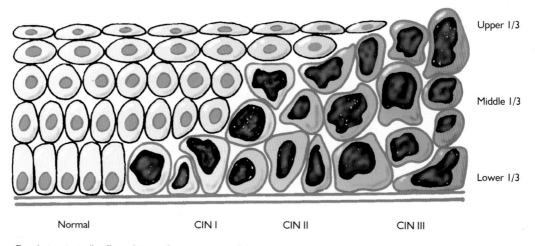

Upper 1/3

Middle 1/3

Lower 1/3

Normal   CIN I   CIN II   CIN III

Dysplasia principally affects the transformation zone of the cervix, i.e. the junction between the columnar epithelium of the endocervix and the squamous epithelium of the ectocervix. It is graded CIN I, CIN II, CIN III, depending on the layers of the epithelium involved. It starts in the basal layer. Dysplastic cells fail to mature and show the nuclear features of malignancy, e.g. ↑nuclear:cytoplasmic ratio and nuclear pleomorphism and mitoses occur above the basal layer

Figure 15.8 Squamous dysplasia in the cervix

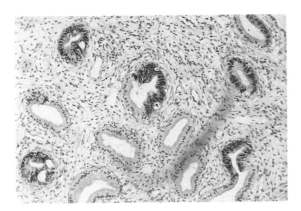

Figure 15.9 Dysplasia involving endocervical glands

and CIN III (replacing severe dysplasia or carcinoma *in situ*) refers to full thickness involvement. Similar terminology can be used for changes in the squamous epithelium of the vulva (VIN) and larynx (LIN), although *glandular* epithelial changes (e.g. of stomach or large bowel) are usually subdivided into mild, moderate or severe dysplasia.

It should not be assumed that dysplasia is irreversible. It is believed that early stages of dysplasia may revert to normal if the stimulus is removed. However, severe dysplasia will often progress to cancer if left untreated and, for this reason, is sometimes referred to as carcinoma *in situ*. If severe dysplasia is cancer confined to the epithelium, what are moderate and mild dysplasia? Fortunately, terminology such as intraepithelial neoplasia helps to clarify our thinking and, in practice, severe dysplasia is treated as a favourable type of cancer, while milder degrees of dysplasia

can be managed slightly less aggressively but followed to ensure that they do not progress to more severe disease.

The concept of dysplasia fits with our current multistep theory of neoplasia (see p. 265) in that it represents a stage between benign hyperplastic proliferation and overt cancer. The concept of dysplasia as a cancer in its early stages has also led to the institution of screening programmes for cervical and breast carcinoma. The logic behind this is that if dysplastic changes precede carcinoma by several months or years and patients with dysplasia can be identified and treated, we can reduce the death toll from that cancer. Obviously, deaths from that cancer must be fairly common to make this worthwhile, and we must be confident that the 'at-risk' group are being screened sufficiently often to detect the early changes. For example, if the progression from CIN II to invasive tumour took only 1 year, it would be of limited value to screen patients every 3 years. Much of the interest in the genetic and immunocytochemical markers of malignancy lies in the hope that they will be able to detect ever-earlier precancerous changes to increase the potential benefits of such screening programmes.

BENIGN NEOPLASMS

A neoplasm is defined as a new and abnormal growth, particularly one in which the cell division

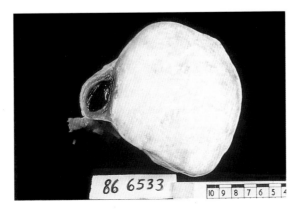

Figure 15.10 Benign leiomyoma

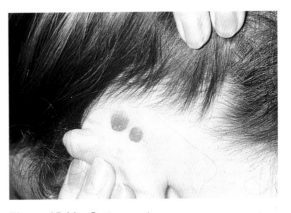

Figure 15.11 Benign naevi

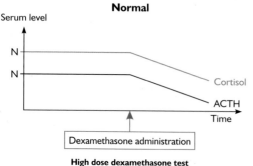

Normal

High dose dexamethasone test
Cortisol and ACTH levels fall in response to administration of high dose dexamethasone

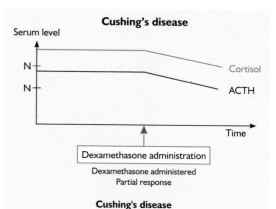

Cushing's disease

Dexamethasone administered
Partial response

Cushing's disease
Pituitary adenoma causes ↑ACTH secretion, stimulating the adrenals to secrete large amounts of cortisol. This does not inhibit further ACTH secretion by the adenoma, which is not under negative feedback control

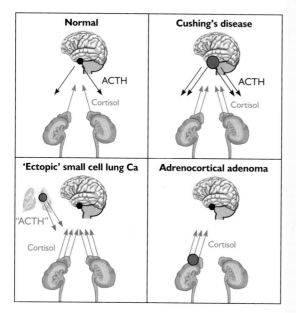

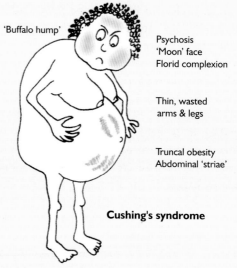

Cushing's syndrome

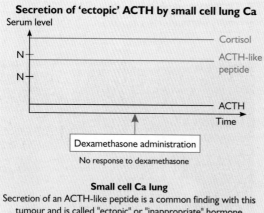

Secretion of 'ectopic' ACTH by small cell lung Ca

No response to dexamethasone

Small cell Ca lung
Secretion of an ACTH-like peptide is a common finding with this tumour and is called "ectopic" or "inappropriate" hormone secretion. The high cortisol output from the adrenal cortex inhibits ACTH secretion by the pituitary, to no effect

Adrenocortical adenoma

No response to dexamethasone

Adrenocortical adenoma
Autonomous cortisol secretion by the adenoma causes ↓ACTH secretion by the pituitary due to negative feedback mechanisms. The lack of ACTH has no effect on the adenoma, which continues to secrete cortisol

Figure 15.12   Endocrine manifestations of benign and malignant neoplasms

is uncontrolled and progressive. Neoplasms may be benign or malignant; the latter will be dealt with in the next chapter. A benign neoplasm, such as an adenoma in the colon, is an uncontrolled focal proliferation of well-differentiated cells that does not invade or metastasise. Unfortunately, the term is sometimes used inaccurately, and some tumours do not quite fulfil these criteria, but it will serve as a working definition. Although benign, these tumours can cause many clinical problems, as discussed in the section on the local effects of tumours (see p. 272). One of the most common benign tumours necessitating removal is the leiomyoma (fibroid) of the uterine myometrium, which may contribute to heavy and painful menstruation. Benign melanocytic tumours of the skin are removed for cosmetic reasons or for fear of malignant change. Endocrine tumours are generally benign but can cause dramatic systemic problems through the excessive production of hormones (Figure 15.12), and some 'benign'

intracranial tumours such as meningiomas can kill the patient because the skull cannot stretch to accommodate the 'benign' expansion. Remember that something which is 'benign' to the pathologist may appear 'malignant' to the patient.

HYPERPLASIA AND HYPERTROPHY VERSUS BENIGN NEOPLASMS

The difference between a benign neoplasm and hypertrophy/hyperplasia is that the neoplasm, by definition, exhibits *uncontrolled cell* proliferation. This is unlike hyperplasia and hypertrophy, in which the growth, because of an increase in either cell number or cell size, is a response to a stimulus, and the removal of this stimulus results in regression.

CHAPTER *16*

MALIGNANT NEOPLASMS

- Clinical case – breast lump
- Clinical features of malignant tumours
- Evaluation in hospital
- Macroscopical features that distinguish malignant tumours
- Microscopical features that distinguish malignant tumours
- Factors influencing prognosis
- Classification of tumours

CLINICAL CASE – BREAST LUMP

A 50-year-old lady presented to her family doctor with a lump in her left breast. She had noticed a recent enlargement in its size, but the mass was not painful. She had no other medical problems, but she had a positive family history, her mother having died of breast cancer 5 years previously. She had two daughters, aged 27 and 25 years, who were both well.

Her family doctor could feel a 2 cm diameter mass below the nipple in her left breast. This was hard, poorly defined and caused dimpling of the overlying skin. It was also fixed to the underlying tissues. The nipple and areola on that side had an eczematous appearance, but the right breast and nipple were normal. The doctor did not find any enlarged lymph nodes in either axilla or supra-clavicular fossa nor any abnormalities in the rest of the body. The family practitioner suspected that this was a malignant tumour so referred her to hospital for further investigation.

But why did the family doctor consider that this mass was malignant?

CLINICAL FEATURES OF MALIGNANT TUMOURS

It should be stressed that it was not a single crite-rion but a combination of factors that allowed him to draw such a conclusion. In this case, the lump was **ill defined, hard** and **involved adjacent tissues and skin**. A characteristic feature of malignant tumours is that tongues of cancer cells infiltrate surrounding tissues, whereas benign tumours tend to grow with a smooth pushing edge.

Thus while benign lumps are generally mobile, malignant tumours are often fixed relative to the surrounding structures. Many malignant tumours induce a proliferation of benign fibroblasts that produce dense collagenous connective tissue. This reaction is termed **desmoplasia** and gives the tumour its hard texture.

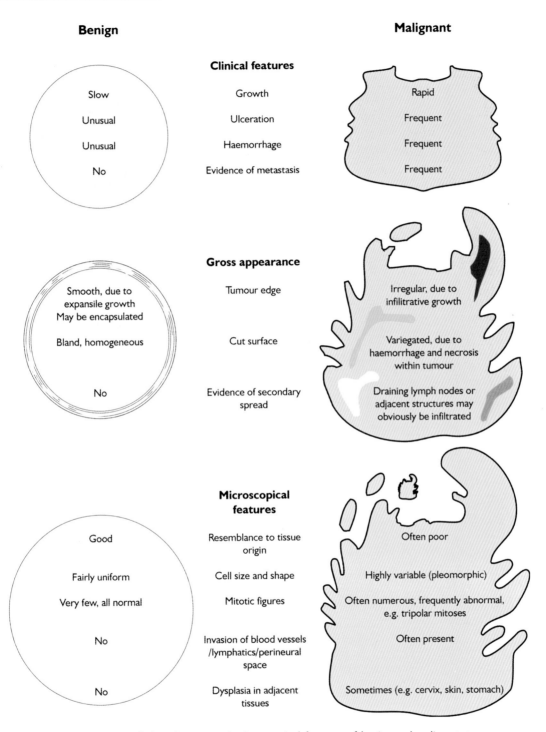

Figure 16.1 Comparison of clinical, gross and microscopical features of benign and malignant tumours

The lesion's **size** was greater than most benign lesions, although this is a variable feature. More importantly, there was a recent **rapid increase in size**, which often indicates malignant growth. In this example, there was one other important clue for the doctor, which is a peculiarity of some breast cancers. The 'eczema' that was noted over the nipple is referred to as **Paget's disease of the**

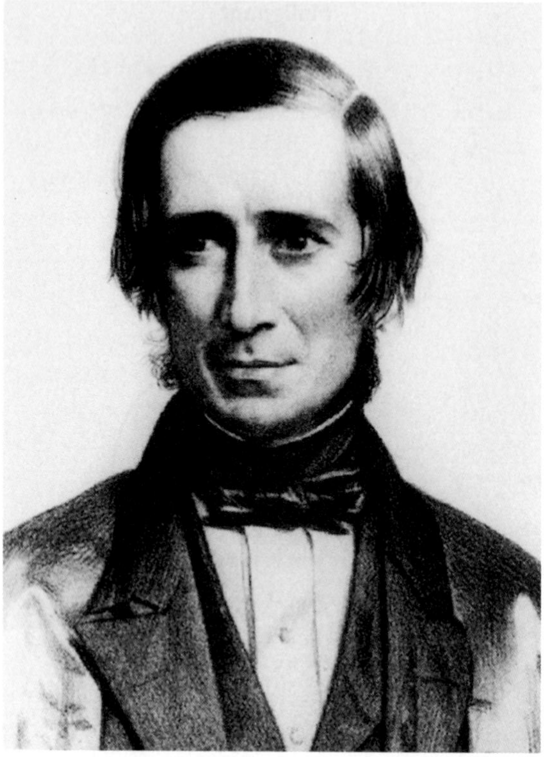

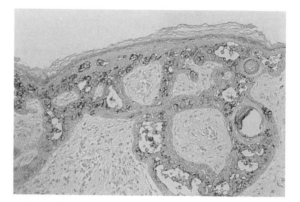

Figure 16.3 Photomicrograph of nipple stained with epithelial membrane antigen (EMA) showing tumour cells (red) within the epidermis

Figure 16.2 Sir James Paget (1814–99) (Courtesy of the Wellcome Institute for the History of Medicine) James Paget was born in Yarmouth, Norfolk. He was apprenticed to a surgeon at the local hospital at the age of 16 and enrolled as a medical student at St Bartholomew's Hospital, London, at the age of 20. In 1837, a year after obtaining his MRCS, he was appointed Curator of the Museum at the Hospital. Paget was an excellent clinical observer and an eloquent lecturer. He is best remembered for his descriptions of Paget's disease of bone (osteitis deformans) and Paget's disease of the nipple. He was elected an FRS in 1851 and Surgeon Extraordinary to Queen Victoria in 1858. He was created a baronet in 1871

nipple. This is caused by carcinoma cells growing along the breast ducts towards the nipple and then into the epidermis of the skin.

Two other factors, had they been present, would have influenced the doctor: **pain** and the presence of **metastases**. Many tumours, both benign and malignant, are painless, but the presence of unremitting pain is suggestive of malignancy. The presence of metastatic disease is the definitive evidence that a tumour is malignant, so it is important to understand possible routes of spread in order that the most likely sites for metastasis can be examined especially carefully. In this lady's case, there was no pain or evidence of metastatic tumour spread, so the doctor suspected that it was a localised malignant growth, and the patient was referred to hospital.

EVALUATION IN HOSPITAL

Here a series of tests were performed to make a more precise diagnosis and to assess the extent of this lady's disease; they included haematological and biochemical blood tests to look for anaemia and changes in liver function that might suggest metastases to bone marrow and liver, mammography (X-ray of the breast) and a chest X-ray and bone scan to look for tumour spread. Mammography showed a 2 cm spiculated mass with linear calcification. The rest of the investigations were unremarkable.

The surgeon must make a definite diagnosis by obtaining some tissue from the breast lump. He has various options. He can:

• insert a needle attached to a syringe to suck out some cells for examination – fine needle aspiration (FNA) cytology

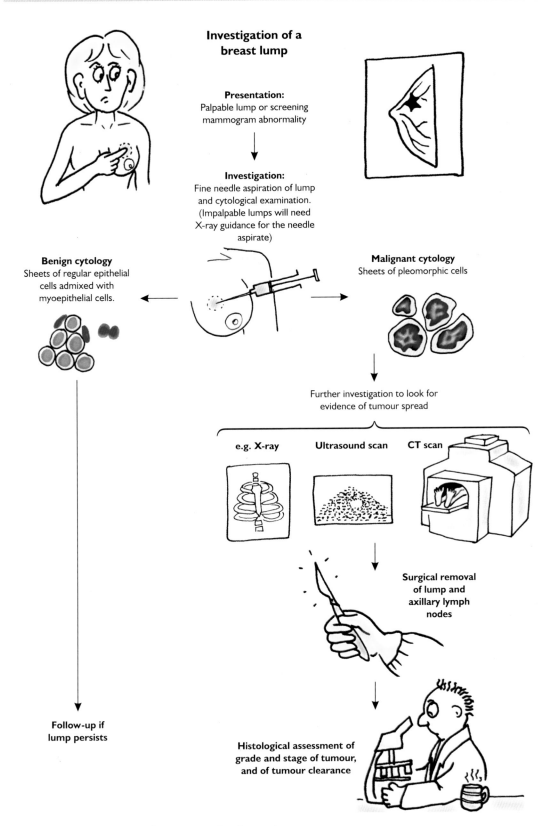

Investigation of a breast lump

Presentation:
Palpable lump or screening mammogram abnormality

Investigation:
Fine needle aspiration of lump and cytological examination. (Impalpable lumps will need X-ray guidance for the needle aspirate)

Benign cytology
Sheets of regular epithelial cells admixed with myoepithelial cells.

Malignant cytology
Sheets of pleomorphic cells

Further investigation to look for evidence of tumour spread

e.g. **X-ray**   **Ultrasound scan**   **CT scan**

Surgical removal of lump and axillary lymph nodes

Follow-up if lump persists

Histological assessment of grade and stage of tumour, and of tumour clearance

Figure 16.4   Investigation of a patient with a breast lump

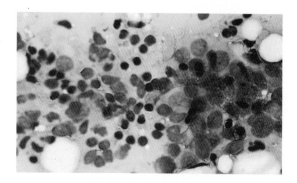

Figure 16.5 Cytological smear showing pleomorphic tumour cells admixed with smaller lymphoid cells

- anaesthetise the patient and remove a part of the lump – excision biopsy
- anaesthetise the patient and remove the whole lump – wide local excision or mastectomy.

In this particular case, the surgeon opted for FNA cytology, which showed malignant cells.

Many centres use this type of 'triple approach' of clinical evaluation, radiology (mammography) and FNA cytology in the initial evaluation of patients. Since all three investigations were positive, the surgeon went on to excise the tumour and sample the axillary lymph nodes. In due course, the surgeon received the pathologist's report on these tissues and used that information to guide his management of the patient. The report is reproduced, and we shall discuss its relevance for patient management and some points it raises about the biology of tumours.

MACROSCOPICAL FEATURES THAT DISTINGUISH MALIGNANT TUMOURS

Let us consider this report in more detail. First, there is the gross appearance, which records points similar to the criteria used clinically by the family practitioner and surgeon for distinguishing malignant from benign lumps. These include the **size**, the **infiltrating margin** and the **consistency** of the tumour. Other features include the presence or absence of **necrosis** and **haemorrhage**. Most importantly, there is an assessment of **excision margins** since incomplete excision will result in

rapid recurrence and an increased opportunity for spread. The report of the microscopic appearances records the pathologist's conclusion, i.e. that it is a primary malignant tumour of breast tissue. Let us consider how this conclusion has been reached.

MICROSCOPICAL FEATURES THAT DISTINGUISH MALIGNANT TUMOURS

Malignant tissues differ from benign tissues in that individual cells have an abnormal appearance and their arrangement is deranged. The **disordered growth pattern** is easy to appreciate providing you know the normal histological appearance of that tissue.

Within the breast, the normal duct–lobule system is composed of an inner epithelial and an outer myoepithelial layer surrounded by basement membrane, which contrasts with the carcinoma shown in Figures 16.10 and 16.11. A crucial factor, which is often essential for diagnosing carcinoma, is that cells should have breached the basement membrane, which marks the boundary between the epithelial and subepithelial tissues. Within the breast, it is possible to identify disordered growth that is still confined within the ducts – an *in situ* carcinoma.

An atypical appearance of individual cells (cytological **atypia**) is a rather more subtle change. The malignant cells differ not only from normal cells but also from each other; this is called **pleomorphism**.

Name: Ida Hopps
Age: 50 years
Ward: Thompson
Consultant: I.M. Surgeon
Specimen: Left mastectomy and axillary dissection
Date of operation: 12.11.96

Macroscopical appearance

A simple left mastectomy specimen, weighing 160 g. It consists of skin, including nipple, which measures 170×90 mm and covers fatty tissue with a maximum dimension of 180 mm. In the tissue beneath the nipple, there is a pale, firm, gritty mass measuring 25×20×20 mm, which has an irregular, poorly defined margin. The closest excision margin (deep) is 15 mm from the mass. There is an area of erythema around the nipple. The axillary dissection measures 80×50×50 mm, and 13 lymph nodes have been identified.

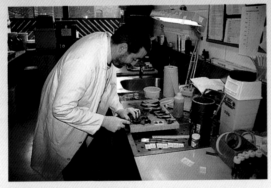

Figure 16.6 Gross examination of mastectomy specimen

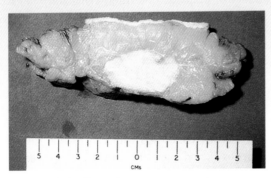

Figure 16.7 Slice of mastectomy specimen showing spiculated tumour close to the deep margin

Microscopical appearance

Sections show high nuclear grade ductal carcinoma *in situ* of comedo type with coarse microcalcification. There is also an invasive adenocarcinoma of ductal type, grade II, exhibiting a moderate amount of tubule formation, moderate nuclear pleomorphism and 5 mitoses/10 hpf. The maximum tumour dimension is 22 mm. There is no evidence of lymphatic or vascular permeation, and both the *in situ* and invasive carcinomas are completely excised by 10 mm (deep margin). The sections of the nipple confirm the presence of Paget's disease. None of the 13 axillary lymph nodes contains tumour. Both oestrogen and progesterone receptor status is positive (ER⁺, PR⁺).

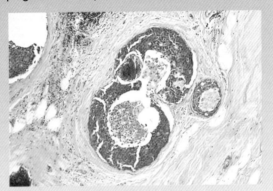

Figure 16.8 *In situ* ductal carcinoma with central necrosis and microcalcification

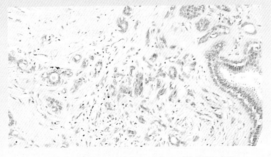

Figure 16.9 Normal breast duct (right) with adjacent tissue showing infiltration by moderately differentiated ductal carcinoma

Conclusion

Left Breast *in situ* and invasive ductal carcinoma grade II

Complete excision

ER⁺, PR⁺

Reported by Dr S. P. Ecimen

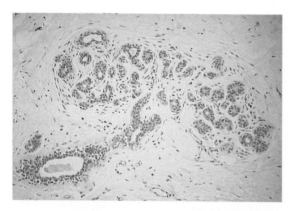

Figure 16.10   Normal terminal duct and lobule of breast

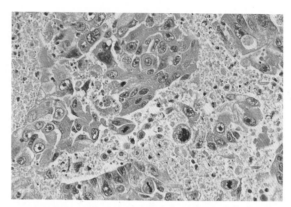

Figure 16.11   Breast carcinoma exhibiting pleomorphism, necrosis and mitotic activity

Pleomorphism may involve both nucleus and cytoplasm. In practice, the term often refers to the nucleus, which may be many times the size of a normal nucleus and may show marked variability in size and shape – **nuclear pleomorphism**. It may also have an altered distribution of chromatin and is a darker colour in stained sections, so-called **hyperchromatism**. These alterations reflect the increased amount and abnormalities of nuclear chromatin, which is common in tumours as they are frequently **aneuploid**.

Aneuploid: an abnormal number of chromosomes that is not an exact multiple of the haploid (23) number

Most normal cells have a small single nucleolus. In malignant cells, there may be many nucleoli of varying sizes or, alternatively, a large single nucleolus. The position of the nucleus within the cell is often abnormal, i.e. it exhibits a **loss of polarity**. Thus the nucleus of, for example, a normal colonic cell is situated at the cell's base, with mucus in the cytoplasm nearer the surface, whereas the nucleus is more central in a malignant cell. There is also an increase in **mitotic activity** as a result of the increase in cell proliferation, and **abnormal mitotic figures** may also be identified. The general appearance of the cells is altered as there is an **increase**

in the nuclear/cytoplasmic ratio, either because the amount of cytoplasm is less, because the nucleus is larger or because of a combination of the two.

The cytoplasmic changes vary depending on the tissue but generally involve a **loss of specialised features**, for example the absence of or a reduction in mucin content in a colonic adenocarcinoma. Ultimately, however, all of these features are only guidelines, and the real test is whether the tumour behaves in a malignant fashion. Of course, we cannot leave patients untreated just to see how the tumour behaves. Pathologists have learnt much about the behaviour of tumours from autopsy studies, and, fortunately, tumours of similar appearance usually show similar behaviour in different patients.

Note that many of the features discussed here are the same as those used for the assessment of dysplasia (see p. 223), and the distinction between grades of dysplasia and frank malignancy is based on both the degree and the extent of the changes.

FACTORS INFLUENCING PROGNOSIS

Here we are concerned with factors that influence prognosis and can be routinely assessed by histopathologists. The important aspects are:

- the type of tumour
- the grade of the tumour
- the stage of the disease.

First, it is essential to decide whether the tumour has arisen locally or whether it is a metastasis. Two points help to make this distinction: whether there are precancerous changes or *in situ* carcinoma present and whether the lesion resembles tumours known to occur at that site.

In situ **carcinoma** is an alteration in the cytological appearance that is similar to that seen in malignant tumours but does not show any invasion through the basement membrane. If the tumour had been entirely *in situ*, it would have an extremely good prognosis because the lack of local invasion would mean that the tumour had no ability to extend into lymphatic or blood vessels and no possibility of metastasis.

Precancerous lesions are harder to define, but are changes (e.g. atypical hyperplasia) that have been shown in large studies to be associated with the subsequent development of cancer and are believed to represent an early, but possibly reversible, stage of malignancy.

In most organs, there is one type of malignant tumour that is far more common than any other,

Table 16.1 Grading of breast cancer

Parameter	Score
Tubule formation	
Majority of tumour >75%	1
Moderate amount 10–75%	2
Little or none <10%	3
Nuclear pleomorphism	
Mild	1
Moderate	2
Severe	3
Mitotic count – count per 10 high-powered fields; varies with type of lens	
0–5	1
6–10	2
>11	3
Total score	**Grade**
3–5	1
6–7	2
8–9	3

and this generally corresponds with the type of tissue that is proliferating in that normal organ. For example, the breast and colon have active glandular epithelium, so the most common malignant tumour at both sites is an adenocarcinoma composed of malignant glandular epithelium. The bladder is lined by transitional epithelium, which gives rise to transitional cell carcinoma, and the oesophagus has squamous epithelium and squamous carcinomas. Remembering the normal histology can be a great help in predicting the most common tumours for a particular site.

To return to our patient; she has an adenocarcinoma that has *in situ* and invasive components. The *in situ* carcinoma tells us that it is locally arising. This is therefore a primary tumour of the breast. Within the breast, there is a large number of different subtypes. Our lady has a ductal carcinoma, which has a poorer prognosis than does a mucinous carcinoma (p. 236).

Although she had an invasive carcinoma, the tumour was not seen in **lymphatic** or **blood vessels**. The most important prognostic feature is the *type* of tumour, but after that, the prognosis is influenced by the grade and stage. The grade of a tumour depends on its histological appearance, whereas the stage of a tumour depends on its size and extent of spread. The **histological grade** is a crude measure of how much the tumour resembles normal tissue, combined with an estimate of its mitotic activity. There is a well-defined scoring system for breast tumours (Table 16.1) based on tubule formation, nuclear pleomorphism and mitotic count, each of which is scored from 1 to 3. The scores are totalled to divide the tumours into three grades, grade 1 tumours having a better prognosis than grade 3 tumours. Many sites have no formal grading system, so the pathologist will merely record whether the tumour is well differentiated, moderately differentiated or poorly differentiated by assessing similar features but in a less objective way.

The **stage of a tumour** is a measure of the extent of disease and depends on pathological, radiological and clinical information. A TNM staging system is often used for breast carcinoma, T standing for the size of the primary tumour, N coding for regional node involvement, and M representing

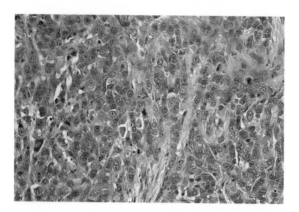

Figure 16.13 High-grade invasive ductal carcinoma

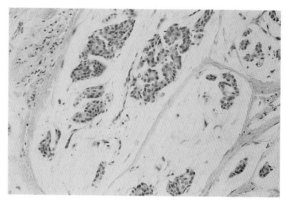

Figure 16.14 Invasive mucinous carcinoma of the breast

metastatic disease. Figure 16.15 illustrates the different pathological staging systems and their links with the TNM classification.

This provides an easy shorthand for indicating the disease stage, which is helpful for deciding

treatment and comparing the outcome of patients treated with new therapeutic regimens. The assessment of a new treatment regimen must obviously take account of the stage of a patient's disease to avoid spurious results.

The pathology report on our patient states that none of the lymph nodes contains tumour, and the clinical investigation did not show metastases. Therefore, she would be categorised as T2 (size 2.2 cm), N0, M0 which translates as stage II disease. This short, coded message tells the doctor that this lady is in a relatively good prognostic group.

When the doctor talks to his patient about these results, she may well ask him a variety of questions about her prognosis, but before we attempt to answer those questions, we should digress to discuss the classification of tumours.

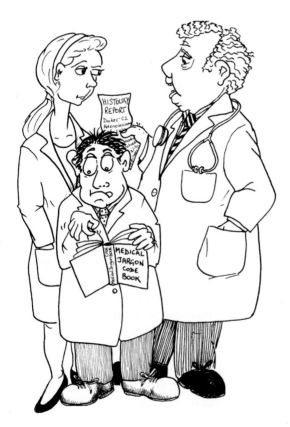

Figure 16.12 'I'm afraid it's a Dukes' C2 – she'll need DXT and chemo.'

CLASSIFICATION OF TUMOURS

The pathological classification of tumours is illustrated in Figure 16.16.

You will recall that a knowledge of the normal structures at a particular site can be of great help in predicting the most common tumours. In most organs, there is one particular type of malignant tumour that is more common than any other, and this generally corresponds with the type of tissue

TNM system, e.g. Ca breast

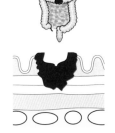

T = Tumour size:
T0: impalpable
T1: 0–2cm
T2: 2–5cm
T3: >5cm±fixation
to underlying
muscle
T4: any size, with
fixation to chest
wall or skin

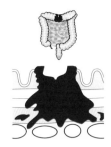

N = Lymph node status:
N1: regional nodes
involved
N2,3: more distant
nodal groups

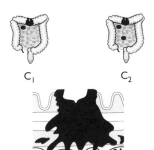

M = Metastases
M0: no detectable
spread
M1: metastases
present (specify
sites)

Dukes' staging of colorectal carcinoma

Comment: 5 year survival figures:
Dukes' A: 80–85%
Dukes' B: 55–67%
Dukes' C: 32–37%

mucosa
m. mucosae
submucosa
m. propria
lymph nodes

Dukes' A: tumour confined within bowel wall; no spread through main muscle layer

Dukes' B: spread through m. propria into serosal fat, without lymph node involvement

C_1 C_2

Dukes' C: tumour spread to lymph nodes.
C1: pericolic nodes involved
C2: involvement of higher mesenteric nodes

Cotswolds revision of Ann Arbor staging system for Hodgkin's Disease

Comment: the presence of "B" symptoms, e.g. fever, drenching sweats, weight loss, adversely affects the prognosis, and is included in the stage, e.g. Stage IIA (no B symptoms), or Stage IIB.

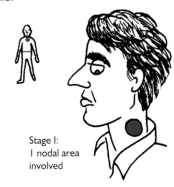

Stage I:
I nodal area involved

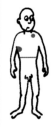 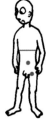

Stage II: ≥2 nodal areas on same side of diaphragm involved (no. of involved sites recorded)

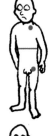

Stage III: nodal areas on each side of diaphragm:
III$_1$ upper abdo,
III$_2$ lower abdo

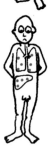

StageIV:
visceral involvement

The spleen is part of the reticuloendothelial system. Splenic involvement does not carry the same staging implications as, for instance, bone marrow or liver

Figure 16.15 Staging of tumours

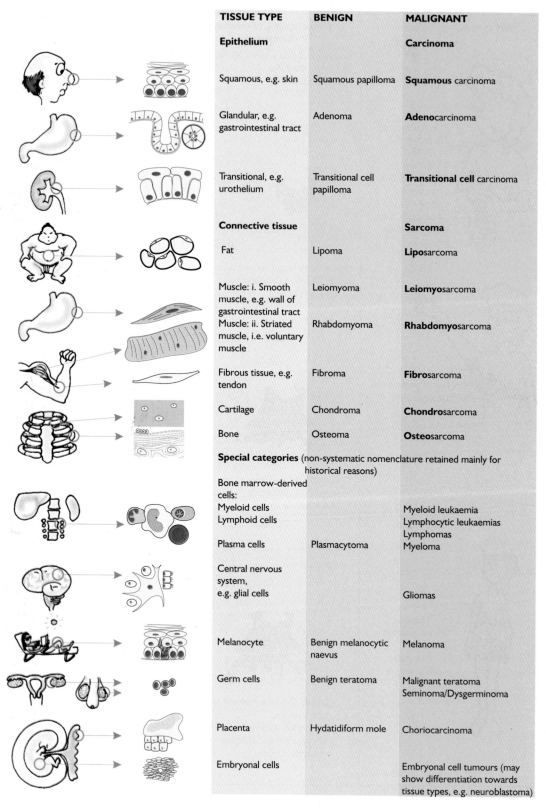

TISSUE TYPE	BENIGN	MALIGNANT
Epithelium		**Carcinoma**
Squamous, e.g. skin	Squamous papilloma	**Squamous** carcinoma
Glandular, e.g. gastrointestinal tract	Adenoma	**Adeno**carcinoma
Transitional, e.g. urothelium	Transitional cell papilloma	**Transitional cell** carcinoma
Connective tissue		**Sarcoma**
Fat	Lipoma	**Lipo**sarcoma
Muscle: i. Smooth muscle, e.g. wall of gastrointestinal tract	Leiomyoma	**Leiomyo**sarcoma
Muscle: ii. Striated muscle, i.e. voluntary muscle	Rhabdomyoma	**Rhabdomyo**sarcoma
Fibrous tissue, e.g. tendon	Fibroma	**Fibro**sarcoma
Cartilage	Chondroma	**Chondro**sarcoma
Bone	Osteoma	**Osteo**sarcoma
Special categories (non-systematic nomenclature retained mainly for historical reasons)		
Bone marrow-derived cells:		
Myeloid cells		Myeloid leukaemia
Lymphoid cells		Lymphocytic leukaemias Lymphomas
Plasma cells	Plasmacytoma	Myeloma
Central nervous system, e.g. glial cells		Gliomas
Melanocyte	Benign melanocytic naevus	Melanoma
Germ cells	Benign teratoma	Malignant teratoma Seminoma/Dysgerminoma
Placenta	Hydatidiform mole	Choriocarcinoma
Embryonal cells		Embryonal cell tumours (may show differentiation towards tissue types, e.g. neuroblastoma)

Figure 16.16 Pathological classification of tumours

that is proliferating at that site. The stomach and colon have active glandular epithelium, so the most common malignant tumour at both sites is an adenocarcinoma, which is composed of malignant glandular epithelium. The bladder is lined by transitional epithelium, which gives rise to transitional cell carcinoma, and the skin has squamous epithelium and squamous carcinomas. Since the tumour resembles part of the parent tissue, the classification is based on the assumed histogenesis: i.e. because a transitional cell carcinoma has some similarities with transitional epithelium, it is assumed to arise from it.

The broad classification divides tumours into those arising from epithelia (carcinomas), connective tissue (sarcomas) and lymphoid tissue (lymphomas) and 'the rest', which includes specialised tissues such as the brain. Included in Figure 16.16 are the benign counterparts arising from the same tissues.

At this point, there needs to be a word of caution because, although this classification originated from ideas on **histogenesis**, it is now apparent that cells of one tissue type may 'differentiate' to resemble cells of another type (a process called metaplasia; see p. 222). For example, bronchial glandular epithelium may become squamous as a result of the chronic irritation from smoking. A tumour arising in such a patient may hence appear squamous, although the original epithelium at this site was glandular. The histogenetic approach to classification is destroyed in such circumstances. Fortunately, we only have to claim that we will classify tumours according to their type of differentiation and we eliminate the problem. Thus a tumour resembling squamous cells is a squamous cell carcinoma regardless of the true origin. You will discover that, although rare, it is possible to get squamous carcinoma in the breast and adenocarcinoma in the bladder. A tumour cell is sometimes very poorly differentiated so that, even to the trained histopathologist's eye, it does not resemble a particular type of normal cell. In this situation, special stains to demonstrate cytoplasmic or surface molecules can be helpful. Thus the presence of intracellular mucins would suggest an adenocarcinoma, and immunohistochemical stains for different intermediate filaments or lymphoid antigens would help to distinguish between a wide variety of tumours. If it is not possible to demonstrate any differentiation, the tumour is referred to as **anaplastic**.

Some of these substances are also released into the blood, which is useful both for diagnosis and for following the patient's response to treatment. For example, prostatic-specific antigen (PSA) levels can be measured in the blood to help screen for prostatic adenocarcinoma, although the levels are also raised in some non-malignant prostatic disorders because the antigen is present on both benign and malignant prostatic cells. The beta subunit of human chorionic gonadotrophin (βHCG) and alpha-fetoprotein (αFP) are also useful markers in patients with teratoma.

Now we must turn to the patient's questions. What causes cancer? How will it behave? What treatments are available? Will there be a lot of pain? If we are not to be stumped by the patient, we have to understand a little more about the natural history of cancer.

CHAPTER 17

What causes cancer?

- Cancer as a disease of genetic material
- Risk factors for cancer

CANCER AS A DISEASE OF GENETIC MATERIAL

The view that cancer originates within single cells as a result of abnormalities within its DNA is now generally accepted. The evidence comes from five main sources:

1. Some cancers have a heritable predisposition. Examples include familial retinoblastoma and familial adenomatous polyposis.
2. Many tumours exhibit chromosomal abnormalities, and karyotypic studies have even identified specific changes in some tumours, for example an 8;14 translocation in Burkitt's lymphoma.
3. A number of rare inherited disorders involve an inability to repair damaged DNA. An example includes xeroderma pigmentosa; these patients have an increased susceptibility to skin cancer following damage to DNA from ultraviolet light.
4. Many chemical carcinogens are also mutagens, i.e. have been shown to cause genetic mutations.
5. DNA recombinant technology has demonstrated that DNA from tumour cells, when transferred into normal cells, can convert them into tumour cells of the same type.

The isolation of genes with a direct role in tumour formation (oncogenes) has firmly established cancer as a disease of genetic material.

We will now consider the many predisposing and aetiological factors that lead to tumour formation. Although it appears that these factors must alter either the DNA structure or its function in some way, the details of many of these processes remain unclear.

One of the patient's concerns will relate to what causes cancer and the risk factors that were important in his or her case.

RISK FACTORS FOR CANCER

AGE

The advent of antibiotics, improved sanitation and good nutrition has extended people's expected life span so that they can now achieve an age at which there is a high incidence of malignant tumours, particularly those of the colon, lung, prostate and bronchus. It is postulated that carcinogens may have a cumulative effect over time, which may explain the increased incidence with age. The ability of carcinogens to induce genetic mutations is well known, and the large number of cell divisions with increasing age may contribute to the neoplastic process. Cell division is itself a risk since each time the DNA is copied, there is a potential to introduce mistakes within the genome. There are elaborate DNA repair mechanisms in place to

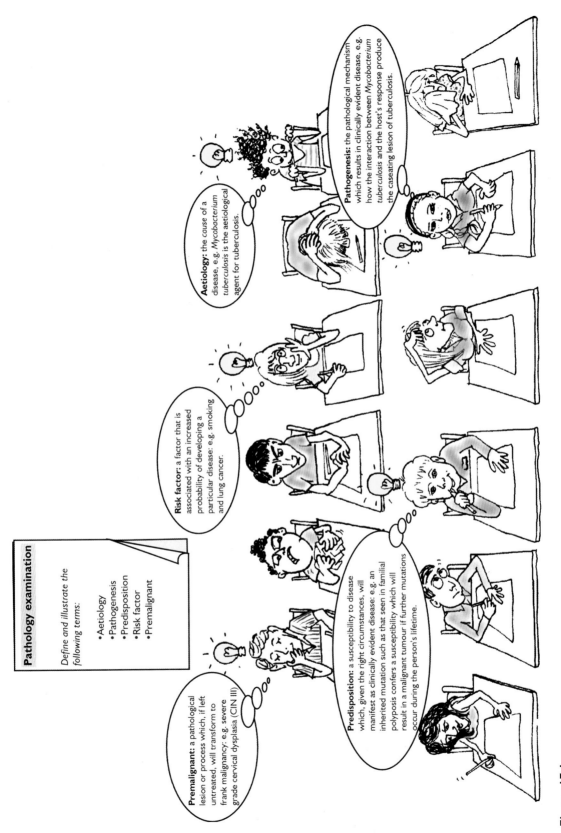

Figure 17.1

correct such errors, but mutations in genes coding for the proteins involved in DNA repair will allow such errors to pass on to the next generation of cells. All these factors, together with age-related metabolic or hormonal changes, may combine to account for the increasing incidence of tumours with age. Tumours are, of course, not just confined to the elderly, some malignancies such as leukaemias being more common in children. In some childhood tumours (e.g. retinoblastoma), heredity plays a major part in the aetiology.

GENETIC FACTORS

In our case of breast carcinoma discussed in Chapter 16, the doctor discovered that the patient's mother had died of breast carcinoma. The patient also had two daughters who, at the time, were both well. This history of malignant disease within close family members is of relevance as there are several tumour types in which the risk of cancer in close family members is increased. How much the risk is increased in individual cases and with different tumours is not easy to specify, but in general it is about two to three times normal. Tumour development is obviously not inevitable, and many other factors such as environmental and dietary influences may modify the risk.

In some tumours, the genetic susceptibility is better understood, and in two autosomal dominant conditions – familial polyposis coli and retinoblastoma – it involves the loss of a **tumour suppressor gene** or **anti-oncogene** (see p. 259). Familial polyposis coli (familial adenomatous polyposis) is a disorder in which individuals develop hundreds of polyps in the gastrointestinal tract. These polyps show varying degrees of dysplasia (see p. 222) and, although benign, should be regarded as premalignant because practically all of these patients will develop a colonic carcinoma if the colon is not removed by the age of 25 years. Retinoblastoma is a malignant tumour of the eye that is most common in children. Between 25 and 30 per cent of cases of retinoblastoma are hereditary, the rest being sporadic. Both the familial and sporadic cases arise as a result of two mutations in the retinoblastoma gene, but the familial cases inherit one mutation through the germ line cells (see p. 260).

GEOGRAPHY AND RACIAL FACTORS

Geographical factors merge with environmental factors, as a geographical factor is only an environmental factor that affects the population of a particular area. This may be a sunny climate, radioactive rock formations or a carcinogen in the water supply.

Let us discuss the increased incidence of stomach cancer in Japan compared with North America. The tumour is seven times more common in Japanese people living in Japan than in Americans living in the USA. Is this a racial difference or an effect of some climatic, geological or dietary factor that operates in Japan? To answer this, we need to know the incidence in Japanese people who move to America and raise families. They will keep their racial (genetic) factors and may import their dietary factors but not their geographical factors. We find that the incidence drops in these immigrants and is halved in their first-generation offspring but is still higher than in white Americans, so we have not achieved a definite answer to our question. Some reports suggest that the incidence drops further in future generations until it equals the American rate. This would appear to rule out a racial (genetic) factor and may imply a cultural dietary change.

A much easier example is the incidence of melanomas in white-skinned Australians. Here, there is a *racial predisposition*, because they do not have sufficient skin pigmentation to protect them from ultraviolet light, and the *geographical factor* of a sunny climate. If the Australian emigrates at birth to a cold, grey country, his risk of melanoma drops dramatically.

ENVIRONMENTAL AGENTS

Numerous environmental agents have been implicated in the causation of cancer. Everybody knows

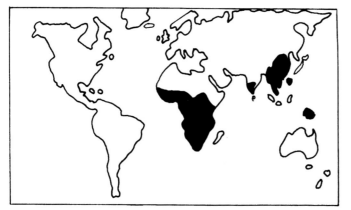

Hepatocellular carcinoma
Sub-Saharan black Africa
Far East

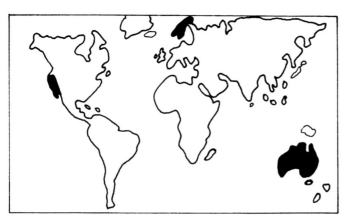

Malignant melanoma
Australia
Scandinavia
North America: Californian whites at highest
risk

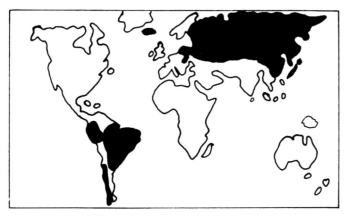

Gastric carcinoma
Japan, China
Brazil, Colombia, Chile
Iceland, Finland,
USSR, Poland, Hungary

Figure 17.2 Geographical variations in tumour incidence

that there is a strong association between smoking and lung cancer. This problem may not only affect the smoker but also the 'innocent bystander' who inhales exhaled tobacco smoke (passive smoking).

Asbestos exposure increases the risk of developing lung carcinoma and malignant mesothelioma of the pleura and peritoneum. Exposure to β-napthylamine, which may occur in the rubber and dye industries, increases the risk of transitional cell tumours of the bladder. Exposure to vinyl chloride in the plastic industry enhances the development of liver angiosarcoma (a malignant tumour of blood vessels).

One of the first examples of an environmental cancer was described in 1775 by Percival Pott, surgeon to St Bartholomew's Hospital, London. He had observed that chimney sweeps had a very high incidence of scrotal cancer and correctly deduced that this was because of chronic contact with soot. In fact, Percival Pott achieved a double, describing an environmental carcinogen and an occupational cancer in one go. He is also remembered for his description of spinal tuberculosis, referred to as Pott's disease.

CARCINOGENIC AGENTS

So far, we have discussed carcinogenesis under the broad headings of age, genetics, race, geography and environment. The next step is to consider what type of agent is operating (the aetiological agent) and to look at ideas on how the agent converts a normal cell to a malignant cell (pathogenesis).

It is worth remembering that, as in the case considered in Chapter 16 of the lady with breast cancer, by the time a patient presents with a tumour, a large number of cellular events and many thousands of cell divisions have already taken place. Consequently, we are looking at a growth that has been in existence for quite some time. Identifying the responsible aetiological factors at this stage can be extremely difficult. There are three major groups of agents involved in carcinogenesis that we need to consider:

- chemical carcinogens
- radiation
- viruses.

These groups should not be viewed in isolation. Chemicals may, for example, interact with ionising radiation or oncogenic viruses. Several different agents within any one group may also interact with each other. Furthermore, all these extrinsic agents may interact with endogenous or constitutional factors in the host, such as genetic susceptibility or hormonal status, emphasising that the carcinogenic process is complex and multifactorial.

Chemical carcinogens

Figure 17.3 illustrates classical experiments of chemical carcinogenesis using mouse skin, which provide the basis for the multistep theory (see p. 265) and lead to descriptions of the process of **initiation** and **promotion**. We now know, however, that tumour development in humans is much more complex than depicted in the figure.

Let us consider Figure 17.3. If you apply a low dose of polycyclic aromatic hydrocarbon (the initiator) to the shaved skin of the mouse and do not do any more, no tumours will result. However, if you later apply another chemical, croton oil (the promoter), to the same skin, local tumours will develop. The important points are that the initiator must be applied before the promoter and that the promoter must be applied repeatedly and at regular intervals. There may be a long time interval between initiation and promotion, which suggests that initiation provokes an irreversible change in the DNA that is fixed by cell division. In contrast, the promoter acts in a dose-related, initially reversible fashion and appears to modify the expression of altered genes. Some chemicals (**complete carcinogens**) can act as both initiator and promoter whereas others (**incomplete carcinogens**) fulfil only one action.

Evidence that certain chemicals are carcinogenic in humans is provided by epidemiological studies. Some chemical carcinogens occur naturally; for example, aflatoxin B_1 is a potent hepatocarcinogen that is a metabolite from the fungus *Aspergillus flavus*, a common contaminant of grain and other crops in the tropics. Several carcinogens occur as complex mixtures as in tobacco smoke. Chemical carcinogens typically take 20 or more years to exert their effects, so there is a long latent period between first encounter with the chemical and the appearance of a tumour. The dose required to induce tumours varies widely. Carcinogens act on a number of fairly specific target tissues, broadly determined by the initial routes of exposure and by subsequent patterns of absorption, distribution and metabolism. Beta-napthylamine is an interesting example. It enters the body mainly via the respiratory system and is inactivated by conjugation with glucuronic acid. Following excretion in the urine,

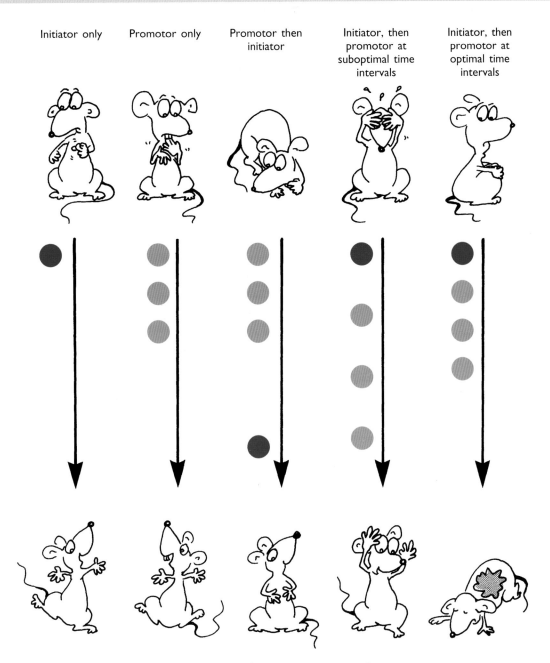

Figure 17.3 Chemical carcinogenesis: the effects of tumour promotors and initiators

it is activated again as a result of the action of urinary glucuronidase, which splits the conjugate, releasing the active molecule. Its carcinogenic effects are hence confined to the urinary tract, where it causes transitional cell tumours.

Chemical carcinogenesis is complex and occurs in several steps, to which both genotoxic and non-genotoxic events contribute. Genotoxic carcino-gens react with DNA. Various types of genetic damage will follow, and if the damage is not lethal to a cell, it will be transmitted to the daughter cells after cell division. The only protection the cell has is its array of DNA repair enzymes, which must reconstitute the DNA before the next cell division or else the abnormality will be 'stamped' in by being transmitted to the daughter cells.

Most genotoxic carcinogens undergo metabolic changes and are converted from inactive procarcinogens to activated ultimate carcinogens that bind to DNA. Some genotoxic chemicals react directly with DNA without previous metabolic activation. The conditions that determine whether a potential genotoxic chemical is activated or detoxified are very complex, but two main groups of enzymes are involved: the family of cytochrome P-450-dependent mono-oxygenase isoenzymes, and various conjugating enzymes that catalyse the formation of water-soluble glucuronides.

The process by which activated genotoxic carcinogens bind to DNA is equally complex. Once an activated carcinogen is bound to DNA, a number of consequences follow, depending on the nature and extent of the DNA damage that has been sustained. If this damage is extensive and irreversible, the cell will die. If less severe, the damage can be restored by the process of error-free DNA repair. The third possibility, mentioned earlier, is that the cell will survive with damaged DNA, which will then be passed on to the daughter cells following cell division.

Non-genotoxic carcinogens, in contrast, do not bind to DNA and do not directly damage it. They appear to act on cells in the target tissues mainly by directly stimulating cell division or by causing cell damage and death (and thus indirectly stimulating cell division through the process of regeneration and repair). Other effects are less clearly understood, but the general mode of action of non-genotoxic chemicals can be thought of as causing the disruption of normal cellular homeostasis. Some non-genotoxic chemicals, such as hormones, act through receptors on the surface of target cells.

One final point should be made. Some genotoxic chemicals exert both genotoxic and non-genotoxic effects on the target tissues. Thus, although genotoxic and non-genotoxic effects are both required for tumour development, they do not necessarily depend on separate genotoxic and non-genotoxic agents.

Radiation

Ionising radiation includes **electromagnetic rays**, such as ultraviolet light, X-rays and gamma rays, and **particulate radiation**, such as alpha particles, beta particles, neutrons and protons. All of these are carcinogenic.

As ionising radiation passes through tissue, it interacts with atoms in its path to destabilise them. This disturbance in the electron shell of atoms may lead to chemical changes. The precise mechanisms for this are still obscure. Radiation causes chromosomal breakage, translocations and mutations. Various protein molecules are also damaged, and there are two principal theories to account for the observations. The **direct theory** states that ionising radiation directly ionises important molecules within the cell, while the **indirect theory** states that ionisation first affects water within the cell, which leads to the production of oxygen free radicals, these causing the damage. Whichever mechanism operates, the end result is that DNA is altered, a process analogous to the initiator effect in chemical carcinogenesis.

The carcinogenic effect of radiation is related to its ability to produce mutations, and it is known that this depends on the type and strength of the radiation and the duration of exposure. Some

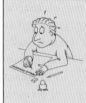

List some examples of chemical carcinogens and the associated tumour types	
Aromatic amines, e.g. β-napthylamine	Transitional cell carcinoma of the lower urinary tract (principally of the bladder)
Polycyclic aromatic hydrocarbons, e.g. benzo(a)pyrene	Skin cancer, lung cancer
Vinyl chloride	Angiosarcoma of the liver
Arsenic	Skin cancers
Aflatoxin B$_1$	Liver cell carcinoma

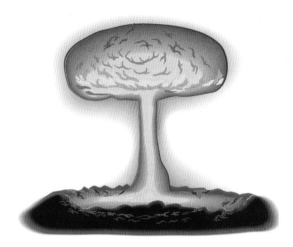

Immediate effects

Death from blast/burn injuries
Acute radiation syndromes:
- Bone marrow depression
- Gastrointestinal tract effects
- Cerebral effects

Delayed malignancies depend on age at time of exposure:

Childhood exposure
- Leukaemias*
- Thyroid cancer
- Breast cancer

Adult exposure
- Leukaemias*
- Lung/breast/salivary gland cancer
- All other cancers increased to some extent

* All leukaemias except chronic lymphocytic leukaemia are increased

Figure 17.4 Effects of irradiation, e.g. nuclear explosion

Which viruses are implicated in human cancers?

Virus	Associated tumour
Oncovirus	
HTLV-1	Adult T cell leukaemia/ lymphoma
Hepadnavirus	
Hepatitis B	Liver cancer
Papovavirus	
Papilloma virus types:	
1, 2, 4, 7	Benign skin papillomas
6, 11	Genital warts
16, 18	Cervical cancer
10, 16	Laryngeal cancer
5	Skin cancer
Herpes virus	
Epstein–Barr (EBV)	Burkitt's lymphoma
	Nasopharyngeal carcinoma
	Immunoblastic lymphoma
Herpes simplex-8	Kaposi's sarcoma

tissues, such as bone marrow and thyroid, are particularly sensitive to the effects of radiation, and children are more susceptible than adults.

Ultraviolet light is particularly important as sun exposure causes vast numbers of melanomas, squamous cell carcinomas and basal cell carcinomas of the skin. Fortunately, squamous cell carcinomas and basal cell carcinomas can generally be cured by complete local excision, but melanomas metastasise early and kill. Many of the pioneers who studied radioactive materials and X-rays developed skin cancers, and miners of radioactive elements have a high incidence of lung cancer. The radiation from the atomic bombs dropped on Hiroshima and Nagasaki in World War II resulted in an increased incidence of leukaemia, especially acute and chronic myeloid leukaemia, and breast, lung and colonic cancers.

Viruses

A large number of viruses has been implicated in the causation of cancer (see below). We will discuss:
- Epstein–Barr virus
- human papilloma virus
- hepatitis B virus
- human T-cell leukaemia virus-1
- Kaposi's sarcoma-associated herpes virus.

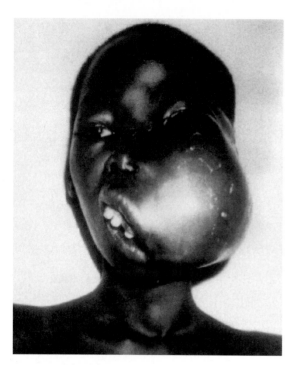

Figure 17.5 Young child with a large maxillary tumour distorting the face. This is a classical presentation of Burkitt's lymphoma

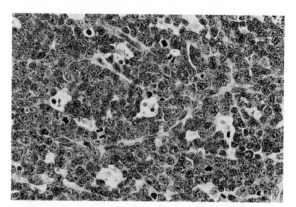

Figure 17.6 Photomicrograph showing classical 'starry sky' appearance of Burkitt's lymphoma

Epstein–Barr virus

Epstein–Barr virus (EBV) is a member of the herpes family. It is implicated in two major types of cancer: **Burkitt's lymphoma** and **nasopharyngeal carcinoma.**

There is a very strong association between EBV and the African variety of Burkitt's lymphoma, since over 98 per cent of the African cases show EBV genome in the tumour cells and all the patients have a raised level of antibodies to EBV membrane antigens. Fortunately, EBV does not inevitably cause cancer, as EBV is a common infection in developed countries, where it causes a 'flu-like illness called infectious mononucleosis or glandular fever. Burkitt's lymphoma can occur without EBV, and few non-African Burkitt lymphomas (15–20 per cent) have the EBV genome. Therefore, EBV must be just one factor involved in the transformation of B lymphocytes to a B cell malignancy.

It is interesting that the African regions where Burkitt's lymphoma is common are also regions where malaria is endemic. It would appear that malaria causes a degree of immunoincompetence that allows the EBV-infected B cells to proliferate and hence gives them an increased risk of mutation. Burkitt's lymphoma exhibits a specific mutation resulting in an 8;14 translocation regardless of whether EBV is involved. This translocation moves the c-*myc* gene from its position on chromosome 8 to be adjacent to the immunoglobulin heavy chain gene on chromosome 14. c-*myc* codes for proteins that control cell proliferation, the effect of this translocation being to increase its transcription, possibly because that zone of chromosome 14 is an area of frequent transcriptional activity.

Human papilloma virus

Human papilloma virus (HPV) is a papova virus that has long been known to be associated with **skin papillomas** (warts). Its role in causing cancer was recognised during the study of the very rare disease epidermodysplasia verruciformis, in which patients have defective cell-mediated immunity and numerous skin papillomas. These papillomas may transform into squamous cell carcinomas, which frequently contain the genome of HPV 5, 8 or 14. HPV is not a single virus but a group of around 65 genetically distinct viruses. Interestingly, some types appear to produce benign tumours, whereas others predispose to malignancy. Thus HPV 16 and 18 are implicated in squamous cell carcinoma of the uterine cervix, while HPV 6 and 11 are common in benign cervical lesions.

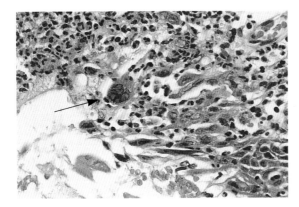

Figure 17.7 Inflamed cervical epithelium with multinucleate giant cell due to HPV infection

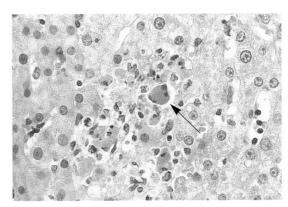

Figure 17.9 Photomicrograph of liver showing inflammation and necrosis due to viral hepatitis

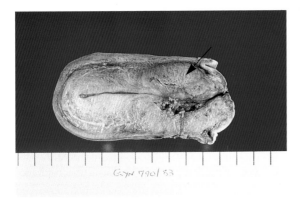

Figure 17.8 Macroscopical picture showing invasive cervical carcinoma

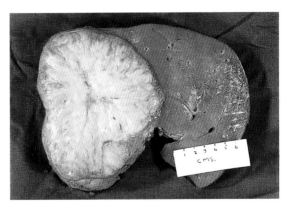

Figure 17.10 Section through the liver showing primary hepatocellular carcinoma

It is not known how HPV alters the cells. HPV can be transmitted by sexual intercourse, and it is noted that there is a high incidence of carcinoma of the cervix in those who begin sexual activity at an early age and in those who are promiscuous. The question is, why doesn't our immune system eradicate the virus? Many people have skin warts on their hands and feet (verrucae) as children but appear to develop immunity so that the warts are less common in later life. Now that we know the viral types involved in some cancers, this opens the door to developing vaccines. Unfortunately, immunising people to prevent cervical cancer is not yet available, but immunisation for the prevention of hepatitis B and its associated hepatocellular carcinoma is already in progress.

Hepatitis B virus
Hepatitis B virus (HBV) is associated with the production of a chronic hepatitis, cirrhosis and **carcinoma of the liver**.

In sub-Saharan Africa and south east Asia, where infection with HBV is endemic, the infection is transmitted vertically from mother to child during pregnancy. These children, therefore, have chronic HBV infection and a high incidence of hepatocellular carcinoma (HCC) at a relatively young age (20–40 years).

The importance of HBV in HCC is apparent from this sort of epidemiological work and also from molecular biological investigation looking for integrated HBV DNA sequences. These have been identified in the hepatocytes of some patients with chronic HBV infection and in some HCC tumour cells. It appears that integration of the viral genome precedes malignant transformation by several years, but no known oncogenic sequences have to date been identified. The HBV genome contains a **transactivating gene**, termed X, which codes for a product that alters the level of transcription of other genes, including the genes in the hepatocytes.

Liver cell carcinomas are also associated with alcoholic liver disease, androgenic steroids and aflatoxins. Aflatoxins are toxic metabolites of the fungus *Aspergillus flavus*, which can contaminate food in the tropics. Aflatoxin B is thought to contribute to the high incidence of liver cancer in parts of south-east Asia and Africa. These agents may act by causing damage that leads to regenerative activity and hence the production of proliferative nodules that are susceptible to further cellular alterations by HBV.

Human T cell leukaemia virus-1

Human T cell leukaemia virus-1 (HTLV-1) is important because it is the only example (so far!) of a retrovirus causing a human cancer. It is implicated in adult T cell **leukaemia/lymphoma** (ATLL), which is a rare tumour of the lymphoid system. HTLV-1 infection is most common in southern Japan, South America and parts of Africa, and precedes the development of malignancy by decades. It has a transactivating gene, *tat*, that increases IL-2 receptor expression in infected T cells, which promotes their growth. The study of **retroviruses** has advanced our knowledge of the role of genes in tumour biology by allowing the identification of specific transforming genes. (This is discussed in greater detail in Part 5.) However they have not to date been shown to be important in common human tumours.

Kaposi's sarcoma-associated herpes virus

Kaposi's sarcoma is an important vascular neoplasm that has come to prominence in HIV-infected patients. Since early 1980 it has frequently been associated with patients who have AIDS. It is an endemic lesion in central Africa, predominantly in healthy men but also in women and children. Evidence is accumulating that this odd vascular tumour is caused by a novel herpes virus. This virus

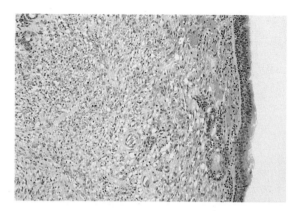

Figure 17.11 Kaposi's sarcoma with slit-like channels within the trachea

has been termed Kaposi's sarcoma-associated herpes virus (KSHV) or human herpes virus-8 (HHV-8).

Even more recently, it has been suggested that the same virus may be involved in the aetiology of multiple myeloma (a tumour of plasma cells). If data from recent research are substantiated, another interesting mechanism of virally induced neoplasia will emerge. Unlike many tumours in which the virus appears to infect the tumour cells, in multiple myeloma, KSHV has been identified in the dendritic (macrophage-derived) stromal cells of the bone marrow. The hypothesis is that the virus stimulates the production of IL6, which stimulates the myeloma cells to proliferate. This hypothesis is still highly speculative, and much more research will be needed to substantiate such a role for the virus in this tumour.

The study of viruses has helped enormously in unravelling the relevance of genes in human cancer. Of particular use are the retroviruses, which normally contain just three genes: two coding for structural proteins (*gag* and *env*) and one (*pol*) for the enzyme reverse transcriptase, which produces DNA from RNA. The addition of a fourth gene can often give the virus acute transforming properties; i.e. infection with the altered virus can produce tumours under experimental conditions, so-called **transfection** experiments. These viruses have acted as tools to enable scientists to identify the genetic sequences that could transform cell lines. Many of the viral oncogene sequences were recognised as variants of cellular genes that the retrovirus had acquired from the human genome. This focused

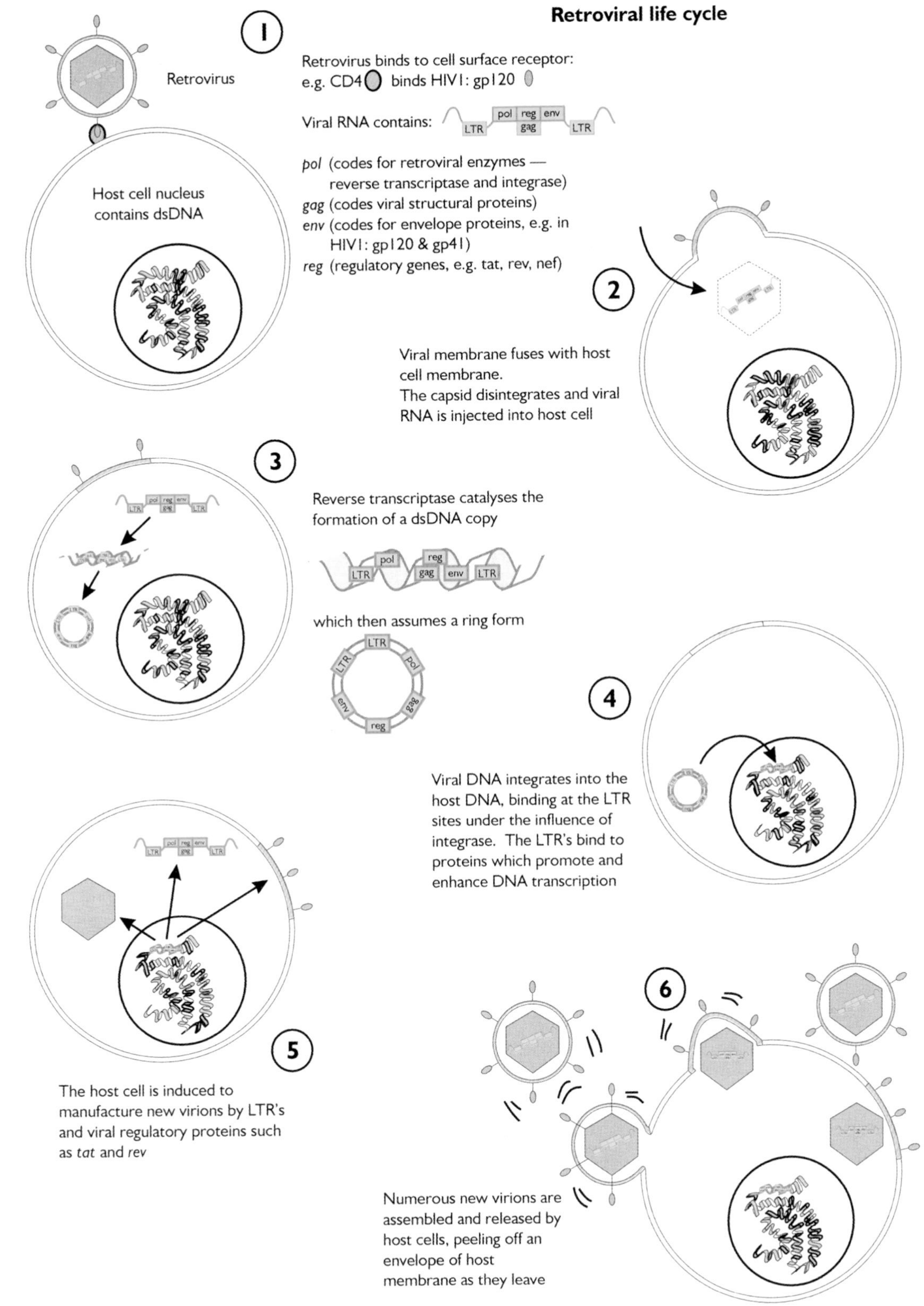
Retroviral life cycle
1
Retrovirus
Host cell nucleus contains dsDNA
Retrovirus binds to cell surface receptor:
e.g. CD4 binds HIV1: gp120
Viral RNA contains:
LTR
pol reg env
gag
LTR
pol (codes for retroviral enzymes — reverse transcriptase and integrase)
gag (codes viral structural proteins)
env (codes for envelope proteins, e.g. in HIV1: gp120 & gp41)
reg (regulatory genes, e.g. tat, rev, nef)
2
Viral membrane fuses with host cell membrane.
The capsid disintegrates and viral RNA is injected into host cell
3
Reverse transcriptase catalyses the formation of a dsDNA copy
LTR
pol
gag
reg
env
LTR
which then assumes a ring form
LTR
pol
gag
reg
env
LTR
4
Viral DNA integrates into the host DNA, binding at the LTR sites under the influence of integrase. The LTR's bind to proteins which promote and enhance DNA transcription
5
The host cell is induced to manufacture new virions by LTR's and viral regulatory proteins such as tat and rev
6
Numerous new virions are assembled and released by host cells, peeling off an envelope of host membrane as they leave

Figure 17.12 Retroviral life cycle

attention on the human cells' proto-oncogenes and led to an understanding of the mutations and translocations that can lead to their activation.

Oncogenic RNA viruses

Oncogenic RNA viruses are all retroviruses, i.e. contain reverse transcriptase, and can be divided into acute transforming viruses, slow transforming viruses and transactivating viruses. The **acute transforming viruses** produce tumours within a few weeks in infected animals and are often capable of transforming cell cultures. The **slow transforming viruses** take months to produce tumours, which are frequently forms of chronic leukaemia.

These two groups of virus alter the infected cell in different ways. The acute transforming viruses are usually incapable of normal replication because they have lost some genes related to replication but gained genes that confer their transforming capabilities. These additional genes are variants of their host's genes, genes that are called proto-oncogenes when in the host and viral oncogenes when in the virus. The proto-oncogene is a normal cell gene that is normally involved in growth or differentiation. The viral oncogene is not identical to the proto-oncogene, although there is quite extensive sequence homology. The viral oncogene is structurally altered, which, in some way, deregulates cell growth. Alternatively, at the time of inclusion into the viral genome, the proto-oncogene may be inserted near a potent viral promoter, resulting in its increased expression. In some cases, acute transforming viruses and normal retroviruses co-infect cells so that the non-transforming retrovirus can provide the replication information that the transforming virus lacks.

Slow transforming retroviruses do not contain oncogenes, have the normal three-gene structure to their genome and are capable of replication. They alter the host cells' behaviour by inserting near to a cellular proto-oncogene, so that they either cause increased activity of the cellular gene or possibly induce a structural change in the gene. This is called **insertional mutagenesis**.

Transactivating viruses do not contain oncogenes but, in addition to the *gag*, *pol* and *env* genes, have a fourth region, which confers trans-

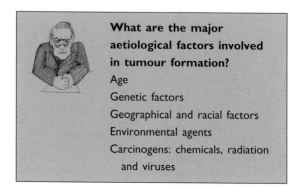

What are the major aetiological factors involved in tumour formation?
Age
Genetic factors
Geographical and racial factors
Environmental agents
Carcinogens: chemicals, radiation and viruses

forming properties. The human T cell leukaemia virus is in this group and its extra genes (*tat*) code for a variety of proteins, one of which activates the host's IL-2 and IL-2R genes, resulting in uncontrolled cell proliferation.

Oncogenic DNA viruses

Oncogenic DNA viruses contain genes that act early in infected cells to increase the expression of a wide variety of genes. The purpose of this is to activate later viral genes concerned with replication and assembly. However, it can also have the effect of inducing an excessive expression of host cell genes responsible for growth regulation. For example, the 'early genes' of the virus can produce proteins (e.g. the T proteins of polyoma and SV40 viruses) that localise in the nucleus and alter the regulation of DNA synthesis. In some cases, this is through binding to the p53 protein, so that its half-life is increased and DNA synthesis remains activated. Some 'growth-enhancing' actions may actually result from inhibiting normal 'growth-inhibiting' proteins.

There is an old wives' saying that 'where God puts disease, he also puts a cure.' Viruses undoubtedly cause infectious disease and can be one step on the road to cancer. However, they may also provide a possible cure for disease as they may be the ideal vehicle for altering the genetic code within human cells. Ultimately, it would be best if patients with single-gene disorders could have their defective gene replaced by the correct gene. This is in theory possible by using retroviruses to introduce the gene, although there are, in practice, many problems to conquer. The most useful practical application of our rapidly expanding knowledge of the genes is in the manufacture of specific proteins.

CHAPTER *18*

MOLECULAR GENETICS OF CANCER

- Cytogenetics
- Cancer-producing genes — oncogenes
- How oncogenes promote cell growth
- Dominant oncogenes
- Tumour suppressor genes/recessive oncogenes
- Other tumour suppressor genes
- Mismatch repair genes and microsatellite instability
- Apoptosis and cancer
- Multistep model of carcinogenesis

CYTOGENETICS

Some of the earliest indications for genetic alterations came from classical karyotypic analysis. This type of study reveals gross abnormalities at the chromosomal level. Classical examples of tumours showing such gross chromosomal abnormalities include chronic myeloid leukaemia and Burkitt's lymphoma. We have already considered Burkitt's lymphoma in Chapter 17. Here, we will briefly consider chronic myeloid leukaemia.

The **Philadelphia (Ph1) chromosome** is present in 90 per cent of cases of **chronic myeloid leukaemia** and can be used as a diagnostic marker. It is produced by a reciprocal and balanced **translocation** between chromosomes 22 and 9. The breakpoint on chromosome 9 occurs at the locus of the *abl* proto-oncogene, and the breakpoint on chromo-

some 22 is in the region termed the breakpoint cluster region (*bcr*). Some recent work suggests that the *bcr* genes code for a protein kinase that could have oncogenic potential. The *abl* proto-oncogene has sequence homology with the tyrosine kinase family of oncogenes, but it is only after translocation to chromosome 22 that it produces a mutant protein with tyrosine kinase activity. This particular tyrosine kinase activity is located in the nucleus, where it is believed to influence the transcription of DNA. Further examples of tumours and the cytogenetic abnormalities are shown in Table 18.1.

Allele: alternative form of the gene found at the same locus in homologous chromosomes

Table 18.1 Chromosomal alterations in human tumours

Tumour type	Chromosomal aberration	Possible action	Gene(s)
Haemopoietic tumours – translocation			
Chronic myeloid leukaemia	t(9;22)(q34;q11)	Alteration of nuclear tyrosine kinase	abl
Burkitt's lymphoma	t(8;14)(q24;q32)	Cell cycle regulation	myc
	t(2;8)(p12;q24)		
	t(8;22)(q24;q11)		
Acute myeloid leukaemia	t(8;21)(q22;q22)		eto
Solid tumours – translocation			
Malignant melanoma	t(1;19)(q12;p13)		?
	t(1;6)(q11;q11)		?
	t(1;14)(q21;q32)		?
Salivary adenoma	t(3;8)(p21;q12)		CTNNB1
Renal adenocarcinoma	t(X;1)(p11;q21)		TFE3
	t(9;15)(p11;q11)		?
Solid tumours – deletions			
Retinoblastoma	del13q14	Loss of oncosuppression	RB
Wilm's tumour	del11p13	Loss of oncosuppression	wt-1
	del11p15		?
	del17q12–21		fwt1
Bladder – transitional cell carcinoma	del11p13		?
Lung cancer – small cell type	del17p13	Loss of oncosuppression	TP53
Colorectal adenocarcinoma	del17p13	Loss of oncosuppression	TP53
	del 5q21	Loss of oncosuppression	apc
Breast cancer	del17p13	Loss of oncosuppression	TP53
	del17q21	Loss of oncosuppression	BRCA1
	del13q12–13	Loss of oncosuppression	BRCA2
Solid tumours – amplification			
Neuroblastoma		Cell cycle control	N-myc
Breast cancer		Increased growth factor activity	CerbB2

CANCER-PRODUCING GENES – ONCOGENES

The term 'oncogene' refers to any mutated gene that contributes to neoplastic transformation in the cell. Two major types of oncogene have been identified: *dominant oncogenes* and *tumour suppressor genes (anti-oncogenes)*.

Some oncogenes involved in carcinogenesis are mutated versions of normal cellular genes (called proto-oncogenes, p-*onc*). The function of these normal genes is enhanced by the mutations and they are hence referred to as 'activating' or 'gain in function' mutations. These genes are also known as 'dominant' oncogenes since the mutation of one allele is sufficient to exert an effect despite the presence of normal gene product from the remaining allele. It is nearly 20 years since such genes were discovered.

In contrast, tumour suppressor genes (TSG) are normal genes whose function is inactivated by

What are the main differences between dominant oncogenes and tumour suppressor genes?

	Dominant oncogenes	Tumour suppressor genes
No. of alleles in normal cells	Two	Two
No. of alleles mutated to exert effect	One	Two
Effect of mutation on the function of the protein product	Enhanced	Reduced
Germline (inherited) mutations identified, i.e. important in genetic predisposition	Only one gene – RET	Many – TP53, RB, etc.
Adjectives to describe mutations	Activating, gain in function, dominant	Inactivating, loss of function, recessive

mutations; hence these are known as 'inactivating' or 'loss of function' mutations. The genes are also known as 'recessive' oncogenes since inactivation of both alleles is required to have an effect at the cellular level. Evidence for the existence of such genes has been largely circumstantial and is based on classical genetics, cytogenetics and molecular genetics. You should beware that the terms 'dominant' and 'recessive' refer to action at the genetic level; confusion sometimes occurs since the terminology has been borrowed from classical Mendelian genetic inheritance patterns.

Where do oncogenes come from? There are both exogenous and endogenous sources. The **exogenous** sources include viral oncogenes (v-*onc*), which may be introduced into cells by tumour viruses. **Endogenous** genes are called cellular oncogenes (c-*onc*), these being genes that are normally present in the cell but have been altered to produce the oncogene. As mentioned above, the normal gene from which the oncogene is derived is called the proto-oncogene.

The viral or exogenous oncogenes can be divided into two types: those which show similarity to normal cellular genes and those which are completely different. This is important because viral oncogenes that resemble cellular genes are actually derived from the cell's genes. This is quite amazing when you think about it. A virus infects a cell and incorporates some of the cellular genes into its own genome. These genes, finding themselves in a new piece of DNA or RNA, become altered in their properties and are then viral oncogenes. When the virus infects another cell, it can introduce the viral oncogene (a process called transduction), which leads to altered growth of the infected cell. **Retroviruses**, which consist of RNA that becomes incorporated into the host DNA through the action of the enzyme reverse transcriptase, can readily 'pick up' some host DNA and thus carry viral oncogenes derived from cellular oncogenes. Oncogenic DNA viruses generally possess gene sequences that are uniquely viral and have no homology with cellular oncogenes.

HOW ONCOGENES PROMOTE CELL GROWTH

There are a number of ways in which the function of oncogenes can be altered, including point mutations, amplification, gene rearrangement/ translocation, deletion of part or the whole of a chromosome, and altered expression. Since most of the mechanisms described apply to both types of oncogene, they are considered here together; however, there are differences in the pattern of alteration between dominant oncogenes, and tumour suppressor genes. In contrast to dominant oncogenes which are mutated in a consistent manner either by

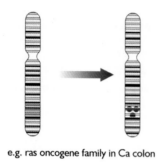

e.g. ras oncogene family in Ca colon

Figure 18.1 Point mutation

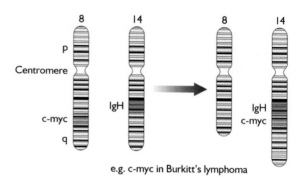

e.g. c-myc in Burkitt's lymphoma

Figure 18.2 Translocation

point mutation (e.g. *ras*), translocation (e.g. *abl*) or gene amplification (e.g. N-*myc*), mutations in tumour suppressor genes tend to be diverse in both type and position within the gene (e.g. *TP53*).

POINT MUTATIONS

These result in the substitution of one base pair by another, e.g. the substitution of G:C by A:T. The effect of the point mutation depends on its position and includes the alteration of the protein structure by a change in the amino acid composition and the insertion of a stop codon, with premature termination of the protein. The clearest example of point mutations in human tumours is found in the *ras* family. Mutations at codons 12, 13 and 61 of H-, K- and N-*ras* contribute to oncogenesis in many of the main types of human tumours. *ras* mutations are encountered in both benign and malignant neoplasms.

GENE REARRANGEMENTS/ TRANSLOCATIONS

This refers to the production of a hybrid chromosome as a result of the joining of part of one chromosome with another. The rearrangement of DNA sequences can lead to the creation of an altered gene (and product) either as a result of structural change or because of a change in the control of transcription. Examples include 8;14 (or 8;22, 2;8) translocation in Burkitt's lymphoma and the 9:22 translocation in chronic myeloid leukaemia (CML).

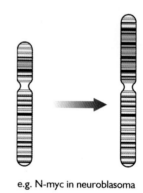

e.g. N-myc in neuroblasoma

Figure 18.3 Gene amplification

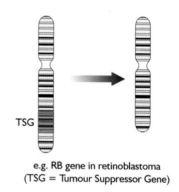

e.g. RB gene in retinoblastoma
(TSG = Tumour Suppressor Gene)

Figure 18.4 Deletion

AMPLIFICATION

The normal genome contains two copies of each gene (the two alleles). In amplification, one copy is multiplied numerous times and may result in increased mRNA and hence increased protein product. At the level of the chromosome, these areas of amplification are seen as double minutes (DMs) or homogeneously staining regions (HSRs).

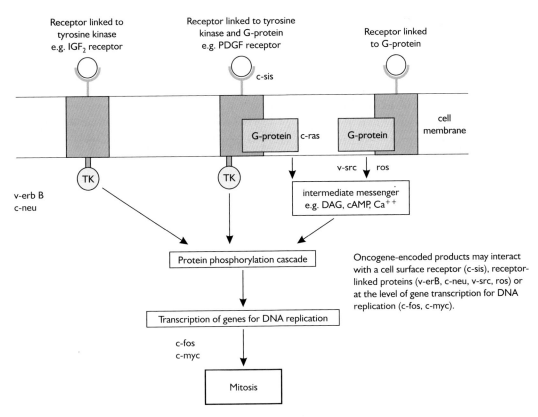

Figure 18.5 Growth factor receptors and signalling pathways: points of interaction of cellular oncogenes

DMs are extrachromosomal chromatin bodies without centromeres that segregate randomly during mitosis. HSRs are expanded chromosomal regions that are linked to the centromere and therefore segregate in the normal way. In many tumours, the overexpression of mRNA and protein is seen in the absence of gene amplification.

Most classes of oncogene have been shown to be amplified in human malignancy. Examples include N-*myc* in neuroblastoma and *Cerb*B2 in breast cancer. Only some of these amplifications have been demonstrated to have pathological significance. N-*myc* amplification is correlated with the advanced stage and recurrence of neuroblastoma, and *Cerb*B2 amplification in breast cancer correlates with poor prognosis.

DELETIONS

These range from the loss of single base pairs to the loss of entire chromosomes. The small intra-

genic deletions have effects (abnormal protein, stop codons) similar to those of point mutations. Larger deletions will, of course, inactivate many genes at a time.

ALTERED EXPRESSION

The inactivation of a gene via deletions or intragenic mutations is now a familiar story. It has recently become apparent that some putative tumour suppressor genes do not exhibit these common phenomena in certain tumours. Instead, changes in the methylation patterns of the promoter region of the gene lead to an altered expression (i.e. translation of protein). This occurs without any mutational event in the gene; hence if the gene were sequenced, no changes would be detected. A good example is the inactivation of the *p16* gene on chromosome 9p21. The protein product of *p16* binds to the cyclin dependent kinase-4 (CDK4) and inhibits interaction with cyclin D1, a cell cycle regulator.

DOMINANT ONCOGENES

Normal cell growth is believed to be influenced by growth factors binding to receptors on the surface of the cell. This produces a stimulus through a 'transducer' molecule that influences the cell's nucleus to produce the instructions for proliferation. Therefore cell growth could be stimulated as a result of:

- increased growth factor production
- an increase in the number of growth factor receptors on the cell's surface
- abnormal growth factor receptors
- abnormal transducers that will act as if growth factor has bound to its receptor
- nuclear acting molecules.

Oncogenes have been identified that act through each of these mechanisms.

GROWTH FACTORS AND GROWTH FACTOR RECEPTORS

Growth factors are polypeptides that act locally to stimulate proliferation and, sometimes, differentiation. If tumour cells produce substances that act as growth factors, they will be continually self-stimulating (**autocrine stimulation**). Several classes of growth factor have been classified according to sequence homology and biological activity. The categories include the epidermal growth factor family (EGF and TGF-α), the fibroblast growth factor family (acidic and basic FGF, hst and int-2), platelet-derived growth factor (PDGF), colony stimulating factors (CSF), interleukins and insulin-like growth factors (IGF). Growth factors act by binding to a receptor residing in the plasma membrane. The binding leads to activation of the receptor and signal transduction to the interior of the cell.

When the normal cell surface receptors are activated by growth factors, there is an increase in their **tyrosine kinase** activity. Some proto-oncogenes code for receptors, and their related oncogenes produce receptors with altered kinase activity. For example, *Cerb*B1 codes for an epidermal growth factor receptor (EGFR) with increased kinase activity. Some tyrosine kinases are not attached to a receptor but are anchored to the plasma membrane and participate in signalling. The c-*src* oncogene alters the activity of one of these **non-receptor tyrosine kinases**.

INTRACELLULAR MESSENGERS – GTP BINDING PROTEINS

Three mammalian *ras* genes – H-*ras*-1, K-*ras*-2 and N-*ras* have been identified. They form one of the most important families of oncogenes identified to date. *ras* genes usually acquire transforming activity as a result of point mutation within their coding regions. These activating point mutations are restricted to certain sites, notably codons 12, 13 and 61. The p21 product of both the *ras* proto-oncogene and transforming genes is located in the inner surface of the cell membrane. They bind guanosine nucleotides (GDP and GTP) and possess intrinsic GTPase activity. These biochemical properties resemble those of the G proteins that are associated with the cell membrane and are implicated in the modulation of signal transduction. It is becoming clear that *ras* proteins function as critical relay switches that regulate signalling pathways between the cell surface receptors and the nucleus.

Overall, point mutation in the *ras* gene is the most common dominant oncogene abnormality in human tumours. It appears to play a major role in colon, pancreatic and thyroid cancers as well as in myeloid leukaemia.

TYROSINE KINASES

The proteins possessing tyrosine kinase activity can be divided into two main groups: receptor and non-receptor tyrosine kinases. The transforming protein of v-*src* was the first oncogene shown to possess kinase activity. Many oncogenes and their products have been shown to possess the ability to phosphorylate themselves and other proteins. These include epidermal growth factor receptor (EGFR) and colony stimulating factor receptor (CSFR).

The second group of kinases is composed of proteins that are associated with the plasma

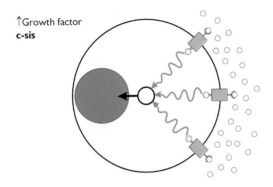

↑Growth factor
c-sis

Permanent activation of receptor
v-erb B

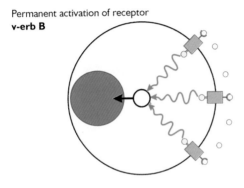

↑Growth factor receptor
c-neu

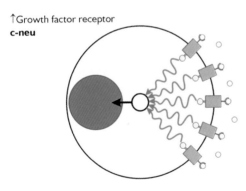

Abnormal signal transduction
c-K-ras

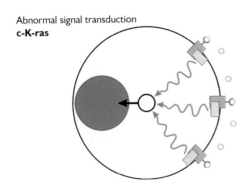

Figure 18.6 Mechanisms of oncogene activation

membrane but which do not have an extracellular domain for ligand binding. The most intensely studied is *src*. These proteins are likely to function as signal transducers. An important example of the role of these non-receptor tyrosine kinases in human tumours is seen in chronic myeloid leukaemia. The 9;22 translocation consists of the translocation of *abl* to the *bcr* gene on chromosome 22q11. The resulting fusion gene usually lacks one 5' exon of *abl*. The loss of the N-terminal part of *abl* protein appears to remove the negative regulatory domain, resulting in constitutive tyrosine kinase activity (i.e. the tyrosine kinase activity is switched on all the time).

NUCLEAR ONCOPROTEINS

These oncoproteins share the feature of nuclear localisation and a proven or suspected ability to bind to specific DNA sequences.

An important family of such genes involved in human malignancy is *myc*. This was originally identified as the oncogene carried by several acutely transforming retroviruses. The *myc* family consists of c-*myc*, N-*myc*, L-*myc*, R-*myc*, P-*myc* and B-*myc*. They have been isolated on the basis of homology to v-*myc* or one of the *myc* proto-oncogenes. c-*myc* is expressed in many tissues and correlates with cell proliferation. Activation due to gene amplification occurs in breast cancer and small cell lung cancer (SCLC). In B and T cell lymphomas, translocation to an immunoglobulin (Ig) or T cell receptor locus is seen.

TUMOUR SUPPRESSOR GENES/RECESSIVE ONCOGENES

Although 'activated' or 'dominant' oncogenes held centre stage 10–20 years ago, it is interesting that there was evidence for yet another type of gene long before that. The successful identification of genes whose proteins are physiological inhibitors

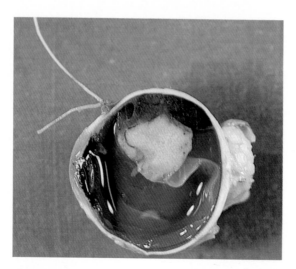

Figure 18.7 Section through the eye showing retinal detachment due to underlying tumour

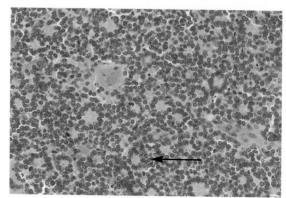

Figure 18.8 Photomicrograph showing characteristic rosettes of retinoblastoma

of growth stemmed from two main types of studies: somatic cell hybrids and genetic studies of inherited cancer syndromes. Furthermore, cytogenetic studies had already shown that many tumours exhibit loss of DNA involving almost all chromosomal arms.

SOMATIC CELL HYBRID STUDIES

This refers to studies in which a normal cell is fused with a transformed ('malignant') cell to form a hybrid cell. The main action of fusion is to produce a non-transformed state. This phenomenon of tumour suppression suggested that the normal cell must replace a defective function in the cancer cell. Since a large amount of genetic material is transferred during fusion experiments, it was difficult to implicate any particular chromosomes in tumour suppression. This was partially circumvented by introducing a single copy of chromosomes into the cell. For example, chromosome 11 was transferred into tumorigenic HeLa-human fibroblast hybrid (lacking chromosome 11). The result was inhibition of the tumorigenicity in the hybrid. It seemed likely therefore that 'tumour suppressor genes' might be involved during the process of oncogenesis. Further collaborating evidence came from the study of cancer susceptibility syndromes.

CANCER SUSCEPTIBILITY SYNDROMES - RETINOBLASTOMA

Retinoblastoma, a tumour arising from the embryonal neural retina, has a worldwide incidence of 1 in 20 000. The tumour is of interest because it has both sporadic and familial forms, approximately 25–30 per cent of the tumours being heritable. These cases tend to present earlier and develop bilateral disease. In contrast, the sporadic cases have unilateral tumours. Advancement in surgery and radiotherapy have led to improved survival, and it has become clear that 50 per cent of the offspring of patients with bilateral tumours were themselves at risk of the disease. Evaluation of family pedigrees clearly shows the inherited form as Mendelian dominant.

In 1971 Knudson proposed his 'two-hit' hypothesis (Figure 18.9). He pointed out that if cancer arises because of a series of somatic events, it is possible that one of these changes is sometimes inherited in the germline and is hence present in every cell of the body. All the cells are therefore already one step along the pathway of carcinogenesis, and this forms the basis for the dominantly inherited cancer susceptibility. In addition, a further mutation occurring somatically during life in the same gene would knock out the function of the gene. Hence, while the susceptibility is dominant, the action at cell level is recessive. This therefore predicted for a class of genes that had to be inactivated or to have 'loss of function'

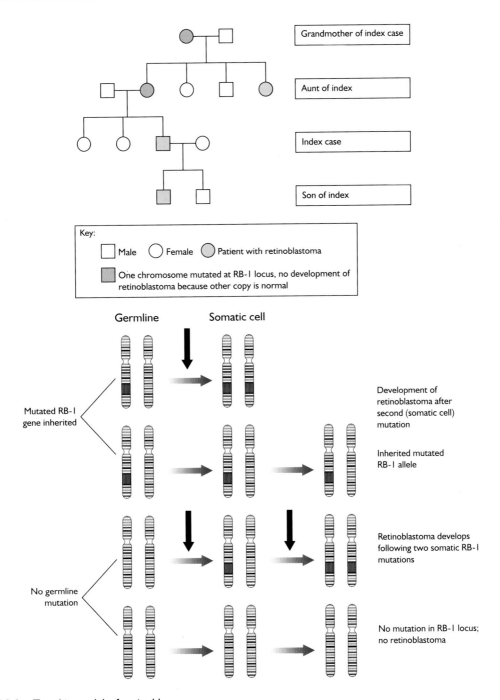

Figure 18.9 Two-hit model of retinoblastoma

in order to provide the malignant phenotype. Knudson examined data relating to the age of first appearance of the tumour in both familial and sporadic cases, and showed that it followed the expected statistical model based on this hypothesis.

Cytogenetic studies had revealed that a few of the familial tumours showed germline deletions of chromosome 13, and careful karyotyping revealed deletions of 13q14. The retinoblastoma gene (*RB1*) was cloned in 1986; it was the first tumour suppressor gene to be isolated. With the cloning of the gene, it could be confirmed that familial retinoblastoma is indeed the result of an inactivating mutation. Further evidence for oncosuppression comes from fusion experiments. Insertion of the 4.7 kb complementary DNA sequence (cDNA) into retinoblastoma and osteosarcoma cell lines lead to reversion of the tumorigenic phenotype, and the introduction of these cells into nude mice failed to produce tumours. Interestingly, mutations of the retinoblastoma gene and expression of the protein product have also been seen in almost every tissue despite the restricted oncogenic effects. Mutations are also found in other types of tumour such as breast carcinoma, although breast cancer does not form part of any syndrome in association with retinoblastoma.

It has been demonstrated that the *RB1* protein exists largely within the nucleus and that it binds to many DNA viruses, including the SV40 large T and E1A of adenoviruses. This binding stops *RB1* protein from functioning. If the region of the viral product that binds to the *RB1* protein is mutated so that no binding occurs, the transforming ability of the viral oncogene is abolished. It seems that part of the action of viral oncogenes is via the removal of *RB1* protein from its site of action. Hence it appears that dominant and recessive oncogenes may well act together in some circumstances to produce tumours.

OTHER TUMOUR SUPPRESSOR GENES

FAMILIAL ADENOMATOUS POLYPOSIS AND COLON CANCERS

Colon cancer is a common cancer in adults and is responsible for 20 000 deaths per year in the UK. Familial adenomatous polyposis (FAP) is an autosomal dominant disorder in which patients develop hundreds of polyps in the colon and rectum. Malignant transformation is inevitable unless the patient has a colectomy, with removal of the whole bowel. The gene for FAP, called the

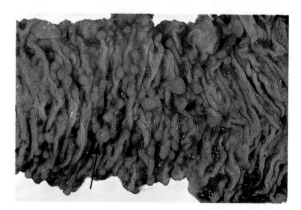

Figure 18.10 Large bowel with numerous polyps in patient with familial adenomatous polyposis

APC (adenomatous polyposis coli) gene, has been identified and is on chromosome 5q21. Another gene that also appears to be a tumour suppressor gene, called DCC (deleted in colorectal cancer), has also been identified on 18q21. Recent work suggests that yet another gene on chromosome 8 is also important in colon cancer.

TP53 AND HUMAN CANCER

p53 is a 53 kD protein that was first identified because it was complexed with the simian virus (SV) 40 large T antigen. There is considerable evidence that *TP53* is a tumour suppressor gene, although it does function in unusual ways in some circumstances. It has been shown that abnormalities of *TP53* are the most common molecular changes in many different types of malignancy. Current data suggest that the p53 protein has a role in sensing and responding to DNA damage. DNA damage leads to stabilisation of the protein, which then blocks further DNA replication. If this happens, there are two possible outcomes: either the DNA will be repaired and the cell will then carry on with its normal activities, or the cell will die by apoptosis. It is, of course, better that the cell with DNA damage dies rather than replicates since this is how tumours develop. This is why *TP53* has been christened 'the guardian of the genome'.

Table 18.2 Tumours and familial predisposition

Syndrome	Principal tumour types	Genetic locus/gene
Familial polyposis coli	Colorectal carcinoma	5q21 (*APC*)
MEN I	Pituitary, parathyroid, thyroid, adrenal cortex, islet cell tumour	11q13
MEN IIa	Medullary carcinoma of the thyroid, phaeochromocytoma, parathyroid tumours	10q11 (*RET*)
MEN IIb	Medullary carcinoma of the thyroid, phaeochromocytoma, mucosal neuromas	10q11 (*RET*)
Von Hipple–Lindau	Haemangioblastoma of the cerebellum and retina, renal cell carcinoma, phaeochromocytoma	3p25 (*VHL*)
Familial retinoblastoma	Bilateral retinoblastoma, osteosarcoma	13q14 (*RB*)
Neurofibromatosis type I	Neurofibromas, neurofibrosarcoma, glioma, meningioma, phaeochromocytoma	17q11 (*NF1*)
Neurofibromatosis type II	Bilateral acoustic schwannomas, multiple meningiomas	22q (*NF2*)
Li-Fraumeni	Breast cancer, sarcoma	17p13 (*TP53*)
Breast–ovarian	Breast cancer, ovarian cancer	17q21 (*BRCA1*)
Breast	Breast cancer, ovarian cancer, prostate cancer	13q12-13 (*BRCA2*)
Hereditary non-polyposis colorectal cancer (HNPCC)	Colorectal carcinoma	2p (*MSH2*) 3p (*MLH1*) 7p (*PMS2*)

MISMATCH REPAIR GENES AND MICROSATELLITE INSTABILITY

Genomic instability plays an important role in the development of tumours in patients with hereditary non-polyposis colorectal cancer (HNPCC). Most HNPCC patients have mutations in the human counterparts of the bacterial mismatch repair genes *mutS* and *mutL*. Mutations in these genes leads to an inability to repair DNA mismatch (mistakes that happen during DNA replication) and hence contribute to neoplastic transformation by allowing mutations to be transmitted to daughter cells.

Microsatellites are repeat units generally found within the non-coding part of the genome. They are highly polymorphic (the two alleles differ in size) and hence they provide a useful tool for the investigation of mutations within the genome. Patients with HNPCC show widespread alterations in these microsatellites and are therefore said to exhibit microsatellite instability (or a mutator phenotype). The implication of finding microsatellite instability is that the mismatch repair genes must be inactivated, otherwise the mismatch repair gene proteins would have corrected the mutations identified in the microsatellites. Hence an analysis of microsatellite instability provides indirect evidence for mismatch repair gene abnormality, and patients with high levels of instability can have direct genetic testing

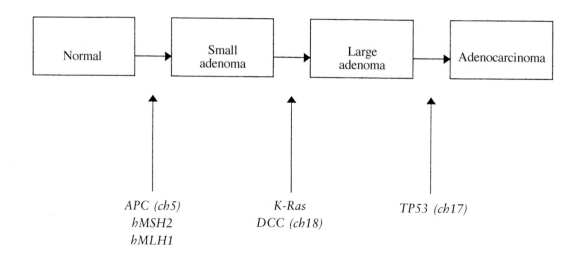

Figure 18.11 Multistep model for colorectal carcinoma

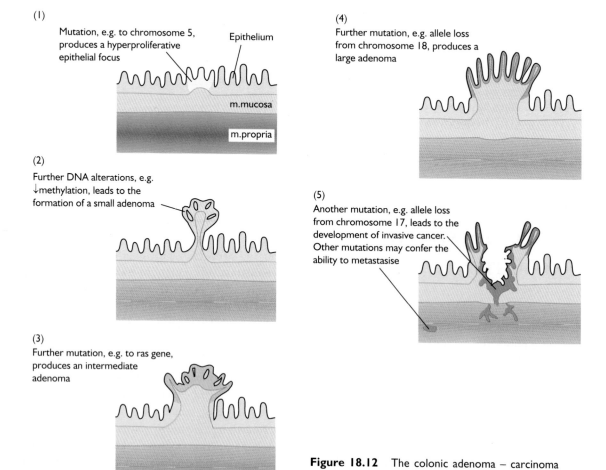

(1)
Mutation, e.g. to chromosome 5, produces a hyperproliferative epithelial focus

Epithelium

m.mucosa

m.propria

(2)
Further DNA alterations, e.g. ↓methylation, leads to the formation of a small adenoma

(3)
Further mutation, e.g. to ras gene, produces an intermediate adenoma

(4)
Further mutation, e.g. allele loss from chromosome 18, produces a large adenoma

(5)
Another mutation, e.g. allele loss from chromosome 17, leads to the development of invasive cancer. Other mutations may confer the ability to metastasise

Figure 18.12 The colonic adenoma – carcinoma sequence

to look for the mutations in the mismatch repair genes.

Table 18.2 lists some of the tumours that show a familial predisposition.

APOPTOSIS AND CANCER

Apoptosis or programmed cell death has been covered in Chapter 12. We have already seen how apoptosis is an important part of the differentiation pathway for many cells. Apart from showing increased proliferation, cancer cells also fail to undergo apoptosis and hence have an increased life span compared with normal cells. The inability of cancer cells to commit suicide is an important contributory factor to tumour growth, both at the primary site and at the sites of metastatic spread. When normal cells are damaged, for example by radiation, there is activation of a series of genetic programmes to promote cell death. This is an important protective mechanism since cells with damaged DNA are prevented from replicating and transmitting the genetic mutations to the daughter cells. In tumours, this protective mechanism is lost by mutations within genes involved in the apoptotic pathway. Two important genes involved in apoptosis are the *TP53* and *bcl2* genes.

MULTISTEP MODEL OF CARCINOGENESIS

In the course of examining malignant tissues, histopathologists frequently encounter lesions that show transitions with appearances half way between normal morphology and frank malignancy. Such lesions are occasionally closely associated with the invasive cancer. This has led to the suggestion that many of these lesions may be precursors of the invasive carcinoma. With the identification of dominant oncogenes and tumour suppressor genes, it became possible to investigate tumours and putative precursor lesions using molecular techniques. The study of colorectal carcinoma with its well-defined preinvasive lesion, the adenoma, has paved the way for this type of investigation (Figure 18.11). The results demonstrate that both activating and inactivating events are involved, and it is the coordinated involvement of both these types of alteration that are important in colon tumour formation. Furthermore, it is not just the timing of the events but the sequential accumulation of genetic damage that is also important in tumour formation. This idea that it is not one event but a sequence of genetic alterations that produces tumours is referred to as the **multistep theory of neoplasia**.

This brings us to the end of this section on the cellular events involved in producing the cancer cell. Of course, we have a long way to go before we have a full understanding, but our knowledge is advancing at an exciting pace, and a whole new language of tumour terminology is emerging. For the scientist, the battle is the biology; for the clinicians and students trying to understand and apply the new knowledge, it is often the terminology!

The next question we need to address, and one that will be in the forefront of the patient's mind, is, how will a given tumour behave?

CHAPTER *19*

THE BEHAVIOUR OF TUMOURS

- Growth of tumours
- How do tumours spread?
- Role of the immune system

The behaviour of a tumour can be considered under a number of headings covering how fast it will grow, whether it is likely to metastasise, which sites are affected and what symptoms and complications the patient is likely to suffer.

GROWTH OF TUMOURS

It is often assumed that tumours grow faster than normal tissues because they expand to compress the surrounding structures. However, this does not mean that the cells are dividing more often but that there is an **imbalance between production and loss**. The time taken for tumour cell division varies between 20 and 60 hours, leukaemias having shorter cell cycles than solid tumours, but, in general, tumour cells take *longer* than their normal counterparts. Cells can be in a resting phase or in growth phase, i.e. in one of the stages of mitosis. Some normal tissues, such as the intestine, have a high turnover of cells, where around 16 per cent of the cells will be in the growth fraction. In contrast, most tumours have only 2–8 per cent of their cells actively dividing. This is important

therapeutically because the cells in the growth phase are most readily damaged by chemotherapy, so tumours with a large growth fraction (e.g. leukaemias, lymphomas and lung anaplastic small cell carcinoma) will respond better than tumours with few cells proliferating (e.g. colon and breast).

Can we predict how fast a tumour is growing? To some extent, yes. The number of mitotic figures present per unit area in a light microscopic section is a crude measure of how active the proliferation is within a tumour. A tumour with a large number of cells in mitosis is likely to behave aggressively, which is why a mitotic count is one of the criteria for grading tumours (see p. 235). However, the number of cells seen to be in mitosis is influenced not only by the growth fraction and the cell cycle time but also by whether they get 'stuck'; i.e. the tumour cell can enter mitosis but, possibly because of an irregularity in chromosome number or in the internal organisation of the mitotic spindle, may fail to complete the mitosis. Thus, on the examination of a tissue section, the tumour appears to be highly proliferative, but it is really 'stuck'. Tumour growth will also be influenced by factors such as the blood supply and, possibly, the host's immune response (see p. 271).

It would also be wrong to assume that every cell in a tumour behaves similarly. The daughter cells of a dividing cell are identical genetically to the parent cell and are said to be a **clone**. However, tumour cells are also prone to developing genetic instability, which results in some cells developing further abnormalities, hence resulting in the formation of multiple **subclones**. These may have certain survival advantages; for example, they may have enhanced angiogenic, invasive or metastatic capabilities. This is referred to as **tumour hetero-geneity**, and it is important to consider when planning treatments because it means that some tumour cells may respond differently to particular chemotherapeutic agents. This is somewhat analogous to bacterial resistance to antibiotics. Just as a combination of antibiotics is most effective against an unknown organism, so a mixture of treatment modalities is often used against a tumour.

HOW DO TUMOURS SPREAD?

Just over a hundred years ago, Stephen Paget (not the man who described Paget's disease – that was Sir James Paget) collected the post mortem records of 735 patients who had died of breast cancer and found that the majority of the metastases were in the liver and brain. He concluded therefore that certain tumours were predisposed to metastasise to certain tissues. He wrote, 'When a plant goes to seed, its seeds are carried in all directions; but they can only live and grow if they fall on congenial soil'. Not surprisingly, it came to be known as the 'seed and soil' theory.

James Ewing, 40 years later, suggested that tumours went to particular organs not because of the seed and soil effect but because of the routes of blood supply to the primary organ. Using his hypothesis, organs directly in line away from the primary site would be targets for metastatic disease.

We know now that they are both partially correct. Tumours of the colon do indeed go to the liver, which is next in line through the portal circu-

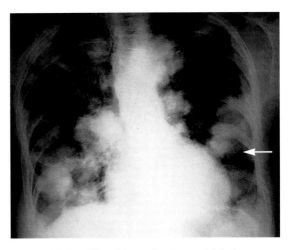

Figure 19.1 Chest X-ray showing multiple 'cannon ball' metastases

lation, but then so do many other tumours much farther away, such as melanomas arising in the eye. We also know that organs such as the heart and skeletal muscle, despite being exposed to large volumes of blood, rarely develop metastases. In broad terms, tumour spread through lymphatics will produce metastases in the anatomically related lymph nodes, while spread through the blood is influenced more by 'seed and soil' considerations, although anatomy is still of some importance.

The main **routes of spread** are via the:

* lymphatics
* veins
* transcoelomic cavities
* cerebrospinal fluid
* arteries.

Lymphatic spread is common in carcinomas (tumours of epithelia), and the nodes that are involved first are the nodes that drain the tumour site. Thus a knowledge of lymphatic anatomy is useful for predicting where the tumour will spread and is the basis for many of the staging protocols (see p. 237). However, lymph nodes near tumours can enlarge as part of an immune reaction that particularly results in the expansion of the macrophage compartment (sinus histiocytosis). This means that the doctor must try to distinguish between soft, mobile nodes, which are likely to be reactive, and the hard, fixed nodes that contain metastatic tumour.

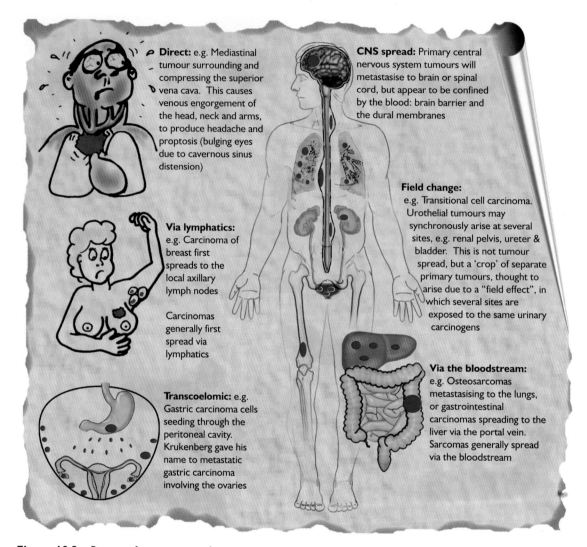

Direct: e.g. Mediastinal tumour surrounding and compressing the superior vena cava. This causes venous engorgement of the head, neck and arms, to produce headache and proptosis (bulging eyes due to cavernous sinus distension)

Via lymphatics: e.g. Carcinoma of breast first spreads to the local axillary lymph nodes

Carcinomas generally first spread via lymphatics

Transcoelomic: e.g. Gastric carcinoma cells seeding through the peritoneal cavity. Krukenberg gave his name to metastatic gastric carcinoma involving the ovaries

CNS spread: Primary central nervous system tumours will metastasise to brain or spinal cord, but appear to be confined by the blood: brain barrier and the dural membranes

Field change: e.g. Transitional cell carcinoma. Urothelial tumours may synchronously arise at several sites, e.g. renal pelvis, ureter & bladder. This is not tumour spread, but a 'crop' of separate primary tumours, thought to arise due to a "field effect", in which several sites are exposed to the same urinary carcinogens

Via the bloodstream: e.g. Osteosarcomas metastasising to the lungs, or gastrointestinal carcinomas spreading to the liver via the portal vein. Sarcomas generally spread via the bloodstream

Figure 19.2 Routes of tumour spread

Venous spread will take tumours of the gastrointestinal tract to the **liver** and tumours from a variety of sites to the **lungs**. It is also the favoured route of spread for **sarcomas** (tumours of connective tissue). Some tumours may even grow along a vein, causing its obstruction – for example renal cell carcinoma in the renal vein.

Arteries are not often penetrated by tumours, but, in the later stages of metastatic spread, tumour nodules can start to develop almost anywhere, and it is likely that this happens after pulmonary metastases enter the pulmonary vein and are then distributed through the systemic arterial system.

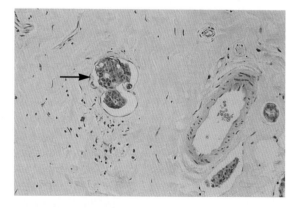

Figure 19.3 Photomicrograph of breast with lymphatic permeation by tumour

It is easy to understand how tumours that reach the pleural or peritoneal cavities can drop into the fluid and be disseminated throughout that **coelomic cavity**. Similarly, the **CSF** provides an easy route of spread for cerebral tumours, which do not generally metastasise outside the central nervous system.

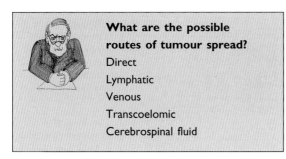

What are the possible routes of tumour spread?
Direct
Lymphatic
Venous
Transcoelomic
Cerebrospinal fluid

One cubic centimetre of tumour can shed millions of cells into the circulation each day – so why are metastases not inevitable? Let us consider the steps required to produce metastases.

First, the tumour has to grow at the primary site and infiltrate the surrounding connective tissue, which may necessitate breaking through a basement membrane and the connective tissues nearby. It may also have to overcome inhibitor substances to the enzymes it produces to break down these connective tissue proteins. Then it can reach the lymphatic and blood vascular channels, which are an important route for dissemination. It has to find a way of attaching to the endothelium and subsequently entering the channels. The vessel wall is traversed, and the tumour cells must detach to float in the blood or lymph and hope to evade any immune cells that might destroy them. Next they must lodge in the capillaries at their destination, attach to the endothelium again and penetrate the vessel wall to enter the perivascular connective tissue, where they finally proliferate to produce a tumour deposit.

What stands between the primary tumour and the vessel? First, there is a variety of extracellular matrix components to break through, for which the tumour may produce a number of enzymes. Loose connective tissue is not much of a barrier, but dense fibrous areas, such as tendons and joint capsules and cartilage, can resist tumour spread. Next is the basement membrane so that the tumour has to be able to secrete a type IV collagenase. Tumours often have collagenases to dissolve collagen but are less able to digest elastic tissue. This may be one of the reasons why arterial walls, which contain much elastic, are less readily penetrated than venous walls. Alternatively, it may be because arterial walls are thicker and contain protease inhibitors. Once in the vessel lumen, tumour cells are prey to immune surveillance by the body's lymphocytes and monocytes. Finally, the tumour must attach to the endothelium at its destination, which may involve specific adhesion molecules (addressins) that 'home' the metastatic tumour to a particular site, analogous to the 'homing' of lymphocytes (see p. 25).

Most of our discussions about tumour cell biology have concentrated on how genetic changes enhance cell proliferation. However, we should now look at how a proliferating tumour cell differs from a proliferating normal cell. Early experiments involving *in vitro* cell cultures demonstrated that normal cells would grow to form monolayers and then stop. This was referred to as contact inhibition. If some cells from this culture were transferred to a new culture vessel (passaged), they would begin to grow again in the same way; however, normal cells would only survive about 30–50 serial passages. Cultures of proliferating tumour cells differed in that they lost contact inhibition, so could grow as disorganised multilayers, and were also immortal, i.e. although each individual cell did not last forever, the clone of cells could be passaged indefinitely. It is now known that tumour cells may show decreased expression of E-cadherin, which normally acts as an adhesion molecule between epithelial cells, and that their increased motility may be influenced by an **autocrine motility factor**, which some transformed culture cells release. Tumour cells can also influence the production of stroma so that **tenascin** may predominate, which does not bind readily to tumour cells. This sort of information suggests not only that it is changes in the tumour cells that produces local invasion and metastasis but that

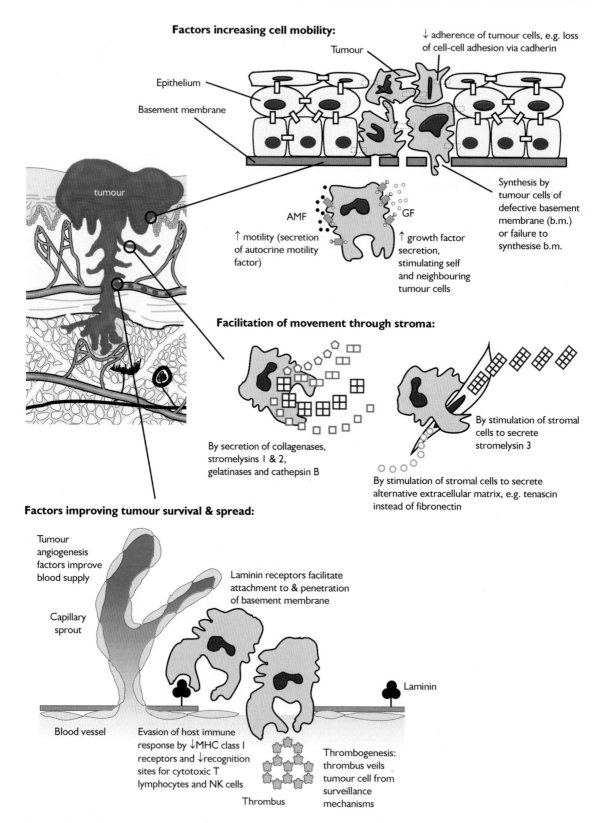

Factors increasing cell mobility:

Tumour

↓ adherence of tumour cells, e.g. loss of cell-cell adhesion via cadherin

Epithelium

Basement membrane

Synthesis by tumour cells of defective basement membrane (b.m.) or failure to synthesise b.m.

tumour

AMF

GF

↑ motility (secretion of autocrine motility factor)

↑ growth factor secretion, stimulating self and neighbouring tumour cells

Facilitation of movement through stroma:

By secretion of collagenases, stromelysins 1 & 2, gelatinases and cathepsin B

By stimulation of stromal cells to secrete stromelysin 3

By stimulation of stromal cells to secrete alternative extracellular matrix, e.g. tenascin instead of fibronectin

Factors improving tumour survival & spread:

Tumour angiogenesis factors improve blood supply

Laminin receptors facilitate attachment to & penetration of basement membrane

Capillary sprout

Laminin

Blood vessel

Evasion of host immune response by ↓MHC class I receptors and ↓recognition sites for cytotoxic T lymphocytes and NK cells

Thrombogenesis: thrombus veils tumour cell from surveillance mechanisms

Thrombus

Figure 19.4 Mechanisms of tumour cell invasion and metastasis

interactions between tumour cells, normal cells and stroma are also important.

ROLE OF THE IMMUNE SYSTEM

We are all aware of the role played by the immune system in defending us against infections, so it is not surprising that questions have been raised of whether it has any role in protection against cancer. It was Paul Ehrlich, in 1909, who postulated that, without the immune system constantly removing the 'aberrant germs', human beings would inevitably die of cancer. Many attempts were made to establish the role of the immune system in cancer, and initial experiments, which transplanted tumours from one animal to another, appeared to support the concept. It was later realised that the destruction of these transplanted tumours was a result not of immunity but of transplant rejection. Now inbred mice can be used experimentally, thus avoiding the factor of transplant rejection. In certain tumours, it has been shown that, if the tumour is removed from a mouse and the animal rechallenged with the tumour, the tumour is rejected. This supports the idea that immunity is involved in tumour rejection, but life is not quite so simple, as we shall see.

You will recall that the cells of the immune system have to be able to distinguish between 'self' and 'non-self' by identifying specific antigens on the cell surface. Malignant tumours are derived from 'self', so if the immune system is to defend against tumours, the malignant cells must acquire antigens that differentiate them from normal cells. These are termed tumour-specific antigens (TSAs), and the whole subject has been highly controversial. In man, such tumour-associated antigens are beginning to be defined, including differentiation antigens (e.g. CD19 and CD29), growth factor receptors such as epidermal growth factor receptor (EGFR) and intracellular proteins such as the MAGE family of proteins, which are highly expressed in melanoma. These antigens have been identified by isolating tumour-reactive T cells from patients with malignancies. While tumours clearly do elicit immune responses, the degree of response does not appear to be sufficient to hold the progression of the malignancy in most cases. It is conceivable that, as tumours progress, clones of cells without the antigens proliferate and escape immune destruction. A whole new area of cancer vaccine is developing rapidly, and initial trials appear encouraging. Vaccination with ganglioside GM2 in melanoma appears to increase survival; however, time will tell whether the effects of immunisation live up to the promise suggested by initial trials.

There is also evidence from animal experiments that surface antigens are altered in some tumours induced by viruses or chemicals. Virally induced tumours in animals can display a new surface antigen (T), which is believed to be a viral peptide associated with the major histocompatibility complex (MHC). This provokes a specific cytotoxic T cell response, and all tumours induced by a particular virus display the same antigen, regardless of the cell of origin. The obvious potential application for this lies in immunising against tumours.

Chemically induced tumours in animals (e.g. by benzopyrene) may also display new surface antigens that induce a specific immune response, but these antigens are very varied, with primary tumours in the same animal exhibiting antigenic differences, so there is no cross-resistance through immunisation.

Of course, the immune response need not be antigen specific. Besides B and T lymphocytes, the body has at its disposal **natural killer (NK) cells** and **macrophages**. NK cells have the capacity to destroy cells without prior sensitisation as well as the ability to participate in antibody-dependent cellular cytotoxicity (ADCC). Macrophages are also involved, either because of non-specific activation or in collaboration with T lymphocytes, and can participate via ADCC or by the release of cytotoxic factors, such as TNF, hydrogen peroxide and a cytolytic protease.

CHAPTER 20

THE CLINICAL EFFECTS OF TUMOURS

- Local effects
- Endocrine effects
- Paraneoplastic syndromes
- General effects
- Management of cancer

LOCAL EFFECTS

The local effects depend on the site of the tumour, the type of tumour and its growth pattern. Some complications, such as haemorrhage, are more common in malignant tumours because of their ability to invade underlying tissues and their vessels, but it must be remembered that even a microscopically benign tumour (e.g. a meningioma on the surface of the brain) can kill the patient because of its local effects.

Local effects can complicate both benign and malignant tumours. They include:

- compression
- obstruction
- ulceration
- haemorrhage
- rupture
- perforation
- infarction.

COMPRESSION AND OBSTRUCTION

A patient with any intracranial tumour (e.g. meningioma, astrocytoma or oligodendroglioma) may present with headaches, nausea and vomiting because the mass growing within the closed cavity of the cranium raises the intracranial pressure. If the tumour is not removed and the pressure continues to rise, the patient will die from pressure effects on the vital respiratory centres.

A more localised example of the effect of compression is when the pituitary gland enlarges in the small cup-shaped space of the sella turcica. Local pressure will cause erosion of the bony sella and compression of the optic chiasma that sits directly above. The patient will then present with visual disturbance, classically a bitemporal hemianopia.

Compression and obstruction have been included in the same section because there is often an overlap. Compression can directly damage

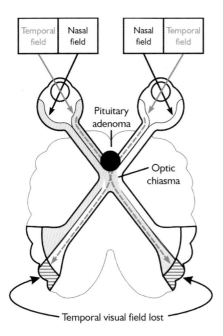

Compression of the optic chiasma by a benign pituitary adenoma damages the optic nerve fibres serving the temporal visual fields, resulting in bitemporal hemianopia

Figure 20.1 Tumour effects: compression

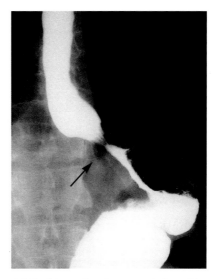

Figure 20.2 X-ray showing constriction of lower oesophagus by oesophageal carcinoma

normal tissue, see Figure 20.1, or it may cause obstruction. This occurs, for example, when a tracheal tumour obstructs a normal oesophagus or vice versa. In the brain, compression of the brainstem structures may obstruct the flow of CSF, and a large prostate (benign or malignant) may compress the prostatic urethra. Alternatively, a tumour can grow into the lumen of the gut or into an airway so that it produces obstruction directly.

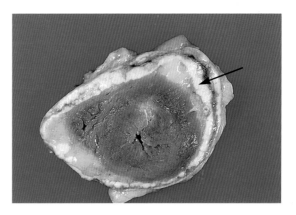

Figure 20.3 Compression of cardiac ventricles by metastatic lung carcinoma infiltrating the pericardium

ULCERATION AND HAEMORRHAGE

An ulcer is defined as a macroscopically apparent loss of surface epithelium and may be benign or malignant. Ulceration of the skin will lead to a crust of dried fibrin and cells covering the area and is unlikely to produce severe haemorrhage. However, ulceration in the gastrointestinal tract, particularly the stomach and duodenum, may result in life-threatening haemorrhage or perforation. Here, the absence of epithelium means the

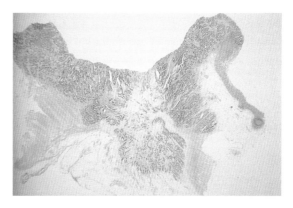

Figure 20.4 Microscopical picture showing rectal ulceration due to adenocarcinoma

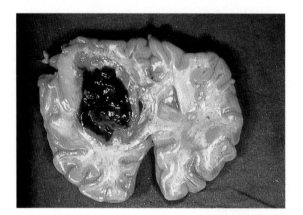

Figure 20.5 Haemorrhage within intracerebral tumour

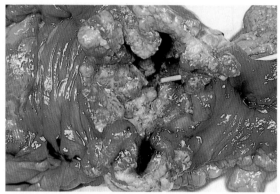

Figure 20.6 Colonic carcinoma with perforation indicated by probe

loss of an important defence mechanism that normally protects the underlying tissue from acid and enzymes. Once the submucosa is exposed to these agents, large vessel walls can be digested, resulting in massive bleeding.

RUPTURE OR PERFORATION

Rupture or perforation typically affects tumours of the gastrointestinal tract and will occur if the intraluminal pressure exceeds the strength of the wall or if the wall is eroded or weakened by tumour, ischaemia, enzymic action, etc. There is obviously a risk of dilatation and rupture when part of the gut becomes obstructed as the gut contents cannot follow their normal route. Rupture may also occur in closed organs, such as the ovary, because the tumour has stretched the capsule, often because of accumulation of fluid or mucin as well as the proliferation of neoplastic cells.

INFARCTION

Many malignant tumours will show necrosis and infarction in their central region, which is believed to result from inadequate blood supply. In experimental models, a tumour can only expand to a diameter of 1–2 mm before it must stimulate new

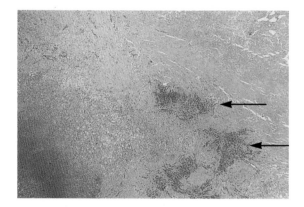

Figure 20.7 Extensive infarction in tumour, leaving small islands of viable cells

blood vessel formation, and, in human tumours, zones of necrosis may be encountered approximately 1–2 mm from a blood vessel. It therefore appears that this is the maximum distance for the diffusion of nutrients. Tumours attempt to solve this by secreting **angiogenic factors** that stimulate capillaries to grow into the neoplasm.

Local anatomy influences the likelihood of infarction related to large vessel obstruction. The bowel, ovaries and testes are particularly liable to **torsion**, i.e. twisting on their vascular pedicle, which occludes the vessels.

Although we often separate the complications of tumours under the headings of local tumour and metastatic tumour, a metastasis can produce any of the local effects mentioned above. In particular, lymph nodes containing metastases can cause obstruction at crucial sites, such as the porta hepatis or the hilum of the lung.

ENDOCRINE EFFECTS

Well-differentiated tumours not only look like their tissues of origin but can also act like them. Thus tumours of endocrine organs can produce hormones that act on the same tissues as their physiological counterparts but are not under normal feedback control.

Cushing's syndrome provides an interesting example of different endocrine tumours producing the same clinical problems. In Cushing's syndrome, the patient suffers from osteoporosis, muscle wasting, thinning of the skin with purple striae and easy bruising, truncal obesity and impaired glucose tolerance. All this is the result of excess glucocorticoids. The same picture can be produced by the prolonged administration of steroids to treat diseases (e.g. chronic asthma), but in this section we are interested in the tumours that can cause it.

The adrenal produces corticosteroids when stimulated by adrenocorticotrophic hormone (ACTH) from the pituitary. The corticosteroids then provide negative feedback to the pituitary, and ACTH levels drop. Cushing's syndrome can result from an adenoma in the pituitary gland, which produces ACTH, or a cortical tumour in the adrenal cortex, which secretes corticosteroids. Normal feedback does not operate as the adenoma cells behave autonomously. However, if very high doses of steroid (dexamethasone suppression test) are given, the pituitary adenoma will reduce its ACTH production and endogenous steroid levels will fall, but excess steroid due to an adrenal adenoma will not be suppressed.

Some non-endocrine tumours can produce substances that have the same effects as hormones – so-called inappropriate production. One of the most common results is Cushing's syndrome when ACTH is produced by oat cell (anaplastic small cell) carcinoma of the bronchus, carcinoid tumours, thymomas or medullary carcinoma of the thyroid. This inappropriate and autonomous production cannot be suppressed with high doses of dexamethasone.

PARANEOPLASTIC SYNDROMES

This refers to symptoms in cancer patients that are not readily explained by local or metastatic disease. Endocrine effects are generally included as a paraneoplastic syndrome if the production is inappropriate (as above) but not if the tumour arises from a tissue that normally produces that hormone.

Hypercalcaemia is a common, clinically important and complex problem with malignant tumours. In a patient with widespread metastases in bone, it may be explained as a local destructive effect of the tumour on bone that releases calcium. However, hypercalcaemia can also occur without metastatic bony deposits, and, in some cases, it appears that a parathyroid hormone-like peptide or TGF-α is secreted by the primary tumour; this is most likely with bronchial squamous cell carcinoma and adult T cell leukaemia/lymphoma.

Clubbing of the fingers and hypertrophic osteoarthropathy are also common with lung carcinoma but can occur in non-neoplastic conditions including cyanotic heart disease and liver disease. It is not clear how it develops nor why sectioning the vagus nerve can lead to its disappearance. Equally mysterious are the skin disor-

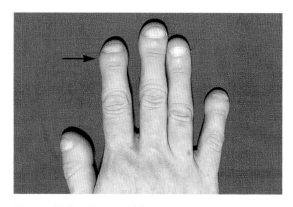

Figure 20.8 Finger clubbing

ders, peripheral neuropathy and cerebellar degeneration that may also occur in association with malignant tumours.

GENERAL EFFECTS

The **general effects** of tumours are not classed as paraneoplastic syndromes, although they are extremely common and must not be forgotten. These include general malaise, weight loss and lethargy, which are due to a combination of metabolic and hormonal influences exacerbated by any malnutrition or infection. This results in the clinical picture known as 'cachexia'. An important chemical factor that may play a role in cachexia is **cachexin**, which is also known as **tumour necrosis factor (TNF)**. This molecule is produced not by the tumour cells but by activated macrophages.

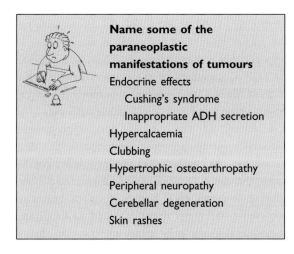

Name some of the paraneoplastic manifestations of tumours
Endocrine effects
    Cushing's syndrome
    Inappropriate ADH secretion
Hypercalcaemia
Clubbing
Hypertrophic osteoarthropathy
Peripheral neuropathy
Cerebellar degeneration
Skin rashes

Anaemia is also common and can contribute to the general malaise. This may be a direct effect of metastatic deposits in bone marrow or an indirect effect of mediators that suppress haemopoiesis.

MANAGEMENT OF CANCER

We will discuss this under individual headings. However, many patients receive a combination of treatment regimens.

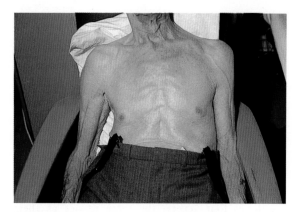

Figure 20.9   Cancer-related muscle wasting (cachexia)

LOCAL EXCISION

Local treatment is aimed either at achieving a cure or providing specific symptomatic relief. Cancers such as squamous and basal cell carcinomas of the skin and cancers arising within polyps in the colon can be cured by local excision. In tumours of the bowel, local excision may relieve an obstruction and provide a good long-term remission of symptoms or even cure.

RADIOTHERAPY

Radiotherapy can be given from an external source or by implanting a small radioactive source into the tissues. Delivery schedules vary from centre to centre, but the general idea is to divide, or fractionate, the doses in order to get the maximum kill of tumour cells with the minimum damage to normal tissues. Implanted radioactive sources are very useful for providing high-dose local radiation and are of particular benefit in cancers of the head and neck, where there are many vital structures close together.

CHEMOTHERAPY

Chemotherapy is a relatively new and rapidly evolving form of treatment. In patients suffering from haematological malignancies (e.g. leukaemia) or disseminated disease, surgery and radiation are not realistic options. You cannot excise a leukaemia, and you cannot irradiate metastases that are widespread in the body.

In the 1950s alkylating agents (e.g. busulphan) and antimetabolites (e.g. methotrexate) were introduced and proved helpful in the management of disseminated cancers. The main problem with such agents is that all of the body's normal tissues are also exposed to the drug, so the challenge is to deliver enough drug to kill the tumour without killing the patient! The mode of action of some chemotherapeutic agents is discussed in Part 3.

ENDOCRINE-RELATED TREATMENT

This often involves giving a drug that inhibits tumour growth by removing an endocrine stimulus. For example, many breast carcinomas have receptors for oestrogen that stimulate tumour growth. A drug such as tamoxifen will block these receptors and reduce progression of the disease. An alternative approach would be to remove the ovaries, which produce oestrogen, much as the testes can be removed in males with prostatic adenocarcinoma to reduce the stimulus for tumour growth from androgens.

IMMUNOTHERAPY

DNA recombinant technology has enabled the production of cytotoxins in sufficient quantities for therapeutic use. The interferons (IFNs) and tumour necrosis factors (TNFs) are of particular interest. IFN-α and IFN-β have been used to treat a variety of tumours with some good effect, although it appears that they may best be used in combination with other treatments. Renal carcinomas, melanomas and myelomas have shown a 10–15 per cent response, various lymphomas a 40 per cent and hairy cell leukaemia and mycosis fungoides an 80–90 per cent response rate. TNF-α has been used in the treatment of melanoma, although the response to date has been disap-

pointing. Lymphokine-activated killer (LAK) cells are a subset of NK cells that have been used in combination with IL-2 to treat renal carcinomas and some melanomas and colorectal cancers.

As previously mentioned, attempts at producing specific tumour antigens is in progress, and initial trials of vaccination seem encouraging. There is also considerable interest in raising monoclonal antibodies to tumour cells. The hope is that it might be possible to attach drugs to these antibodies so that they will be delivered specifically to the tumour cell – the concept of the 'magic bullet'. Many questions remain unanswered, but the field of immunisation and targeted treatment is bound to create excitement over the next decade.

PALLIATIVE TREATMENT

The treatment of cancer has a wider role than merely providing a cure, and cancer physicians are not interested in simply achieving a response to the administered treatment. Palliative treatment does not just refer to treatment that is given to patients in order to make them comfortable prior to death. It is and should be part of the oncological support given to all cancer patients, not only including medication for the control of pain and nausea but also chemotherapy and radiotherapy for the relief of local symptoms. The term 'continuing care' is sometimes used for this multidisciplinary approach, starting with diagnosis and extending to the patient's death. The important point is that our knowledge of all modalities of treatment, including pain control, has advanced considerably in recent years, and the pessimistic view that if one has cancer one must pass one's last hours either conscious but in agony, or pain-free but unconscious, is no longer justified.

In conclusion, science, like most aspects of life, has its fashions. Much of this chapter has concentrated on our evolving understanding of the role of the genetic code in producing cancer. Current fashion lies very much with the identification and cloning of genes that cause a familial predisposition to malignancy. Recently, two breast cancer predispo-

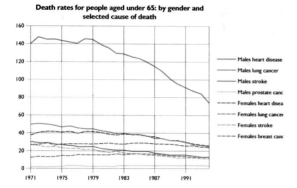

Figure 20.10 Death rates for people aged under 65, by gender and selected cause of death. (Data from Social Trends 1996, the Office for National Statistics, Crown copyright)

sition genes called *BRCA1* and *BRCA2* have been cloned. Both these genes are large, and mutations in almost every part of the gene have been identified in patients with cancer. This has highlighted many ethical and social implications of genetic testing for cancer susceptibility. It has brought to the forefront the financial considerations as private organisations fight for patency rights for genetic sequences. Millions of pounds and dollars have been invested in the search; billions will be reaped in screening tests.

FURTHER READING

Cooper, G.M. 1997: Cancer. In *The Cell. A Molecular Approach*. Washington: ASM Press, Ch. 15.

Cotran, R.S., Kumar, V., Robbins, S.L. 1994: Neoplasia. In *Robbins' Pathologic Basis of Disease*, 5th edn. Philadelphia: W.B. Saunders, Ch. 7.

Neal, A., Hoskins, P. 1994: *Clinical Oncology. A Textbook for Students*. London: Edward Arnold.

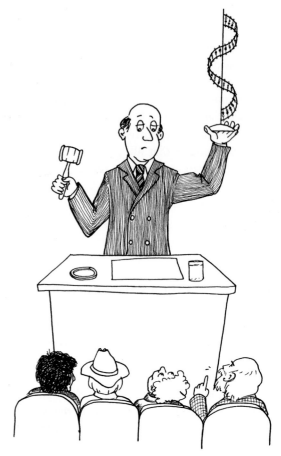

Figure 20.11 'Shall we start the bidding for Lot 1 ... a 200 kb segment from the short arm of chromosome 13. This is believed to incorporate the gene for eternal youth, the ultimate anti-oncogene and the anti-baldness gene ... shall we say £5 billion?'

Scientific American 1996: What you need to know about Cancer, Sept.

Underwood, J.C.E. 1996: Carcinogenesis and neoplasia. In *General and Systemic Pathology*, 2nd edn. Edinburgh: Churchill Livingstone, Ch. 11.

CLINICOPATHOLOGICAL CASE STUDY

Clinical

A 38-year-old lady came to the surgery for a cervical smear.

She was single and had been living with her boyfriend for the past 6 months. She divorced her husband 2 years before and since then had had a number of casual relationships. Her first sexual contact was at the age of 16.

Four years ago, her smear showed warty change, and the last one, 1 year ago, again showed extensive warty change with possible dyskaryosis. The hospital had asked for a repeat smear as the epithelial cells were obscured by inflammatory debris.

Pathology

Carcinoma of the cervix is an important cause of death, and the cervical screening programme has been instituted to try to reduce this toll. The idea is that, if the disease can be picked up at an early stage, it should be possible to cure it.

The risk factors for cervical cancer include: smoking, early onset of sexual intercourse, multiple sexual partners, a sexual partner with a history of promiscuity and infection with the human papilloma virus (HPV). Her history reveals that she had a number of risk factors, including wart virus change on her previous cervical smears.

She initially ignored the recall due to social problems.

The normal routine recall for cervical smears is 3 years, but early recall is instituted for suspicious or abnormal smears.

The result of the repeat smear showed warty change and severe dyskaryosis and she was referred for a colposcopic biopsy.

The cervical biopsy confirmed the above findings and she was booked in to have a cervical cone biopsy.

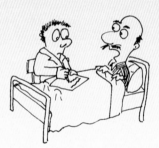

Severe dyskaryosis is the cytological equivalent of severe dysplasia on histological examination.

Dysplasia is a premalignant condition in which there are cytological features of malignancy, i.e. increased nuclear:cytoplasmic ratio, nuclear pleomorphism, hyperchromatism, loss of maturation and mitotic activity. Dysplasia can be graded into mild, moderate and severe. Severe dysplasia implies a full-thickness abnormality, the feature distinguishing this from carcinoma being the presence of invasion through the basement membrane. Metaplasia, on the other hand, is entirely benign. It is a form of adaptation to injury in which one type of epithelium is replaced by another. In the cervix, the glandular epithelium, after repeated bouts of inflammation, changes to a more resistant squamous epithelium.

The results of the cone biopsy came as a shock. The report read that she had extensive squamous metaplasia with wart virus change, together with severe dysplasia between 3 and 5 o'clock and a focus of invasive squamous cell carcinoma, which was completely excised. Invasive tumour did not involve deep tissues or invade blood vessels. The dysplastic epithelium extended to the endocervical excision margin and was therefore not completely excised.

The cone biopsy is a way of performing a local excision of the cervix; the tissue removed is in the form of a cone. A suture is usually put at 12 o'clock to orientate the specimen. The role of the pathologist is to map the abnormal areas, to assess the abnormality in terms of severity and to comment on the completeness of excision.

The report was discussed with the patient and she was advised to have a hysterectomy.

She was 38, and still capable of having children. The decision to have a hysterectomy can be a difficult one, although she had very little choice.

The examination of the hysterectomy specimen showed residual foci of severe dysplasia but no invasive carcinoma. The excision was complete, and she was discharged after an uneventful recovery.

The hysterectomy specimen did not reveal any more areas of carcinoma and the single focus of carcinoma was completely excised, so she should be cured.

PART 5

GENES AND DISEASE

CHAPTER *21*

OVERVIEW OF GENETICS

- Mendel and his peas
- Clinical case – Turner syndrome

> 'In considering the Origin of Species, it is quite conceivable that a naturalist, reflecting on the mutual affinities of organic beings, on their embryological relations, their geographical distribution, geological succession, and other such facts, might come to the conclusion that each species had not been independently created, but had descended, like varieties from other species.'
>
> *Charles Darwin*

SHE	HAD	ONE	MAD	CAT	AND	ONE	SAD	RAT
SHE	HAD	ONE	BAD	CAT	AND	ONE	SAD	RAT
THE	MAD	BAD	CAT	ATE	THE	ONE	SAD	RAT
THE	MAD	SHE	CAT	ATE	THE	ONE	SAD	RAT
THE	MAD	HEC	ATA	TET	HEO	NES	ADR	AT

It is a common misconception among medical students that pathology is an exact science. It is sometimes difficult to see why the examination of tissues at post mortem, both grossly and micro-scopically, cannot give a precise answer. Yet a short time in a laboratory will reveal that the terms 'possibility' and 'probability' are well known to the pathologist. If you encounter a patient with metastatic tumour in the liver, it is *possible* that the primary tumour may have arisen in the nose, but it is much more *probable* that it arose in the colon. The study of genetics involves appreciating how the inheritance of genes produces diseases so that the *probability* of a particular individual developing a disease can be calculated.

Most of us take our existence for granted, but life really is a source of constant wonder, and it has occurred against probability. Let us begin when there was no life on earth. At some stage, molecules must have come into existence that were capable of self-replication, and these molecules multiplied. If you have two molecules – one that manages to replicate and make copies without any mistakes, the other making many mistakes each time it is copied – the correctly copied molecule is more likely to increase in number. Ironically, the molecule that copies perfectly will never change, and it will still be the same molecule after 1 year, after 50 years and after a billion years. If a random mistake happens in the copying, there is the oppor-tunity for change – possibly for the better, proba-bly for worse. This is the basis for evolution recognised by Darwin in 1838. The other impor-tant factor is that there should be a 'struggle for

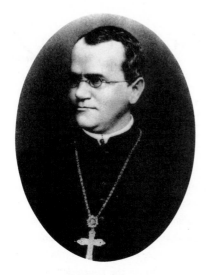

Figure 21.1 Gregor Mendel was born in Heizendorff, Moravia, on 22 July 1822. He joined the Augustine order in 1843 and, 10 years later, after studies at the University of Vienna, he went to the monastery at Brunn. His famous work with the peas began in 1856, but it was not until 1865 that he communicated the results to the Brunn Society of Natural Science. They remained in the archives until they were discovered in 1900, 35 years after publication, by three botanists pursuing a similar path. Mendel died in 1884. (Courtesy of the Wellcome Institute for the History of Medicine)

survival', an evolutionary pressure that gives an advantage to the molecules or animals best adapted to the prevailing conditions.

MENDEL AND HIS PEAS

The probability of inheriting characteristics from parents was studied by Gregor Mendel. Mendel took garden peas with contrasting characteristics, seven to be exact, and bred from the plants that differed in only one characteristic. For the sake of discussion, let us consider violet and white flowers. He crossed plants with violet flowers with those bearing white flowers to produce the next generation, called the F1 generation. He found that the F1 generation plants all had the same colour flowers. Let us say that they were all violet. The

F1 plants were then self-pollinated (inbred) to produce the next generation, called F2. Interestingly, there were three plants with violet flowers for every one plant with white flowers. He took this process one step further and self-pollinated the white plants, which gave rise to an F3 generation of plants that all had white flowers. Self-pollination of the violet plants produced an intriguing result: some plants produced only violet plants, while others produced a mixture of white and violet plants in the ratio of 1:3 (Figure 21.2).

As Mendel correctly deduced, although the violet plants in the F2 generation all looked the same, they had different inheritance factors. He postulated that each plant must possess two factors that determine a given characteristic, such as colour of the flower. If two plants are crossed, each will contribute one factor to the next generation, and it is purely random which factor is passed on. This is the **law of segregation**, also known as Mendel's first law. We now know that these 'factors' are genes on chromosomes that are paired, the two genes on the two chromosomes being **alleles** of each other. In Mendel's experiment, violet is the **dominant** allele and white the **recessive** one. The F1 generation has one white plant, which is **homozygous** for the white allele, one violet plant that is homozygous for the violet allele, and two violet plants that are **heterozygous**, i.e. they have one white and one violet allele, the violet one dominating.

In simple examples like this, one allele dominates; i.e. if the plant has at least one violet allele, all the flowers will be violet. Sometimes the situation is more complicated as there will be **variable penetrance**, i.e. the 'dominant' allele only dominates in a percentage of cases.

It was later appreciated by Morgan (1934) that cell differentiation might depend on variation in the action of genes in different cell types. In the later part of the nineteenth century, DNA, RNA and histones were discovered, and it was originally believed that the histone proteins were genes. However, in 1944 Avery, MacLeod and McCarty recognised that DNA was the structural component of the gene. In 1953 Watson and Crick elucidated the double helical structure of DNA that provides the basis for its ability to replicate.

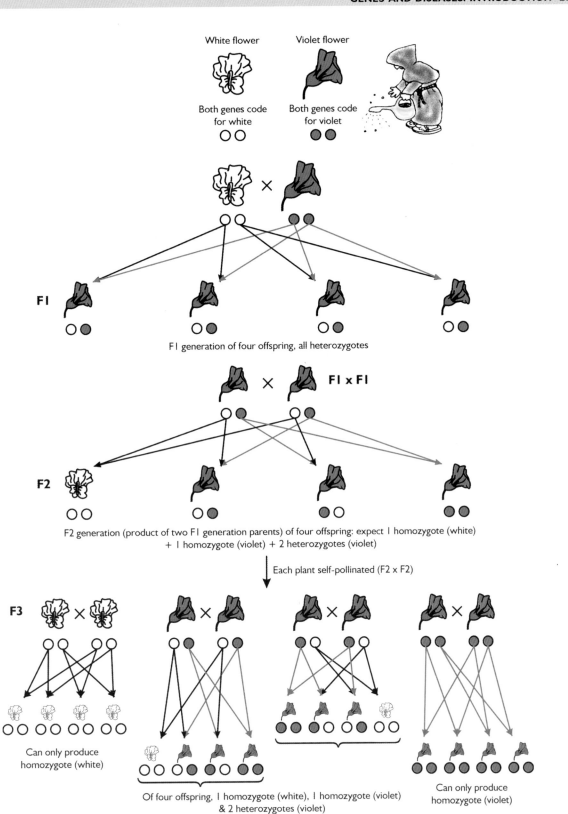

Figure 21.2 Mendelian inheritance

Name:	Fetus of A. Smith
Consultant:	Mr. I.M. Obs
Date of operation:	12.5.97
Gestation:	20 weeks

External examination

The body was that of a female fetus, and external measurements were consistent with a gestation of 18 weeks. There was generalised subcutaneous oedema, and a cystic hygroma (benign cystic tumour of lymphatic vessels) was noted in the posterior aspect of the neck. The placenta was pale and bulky.

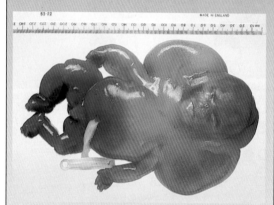

Figure 21.3 Hydropic fetus at 18 weeks – Turner syndrome (Courtesy of R. Scott, UCLMS)

Internal examination

The organ weights were consistent with a gestation of 18 weeks. The main abnormality was in the cardiovascular system. The left ventricle was small and the aorta proximal to the ductus arteriosus was narrowed – a severe infantile coarctation.

Special investigations

Placental tissue was sent for cytogenetic analysis. Chromososmal analysis revealed the karyotype 45,X confirming a monosomy X – i.e. Turner syndrome.

Obstetrics forms a major part of the medical curriculum, and during your training, you will meet pregnant women who are naturally concerned about their unborn baby. Let us briefly consider a clinical scenario to illustrate a possible problem you might encounter.

CLINICAL CASE – TURNER SYNDROME

A 34-year-old lady was seen in the antenatal clinic complaining of abdominal pain and 'spotting' of blood. This was her first pregnancy, and examination revealed a uterus of approximately 20 weeks size. The gestation should have been 22 weeks according to her estimated date of delivery. The doctor failed to hear a fetal heart sound and arranged an ultrasound scan of her abdomen. This revealed an intrauterine death, and evacuation of the fetus was carried out.

PATHOLOGICAL EXAMINATION

Post mortem examination of the aborted fetus was carried out to elucidate the cause. The report is illustrated on the left.

In the following chapters, we will consider some of the questions you may be faced with; after all, you will need to be able to answer them!

- What are the risks of having an abnormal baby?
- How soon can any abnormality be detected?
- What are the most common genetic diseases?
- How are they caused?
- Are all inherited abnormalities apparent in infancy?
- Can genes change after birth?

CHAPTER 22

WHAT ARE THE RISKS OF HAVING AN ABNORMAL BABY?

- Family history
- Maternal age
- Infections and environmental hazards during pregnancy

FAMILY HISTORY

Here, we are concerned principally with inherited diseases, so any family history of abnormality will be important. The problem is to decide which of the enormous range of diseases result from a genetic abnormality that can be transmitted to the offspring. This requires careful observation of the incidence of a disease in the general population and within a family group. Many disorders are, however, multifactorial in nature, both genetic predisposition and environmental agents influencing the outcome. We have already encountered this in our discussion on breast cancer in Part 4. In many cancers, there is an increased risk in close relatives, but, at least in the antenatal clinic, the main concern will be non-neoplastic conditions that are known to be inherited in a Mendelian fashion. Although many of these conditions are rare, over 4000 separate types have been identified.

We will illustrate the importance of family history by considering the example of sickle cell disease.

SICKLE CELL DISEASE

Patients with this recessive haemoglobin disorder may present clinically with abdominal pain, joint pains, cerebral symptoms, renal failure and cardiac failure, which result from thrombotic and ischaemic damage. This occurs because the red cells 'sickle', thus altering their shape and occlud-

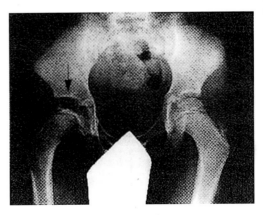

Figure 22.1 Pelvic X-ray with avascular necrosis of the right femoral head in a patient with sickle cell disease

ing capillaries. The red cells have an abnormal haemoglobin that, under hypoxic conditions, polymerises and alters the cell's shape.

In 1949 Pauling analysed the haemoglobin from patients with sickle cell anaemia and discovered that its mobility on electrophoresis differed from that of normal haemoglobin. He called it haemoglobin S (HbS). Later, family studies suggested that the gene for sickle cell haemoglobin was an allele of the normal gene on chromosome 11 for the beta chain of the haemoglobin molecule, i.e., an alternative gene at the same locus on the chromosome. The difference between the normal haemoglobin gene and the sickle cell gene is a change in one base pair: GAG becomes GTG. This causes valine to replace glutamic acid in position 6 of the beta chain. That's it – a **point mutation** changing just one nucleotide leads to the translation of one different amino acid, which entirely changes the property of the protein.

Fortunately, genes are paired, and people who are heterozygous (i.e. have one normal allele and one sickle cell allele) do not usually have any problems unless they become unusually hypoxic (e.g. at surgical operation). They have a mixture of the normal and abnormal haemoglobin.

For practical purposes, we can regard sickle cell disease as an **autosomal recessive** disorder. How should we counsel a healthy pregnant woman who has a family history of sickle cell disease? The problem lies in deciding which members of the family are carriers of the gene because two people with sickle cell trait (heterozygotes) are likely to produce one healthy child, one sick child and two carriers.

Carriers of the sickle cell gene can be identified by adding a reducing agent to the blood *in vitro*,

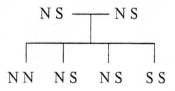

Figure 22.2 Possible outcomes of the offspring of two people with sickle cell trait. N = normal gene; S = sickle cell gene

which induces the red cells to sickle. More recently, techniques have been developed to analyse the DNA itself. This is particularly useful in prenatal diagnosis for testing the fetus before it has switched on to full production of the beta chains. It is not possible to detect the abnormal beta chains in fetal red blood cells because the fetus is relying on haemoglobin produced from alpha and gamma chains, i.e. HbF. However, it is possible to remove a small piece of placenta (chorionic villus sampling) for DNA analysis, relying on the point mutation to alter the binding of specific oligonucleotide probes or interfere with restriction enzyme digestion (see below).

How did sickle cell disease arise?

Let us digress to consider the evolutionary aspects of sickle cell disease. If two hypothetical parents with sickle cell trait have four children, one should die before being able to reproduce. That child will be homozygous for the abnormal gene, and so we might expect the incidence of that gene to reduce in the population because of its disadvantage for survival. However, the gene has not died out but is very common in areas where malaria is endemic. This suggests that the sickle cell carriers have a survival advantage in malaria-infected areas. How would this operate? Let us consider the life cycle of malaria.

The malarial parasite has to transfer from a mosquito into a human's blood stream and then invade the red blood cells to complete its reproductive cycle. The infected red cell has a lower oxygen tension, so, if the patient has sickle cell trait (i.e. some HbS), the cell will collapse and the parasite will die.

The fascinating thing is that when this mutation first appeared in one gene, the corresponding allele would have been normal and the patient would have a 'perfect' genetic combination that protected against malaria and left the person in good health. As the survival of these patients was enhanced, so was the spread of this new gene as carriers of the allele married each other and passed it on to their offspring. Some unfortunate children received double doses of the allele (one from each parent) and hence developed full-blown sickle cell disease. The geographical distribution of sickle cell disease, not surprisingly, correlates with the distribution of malaria, after allowing for the effects of emigration.

Sickle cell trait is not the only method that evolution has devised for defending against malaria. There are other haemoglobinopathies, such as thalassaemia, that provide protection or conditions where the red cell surface markers necessary for entry of the parasite are altered.

MATERNAL AGE

There is a dramatic increase in the number of chromosomally abnormal fetuses in women over the age of 35 years. This produces a wide variety of disorders, the most common being trisomy 21 or Down syndrome.

People with **Down syndrome** are mentally retarded and may have congenital heart disease and an increased incidence of infections and leukaemia. In 1959 Lejeune and his colleagues showed that these patients have an extra chromosome 21. This most commonly arises because of **non-disjunction** of chromosome 21 during meiosis in one of the parents, so that either the egg or the sperm carries two copies of chromosome 21. In about 5 per cent of cases, there is a translocation of chromosome 21 to 14 and occasionally translocations of chromosome 21 to chromosome 22, or of 21 to 21.

A **translocation** is the transfer of part of one chromosome to another. Translocations occur because the repair mechanism for breakages in the chromosomes can join the wrong pieces together. If this results in pieces of chromosomal material being exchanged between chromosomes with no loss of genetic material, or joining of one entire chromosome with another, the individual is said to have a **balanced translocation**. The person is generally clinically normal. However, the genes are only 'balanced' in diploid cells, and the haploid gametes will have an abnormal amount of the translocated segment. Therefore, sperm or ova

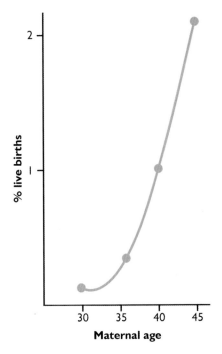

Figure 22.3   Incidence of Down syndrome with increasing maternal age

from individuals with balanced translocations have a high risk of subsequently producing an abnormal child. For Down syndrome, the risk is 10 per cent when the mother is the carrier of the translocation and 2.5 per cent if the father is the carrier. It is obviously important to investigate the parents of children with such inherited disorders to look for balanced translocations, although non-disjunction is the most common cause.

About half of all fetuses affected by Down syndrome do not survive to term. The incidence in live births is 1 in 650, but that is an average figure for all ages. The risk at maternal age 30 is 1 in 900, which doubles by age 35, stands at 1 in 100 at age 40 and 1 in 40 at age 44. This age distribution makes it sensible to screen women over 35 years by examining chromosomes cultured from amniotic cells and measuring α-fetoprotein levels, which are *lowered* in Down syndrome. (N.B. They are *raised* in many other abnormalities, e.g. neural tube defects.) The purpose of screening is twofold. First, it allows the parents to undergo genetic counselling, and second, it offers the possibility of

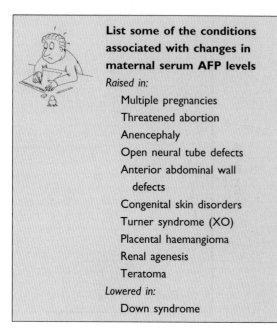

List some of the conditions associated with changes in maternal serum AFP levels

Raised in:

    Multiple pregnancies

    Threatened abortion

    Anencephaly

    Open neural tube defects

    Anterior abdominal wall defects

    Congenital skin disorders

    Turner syndrome (XO)

    Placental haemangioma

    Renal agenesis

    Teratoma

Lowered in:

    Down syndrome

Table 22.1 Consequences of intrauterine infection

Agent	Effects
Rubella	Cataracts, retinopathy, mental retardation, deafness, cardiac defects
Cytomegalovirus	Growth failure, microcephaly, mental retardation, deafness
Toxoplasmosis	Hydrocephalus, microcephaly, chorioretinitis, mental retardation

termination of the pregnancy. The latter option may or may not be taken up by the family. You will realise that, since termination of pregnancy is an option, there may be distortion of the incidence of live births quoted above.

INFECTIONS AND ENVIRONMENTAL HAZARDS DURING PREGNANCY

Infections during the first trimester may cause intrauterine death or a variety of abnormalities (Table 22.1).

Important infections include rubella, cytomegalovirus (CMV) infection, syphilis and toxoplasmosis. Rubella and syphilis are routinely screened for in

Name some of the organisms that may cause intrauterine infection

Rubella

Cytomegalovirus (CMV)

Treponema pallidum – syphilis

Toxoplasma gondii

HIV

Plasmodium – malaria

Chickenpox (*Varicella zoster*)

Hepatitis B

Listeria

Note: Not all agents that cause intrauterine infection lead to malformations. Rubella, CMV, toxoplasmosis, syphilis and chickenpox do; listeria, hepatitis B and malaria do not. There is, to date, no information that HIV causes malformation

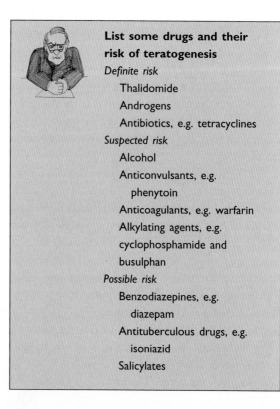

List some drugs and their risk of teratogenesis

Definite risk

    Thalidomide

    Androgens

    Antibiotics, e.g. tetracyclines

Suspected risk

    Alcohol

    Anticonvulsants, e.g. phenytoin

    Anticoagulants, e.g. warfarin

    Alkylating agents, e.g. cyclophosphamide and busulphan

Possible risk

    Benzodiazepines, e.g. diazepam

    Antituberculous drugs, e.g. isoniazid

    Salicylates

the population. Although toxoplasmosis is a serious infection during pregnancy, it does not appear to be a significant problem within the UK. Women of childbearing age may be at risk when they travel to high-risk areas such as North Africa and are exposed for the first time as adults. Environmental hazards, such as radiation, industrial chemicals, alcohol and tobacco, may retard growth and predispose to spontaneous abortion. Generally, neither infections nor environmental agents induce transmissible changes in the parent's genome, so there is no risk of recurrence providing that the agent is not encountered in future pregnancies.

Thalidomide, a drug that was given to pregnant women to prevent nausea and vomiting, resulted in developmental defects such as limb deformity. There has recently been a suggestion that children born to victims of Thalidomide have defects similar to those of their parents, implying that the drug has indeed produced a transmissible defect in the genome. It remains to be proved whether this is indeed the case. Stilboestrol is another agent that has been implicated in the development of genital malformations and malignancies in children born to mothers exposed to the drug.

CHAPTER 23

HOW SOON CAN ABNORMALITY BE DETECTED?

- Non-invasive tests
- Invasive procedures
- Methods of genetic analysis

NON-INVASIVE TESTS

Fortunately, the majority of pregnancies progress without any problems to produce a normal healthy baby after approximately 40 weeks' gestation. It would be unreasonable to subject all pregnant women to the stress and possible hazards of the many investigations that are available to detect fetal abnormalities. Instead, it is sensible to make only simple observations on those women who are expected to have a trouble-free pregnancy. These include recording the increase in body weight, assessing the size of the uterus at each visit as an indicator of fetal growth, listening to the fetal heart and enquiring about fetal movements.

In recent years, the quality of **ultrasound scanning** has achieved a standard that makes it useful for detecting internal and external fetal malformations as well as giving accurate information on the rate of fetal growth through head circumference and body length measurements. In practice, early ultrasound (at 8–10 weeks) can be used to date the pregnancy and identify anencephaly. Spina bifida can be identified on ultrasound after 16 weeks' gestation and the scan is usually carried out between 17 and 20 weeks.

The tests mentioned so far are non-invasive and no risks have been identified to either mother or baby.

INVASIVE PROCEDURES

There are also invasive tests, one of the simplest of which is to measure the **mother's serum α-fetoprotein (AFP)** concentration. Ultrasound is very good at picking up neural tube defects, so the AFP test is useful mainly for small defects that are missed. It is measured at about 16–18 weeks' gestation and will be raised in 90 per cent of mothers bearing children with open neural tube defects and 95 per cent of anencephalic cases. This obviously means that 5–10% of cases will remain undetected, so it is essential to offer more sensitive techniques to mothers at particularly high risk. AFP is also increased in multiple pregnancies, threatened abortions and a variety of fetal malformations. Its level is lowered in Down syndrome.

Screening for fetal well-being has developed rapidly over the past decade, and many centres use a 'triple test' for Down syndrome. This includes AFP, human choriogonadotrophic hormone (hCG) and oestriol. Such screening tests are particularly useful in detecting Down syndrome in younger women who do not have any particular risk factors for fetal abnormalities.

Amniocentesis can be performed between 15 and 16 weeks' gestation and involves removing about 20 ml amniotic fluid, which contains small numbers of amniotic cells that can be cultured. The fluid can be tested for AFP and acetylcholinesterase activity to detect neural tube defects or more specialised tests can be employed for detecting rare inborn errors of metabolism. The cells are cultured and used for karyotypic (chromosome) analysis.

Fetoscopy, which involves introducing a scope into the amniotic cavity, has also been used to perform fetal blood sampling and for therapeutic procedures such as intrauterine transfusion. It does have the risk of inducing an abortion.

METHODS OF GENETIC ANALYSIS

CYTOGENETICS

The human nucleus contains 23 pairs of chromosomes: 22 pairs of autosomes and one pair of sex chromosomes. It has been apparent for some time that certain diseases are associated with specific chromosomal abnormalities, and it is logical to divide these into those affecting the *autosomal chromosomes* and those affecting the *sex chromosomes*. As we shall see, these groups can also be divided into those affecting the *number* of chromosomes and those affecting their *structure*.

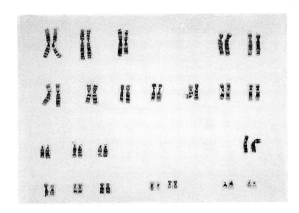

Figure 23.1   Normal female karyotype

Disorders affecting the number of chromosomes are most commonly **aneuploid**; i.e. the chromosome number is not an exact multiple of the haploid set. This may involve extra chromosomes or the loss of chromosomes. Structural changes to individual chromosomes can be deletions, inversions, duplications, translocations, ring chromosomes or fragile sites (Fig. 23.2).

Chromosomal analysis is most commonly performed on cells from the skin, bone marrow or peripheral blood in postnatal life, but, prenatally, cultured amniotic cells or samples of chorionic villi can be used. Colchicine is added to arrest the cells in metaphase, and hypotonic saline causes the cells to swell and disperse the chromosomes. Analysis involves staining the chromosomes to show up the bands as alternating light and dark areas and then photographing them under a light microscope. The photographs of the chromosomes are cut up and the chromosomes rearranged in pairs. This simple method allows identification of the individual chromosomes and will reveal gross changes, such as loss or addition of a whole or large part of a chromosome.

At metaphase, the two chromatids of each chromosome are joined by a centromere, the long arm being termed 'q' and the short arm 'p'. There is a convention for reporting karyotypes so that the total number of chromosomes is given first, followed by the sex chromosomes. Examples are illustrated in Table 23.1.

The child with mosaicism (see Table 23.1) has two genetically different cell types distributed in its

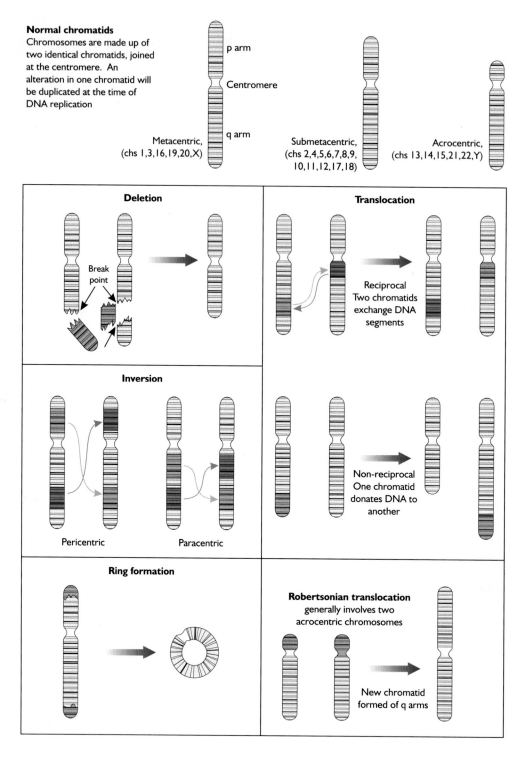

Figure 23.2   Structural chromosomal abnormalities

Table 23.1 Examples of karyotypes

46XY	Normal male
46XX	Normal female
47XXY	Male with Klinefelter's syndrome

If there is a change in chromosomal number, the affected chromosome is indicated with a + or −, e.g.:

47XX +21	Female with Down syndrome

If there is a structural rearrangement, the karyotype indicates the precise site affected and the nature of the abnormality, e.g.:

46XX del 7 (p13–ptr)	Deletion of the short arm of chromosome 7 at band 13 to the end of the chromosome
46XY t (11;14) (p15.4;q22.3)	A translocation between chromosome 11 and 14 with the break points being band 15.4 on the short arm of chromosome 11 and band 22.3 on the long arm of chromosome 14

Mosaicism indicates that two different cell lines have derived from one fertilised egg and the karyotype specifies both cell lines:

46XX/47XX + 21	Down mosaic
46XX/45X	Turner mosaic

tissues. These are not distributed evenly, and some affected individuals may demonstrate only a normal phenotype in their peripheral blood lymphocytes. It may therefore be necessary to culture from other organs, such as the skin, to confirm a suspected abnormality. Patients with mosaicism are generally less severely affected than those with the full disorder. This makes prenatal counselling difficult if mosaicism is detected in a fetus as the clinical effects could be mild. There is also the complication that any mosaicism detected in chorionic villus samples may only indicate an abnormal genotype in some placental cells, and the fetus need not be affected.

 Mosaicism: the presence of two or more cell lines that are both karyotypically and genotypically distinct but are derived from the same zygote

Chorionic villus sampling has some advantages over amniocentesis in that it can be performed between 8 and 12 weeks' gestation so that a diagnosis can often be made by 12–14 weeks' gestation, when termination is easier. It also provides material suitable for DNA analysis, which is necessary when the genetic changes are too small to be seen on light microscopic chromosomal preparations. It does however, carry a greater risk of miscarriage.

FLUORESCENCE *IN SITU* HYBRIDISATION

Recent advances in molecular biology have led to novel technologies for the assessment of chromosomes and genes. One such technique is fluorescence *in situ* hybridisation (FISH). This technique has been used extensively in research as well as in clinical diagnosis.

The idea behind the technique is very simple. DNA probes labelled with fluorescence dyes are hybridised to the chromosomes to reveal their structure and number. 'Whole chromosome painting' is used to identify structural abnormalities, while probes specifically aimed at the centromeres of the chromosomes are used to identify chromosome numbers. More recently, a further level of sophistication has been added by labelling the probes with different dyes and hence performing a multicoloured FISH. This allows the detection of multiple genetic alterations within the same chromosomal spread. Another advantage of this method is that, unlike classical karyotyping, it can also be used on interphase nuclei. This is particularly important for diagnosis in certain tumour types, e.g. leukaemias, in which metaphase chromosomal spreads are difficult to obtain.

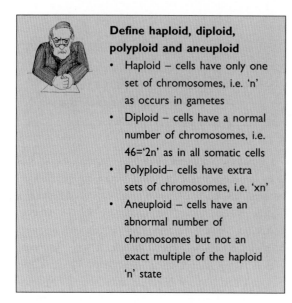

Define haploid, diploid, polyploid and aneuploid

- Haploid – cells have only one set of chromosomes, i.e. 'n' as occurs in gametes
- Diploid – cells have a normal number of chromosomes, i.e. 46='2n' as in all somatic cells
- Polyploid– cells have extra sets of chromosomes, i.e. 'xn'
- Aneuploid – cells have an abnormal number of chromosomes but not an exact multiple of the haploid 'n' state

Comparative genomic hybridisation (CGH) is yet another adaptation of the FISH technique, which allows a global view of DNA copy number changes within a single hybridisation. This has opened up avenues not only in tumour research but also in assessing genetic alterations in a clinical setting.

DNA ANALYSIS

First, let us remind ourselves of some basic facts about DNA (deoxyribonucleic acid). DNA consists of two antiparallel strands that have a backbone of deoxyribose sugars from which project **purine** and **pyrimidine** bases. The sequence of these bases determines the genetic code. It is estimated that there are approximately 6 billion bases in the human genome. The purine bases are adenine (A) and guanine (G), and the pyrimidine bases are cytosine (C) and thymine (T). The two strands form a right-handed double helix with about 10 nucleotide pairs per helical turn. They are linked through these purine and pyrimidine bases, G always pairing with C and A with T. This point is fundamental to the use of probes for analysing DNA.

The binding of complementary purine and pyrimidine bases also allows DNA to act as a

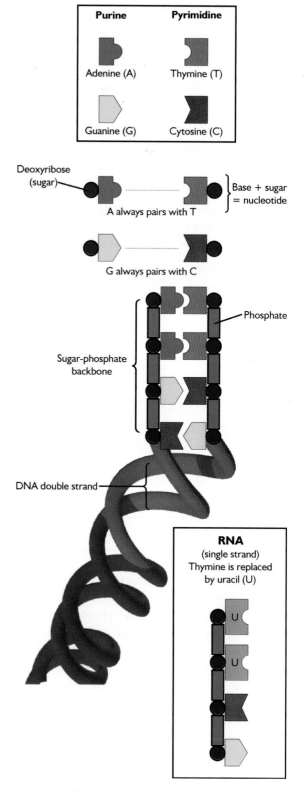

Figure 23.3 DNA – the bases

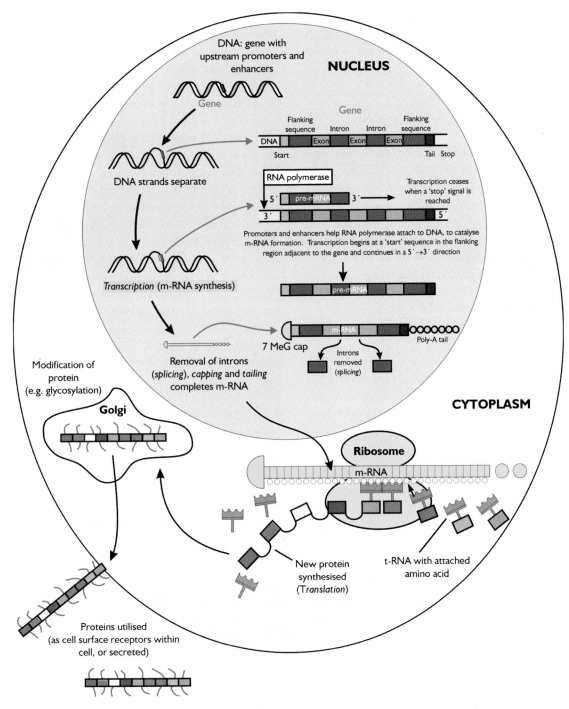

Figure 23.4 Gene expression

template for the production of mRNA. This process is called **transcription**. The mRNA moves to the cytoplasm, attaches to a ribosome and is then used for protein production. This is termed **translation** and involves the binding of transfer RNA (tRNA) carrying a specific amino acid. The amino acids then combine to form a polypeptide chain and are released (Figure 23.4). RNA differs from DNA in three respects: it is a single-stranded molecule, it contains ribose sugar instead of deoxyribose, and the base thymine (T) is substituted by uracil (U).

Restriction fragment length analysis

There have been two major advances that have made DNA analysis possible: the ability to cut DNA and the ability to sort the resulting fragments. Certain bacteria can produce enzymes that are capable of cutting DNA at specific sites and only at those sites. These enzymes are called **restriction endonucleases**, and the DNA fragments are known as **restriction fragments**. Different bacteria produce enzymes that cut DNA at different sites. How is this useful in diagnosis? If you consider the sentence below, there are two identical sentences.

> The capacity to blunder slightly is the real marvel of DNA; without this special attribute, we would still be anaerobic bacteria and there would be no music.

> The capacity to blunder slightly is the real marvel of DNA; without this special attribute, we would still be anaerobic bacteria and there would be no music.

One has been cut whenever a 'be' appears and the other whenever 'is' appears. You can see that the fragments produced are of different lengths. In the first case, there are three fragments, the smallest comprising 'no music'. In the second case, there are two large fragments.

The same principle applies to the endonucleases. Once fragments of different sizes are produced, they are run on an electrophoretic strip, which separates the fragments according to their size, and are then 'stained' with a DNA probe. The details of these electrophoretic methods are not important; suffice it to say that the method used for DNA fragments is called **Southern blotting**, after its inventor, and the corresponding technique for RNA is **Northern blotting**. The technique for the

analysis of proteins is called **Western blotting**. There is no Eastern blotting! The binding of the probe to its complementary sequence is called **hybridization**. The **DNA probes** or **oligonucleotides** are short lengths of DNA whose nucleotide sequence is known. These are labelled, for example with a radioactive element, so that their position on an electrophoretic strip can be identified by autoradiography. Their importance lies in their ability to bind only to a specific section of the patient's DNA, i.e. to a piece with an identical sequence of complementary bases.

The restriction endonuclease technique can be used for detecting heterozygous and homozygous carriers of the sickle cell gene, which, as we mentioned above, is due to a point mutation changing GAG to GTG. There is a restriction enzyme called *MstII* that recognises the area including GAG in the normal genome and will digest the DNA at this point. As Figure 23.5 shows, those with the normal gene will produce a fragment 1.15 kb long, while those with the abnormal gene will not digest at that position and the fragment will be longer.

To 'stain' these on a strip requires a probe that will bind anywhere on this fragment. It is more common now in practice to look for the sickle cell gene by the polymerase chain reaction (see p. 300).

This use of restriction endonucleases relies on the enzyme digesting at exactly the point that mutates to cause the disease. Often, we do not know the precise mutation responsible for an inherited disease, but it may be possible to identify which section of DNA it is in by comparing the DNA of affected family members with that of healthy family members. The human genome has approximately 6 billion bases, so how do we start looking for differences?

We can look for **restriction fragment length polymorphisms (RFLPs)**. These are variations in DNA fragment length that can be produced by using a restriction endonuclease and probe appropriate for detecting a particular disease. For example, the DNA from family members with Huntington's disease has been investigated with an enormous range of enzymes and probes. It was discovered that digestion with an enzyme called

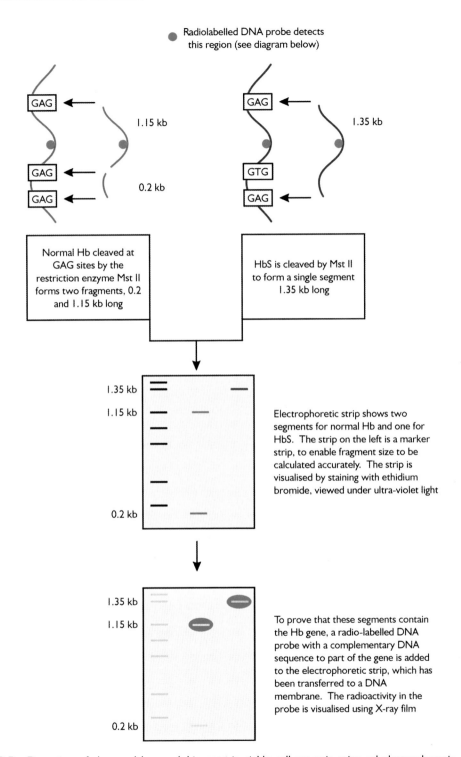

Radiolabelled DNA probe detects this region (see diagram below)

GAG   1.15 kb

GAG   0.2 kb

GAG

GAG   1.35 kb

GTG

GAG

Normal Hb cleaved at GAG sites by the restriction enzyme Mst II forms two fragments, 0.2 and 1.15 kb long

HbS is cleaved by Mst II to form a single segment 1.35 kb long

1.35 kb
1.15 kb

0.2 kb

Electrophoretic strip shows two segments for normal Hb and one for HbS. The strip on the left is a marker strip, to enable fragment size to be calculated accurately. The strip is visualised by staining with ethidium bromide, viewed under ultra-violet light

1.35 kb
1.15 kb

0.2 kb

To prove that these segments contain the Hb gene, a radio-labelled DNA probe with a complementary DNA sequence to part of the gene is added to the electrophoretic strip, which has been transferred to a DNA membrane. The radioactivity in the probe is visualised using X-ray film

Figure 23.5 Detection of abnormal haemoglobin gene in sickle cell anaemia using gel electrophoresis

Hind III, combined with hybridisation with a probe called G8, identified variations in the short arm of chromosome 4 that segregated with the disease. What is the principle behind this technique? It relies on variations in the genetic code that influence restriction endonuclease diges-

Discuss the techniques used for antenatal investigation and their risk to the fetus

Method	Use	Risk	Performed in
Ultrasound	Structural abnormalities	Safe	2nd trimester
Maternal blood sample: AFP, hCG, oestriol	Neural tube defect	Safe	2nd trimester
	Down syndrome		
Amniocentesis	Chromosomal analysis	0.5%	2nd trimester
	Biochemical analysis: AFP		
Chorionic villus sampling	DNA analysis	2%	1st trimester
	Chromosomal analysis		
	Biochemical analysis		
Fetoscopy	Fetal material sampling	3%	2nd trimester
	Direct examination		

tion but do not cause any clinical problems. We have already seen that a change of just one base causes sickle cell disease, so why do other common mutations have no effect? It is because only about 10 per cent of DNA codes for proteins, while the rest has no clearly defined function. The coding regions (structural genes) are fairly constant from person to person, and mutations in these regions generally cause disorders. The non-coding regions can vary from person to person, and this diversity is useful for producing the 'DNA fingerprint'.

If a mutation has occurred in a non-coding region that is fairly close to the gene responsible for a disease, it will be inherited with the disease gene. Obviously, the same mutation must not have occurred near to the normal gene or no difference will be detected. Provided that an enzyme exists that digests at the altered non-coding area, the disease gene can be tracked. There is the inevitable problem of new mutations or cross-over of chromosomal material that might 'unlink' the mutant non-coding region from the disease gene, but this technique is useful for counselling families for future pregnancies *after* an affected child has been born.

So far, we have only mentioned the use of oligonucleotide probes as 'stains' for the altered fragment produced by restriction endonuclease digestion. They can also be used on DNA without digestion to demonstrate **deletions** that are too small to see on light microscopic chromosomal preparations. Haemophilia A, Duchenne muscular dystrophy, alpha thalassaemia and some cases of beta thalassaemia can be detected in this way.

Their most sophisticated use, however, is for 'staining' the gene that causes the disease. Provided that the same genetic change is always responsible for the disease, this approach can be used without the need for family studies. In sickle cell disease, an oligonucleotide probe has been produced that detects the normal beta-globin gene sequence, and another probe detects the mutant sickle gene. Each probe binds only to its specific complementary nucleotide sequence, so the 'normal' probe binds to the normal gene, the 'sickle' probe binds to the mutant gene and, in heterozygous people, both probes will bind – one to each chromosome 11. How do the oligonucleotide probe sequences differ? Since we know that sickle cell disease involves a change from GAG to GTG, then the probes must be:

normal probe   xxxxxx CTC xxxxxx
sickle probe   xxxxxx CAC xxxxxx

Polymerase chain reaction

One of the problems of analysing DNA by the means so far described is that a relatively large amount of material is required. An ingenious technique that harnesses DNA's normal role – to act as a template for producing complementary

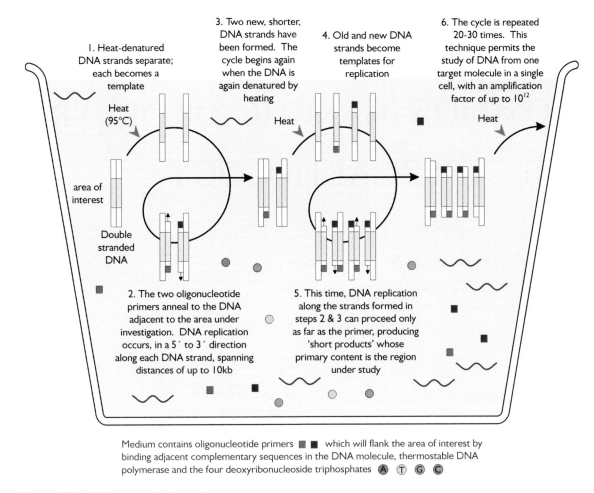

1. Heat-denatured DNA strands separate; each becomes a template

Heat (95°C)

area of interest

Double stranded DNA

3. Two new, shorter, DNA strands have been formed. The cycle begins again when the DNA is again denatured by heating

Heat

4. Old and new DNA strands become templates for replication

Heat

6. The cycle is repeated 20-30 times. This technique permits the study of DNA from one target molecule in a single cell, with an amplification factor of up to 10^{12}

Heat

2. The two oligonucleotide primers anneal to the DNA adjacent to the area under investigation. DNA replication occurs, in a 5′ to 3′ direction along each DNA strand, spanning distances of up to 10kb

5. This time, DNA replication along the strands formed in steps 2 & 3 can proceed only as far as the primer, producing 'short products' whose primary content is the region under study

Medium contains oligonucleotide primers ■ ■ which will flank the area of interest by binding adjacent complementary sequences in the DNA molecule, thermostable DNA polymerase and the four deoxyribonucleoside triphosphates Ⓐ Ⓣ Ⓖ Ⓒ

Figure 23.6 Polymerase chain reaction

DNA or RNA strands – has been developed. It is called the **polymerase chain reaction** (**PCR**). It is without doubt one of the most significant technological advances of the last decade. The method involves amplifying a specific segment of DNA through successive rounds of replication (Figure 23.6).

This amplified segment, which must contain the area suspected of containing the mutant code, is then cut with the appropriate restriction enzyme and run on an electrophoretic agarose gel. It is not necessary to use a specific probe to stain the digested fragments because it is the relevant area that has been amplified. Instead, the DNA bands themselves can be viewed under ultraviolet light after staining with ethidium bromide. This is much faster than using autoradiography and can provide a result within 2 days of taking the sample. PCR is also used in forensic work to produce the well-known 'DNA fingerprint' from small samples of blood, semen or hair left at the scene of the crime.

CHAPTER 24

COMMON GENETIC DISORDERS AND THEIR AETIOLOGY

- Incidence
- How does the genetic abnormality produce disease?
- How does the genetic abnormality arise?

INCIDENCE

Table 24.1 lists the incidence per 1000 live births of the most common genetic disorders. It is helpful to subdivide them into **single gene disorders**, which will be inherited in a Mendelian fashion, and **chromosomal disorders**.

There are several points to highlight. The first is that the incidence quoted in Table 24.1 relates to live births, which means that genetic abnormalities causing intrauterine death will be underreported. This principally influences the figures for the chromosomal abnormalities, as their incidence in spontaneous abortions and stillbirths is 50 per cent, whereas the incidence in live births is 6.5 per 1000. In spontaneous abortions with chromosomal abnormalities, around 50 per cent will have a trisomy, 18 per cent will be Turner syndrome (XO) and 17 per cent will be triploid.

The most common condition is X-linked red–green colour blindness, which, fortunately, is only a very minor handicap (and is not an excuse for avoiding histology sessions!). **Klinefelter's syndrome** is due to an extra X chromosome in males (47,XXY). Affected individuals are generally of normal intelligence and are tall, with hypogonadism and infertility. **XYY syndrome** also produces tall males. They may have behavioural problems, especially impulsive behaviour.

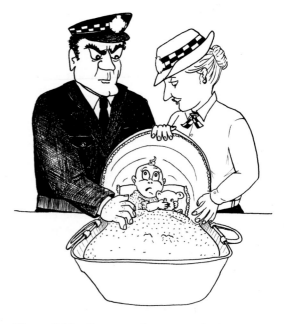

Figure 24.1 'I suspect that you are harbouring a dangerous gene'

Table 24.1 Common genetic disorders

Condition	Estimated frequency/1000 live births	Abnormality
Red–green colour blindness	80*	X
Total autosomal dominant disease	10	AD
Dominant otosclerosis	3	AD
Klinefelter's syndrome (XXY)	2*	C
Familial hypercholesterolaemia	2	AD
Total autosomal recessive disease	2	AR
Trisomy 21 (Down)	1.5	C
XYY	1.5*	C
Adult polycystic kidney disease	1	AD
Triple X syndrome	0.6†	C
Cystic fibrosis	0.5	AR
Fragile X-linked mental retardation	0.5*	X
Non-specific X-linked mental retardation	0.5*	X
Recessive mental retardation	0.5	AR
Neurofibromatosis	0.4	AR
Turner syndrome (XO)	0.4†	C
Duchenne muscular dystrophy	0.3*	X
Haemophilia A	0.2*	X
Trisomy 18 (Edward's)	0.12	C
Polyposis coli	0.1	AD
Trisomy 13 (Patau's)	0.07	C

AD = autosomal dominant; AR = autosomal recessive; X = sex-linked disorder; C = chromosomal disorder.
*per 1000 male births; †per 1000 female births.

In **familial hypercholesterolaemia** patients have increased plasma LDL levels and a predisposition for developing atheroma at an early age, which gives them an eight-fold increased risk of ischaemic heart disease. The primary defect is a deficiency of cellular LDL receptors so that the liver uptake is reduced and plasma levels are two to three times normal. Around 30 different mutations of the LDL receptor gene have been identified. About 1 in 500 people are affected, and they are heterozygotes who have half the normal number of LDL receptors. One person in a million is a homozygote, and they usually die from cardiovascular disease in childhood.

Adult polycystic kidney disease results from a defect on the short arm of chromosome 16 that is inherited in an autosomal dominant fashion. Both kidneys are enlarged, with numerous fluid-filled cysts, and may weigh a kilogram or more (normal

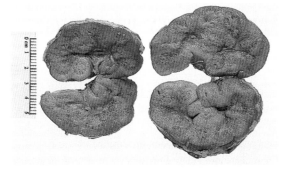

Figure 24.2 Autosomal recessive polycystic kidney disease. Smaller normal kidneys are included for comparison – 37 weeks' gestation (Courtesy of R. Scott, UCLMS)

= 150 g). The patients develop symptoms of renal damage and hypertension in their third or fourth decade.

Triple X syndrome produces tall girls who may have below-average intelligence, and, although gonadal function is usually normal, there may be premature ovarian failure. **Fragile X syndrome** was first described in 1969 and is now recognised as the second most common cause of severe mental retardation after Down syndrome. Affected males have a reduced IQ, macro-orchidism and a prominent forehead and jaw. Heterozygote females can show mild retardation, but counselling is difficult because not all female carriers show the chromosomal abnormality on testing. **Turner syndrome** (monosomy X, i.e. 45,X) is a common cause of fetal hydrops and spontaneous abortion. About 95 per cent of affected pregnancies will abort. Those surviving to delivery will be less severely affected and generally show short stature, webbing of the neck, normal intelligence, infertility, aortic coarctation and an altered carrying angle of the arm (cubitus valgus).

Although we have listed the common genetic disorders and their karyotype, this does not answer the question, 'How are they caused?' This is really two questions:

- How does the genetic abnormality produce disease?
- How does the genetic abnormality arise?

HOW DOES THE GENETIC ABNORMALITY PRODUCE DISEASE?

From our list so far, we have explained only the pathophysiology of familial hypercholesterolaemia. Now we shall discuss the recent discoveries that have increased our understanding of cystic fibrosis.

Patients with **cystic fibrosis** present in infancy with pancreatic insufficiency, malabsorption and lung damage. This is an autosomal recessive disease and occurs in about 1 in 2000 live births. Approximately 1 person in 25 is a heterozygote. The pathological manifestations result from thickened secretions that lead to obstruction, inflammation and scarring. The tenacious secretions are an indicator of a fundamental problem in water and electrolyte handling.

This has been recognised for a long time and used as a diagnostic test – the **sweat test** – that looks for elevated levels of sodium in the sweat.

The reason for the increased electrolyte level in sweat is that there is defective, cyclic-AMP-mediated regulation of chloride channels. The gene has now been identified on the long arm of chromosome 7 (7q31) and called the **cystic fibrosis transmembrane conductance regulator (CFTR)**. The CFTR gene codes for a protein of 1480 amino acids where structure is similar to that of the family of ATP binding proteins. It is not clear yet whether the CFTR protein transports chloride directly or regulates chloride indirectly via another protein, but it is clear is that a change in CFTR protein will affect electrolyte transport.

In about 70 per cent of cases of cystic fibrosis, there is a mutation referred to as the Delta F508 mutation. This is a deletion in the codon at position 508 that leads to loss of a phenylalanine molecule in a highly conserved region of the CFTR protein. This is thought to alter the folding of the protein. The abnormal protein that is produced is unable to respond to cyclic AMP. In the pancreas and lungs, this leads to reduced chloride and water secretion, so the mucus is thick. In the sweat test, the sweat glands secrete water and chloride normally, but the secretory coil does not respond to beta-adrenergic stimulation and does not reabsorb the chloride ions, hence allowing increased chloride and sodium in the sweat.

HOW DOES THE GENETIC ABNORMALITY ARISE?

We need to consider abnormalities of chromosome number separately from abnormalities in chromosome structure or single gene disorders, as different mechanisms operate.

ABNORMAL CHROMOSOME NUMBER

This occurs because of problems at the anaphase stage of meiosis, leading to unequal sharing of the

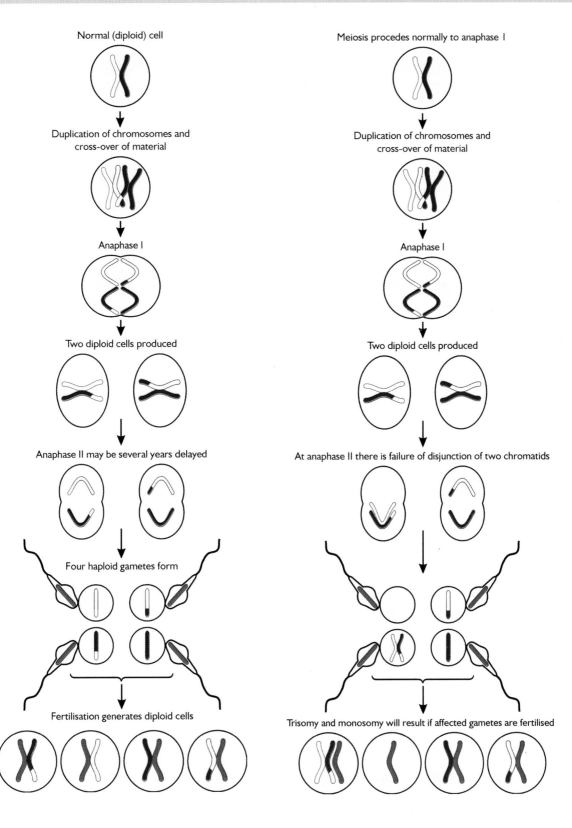

Normal (diploid) cell

Duplication of chromosomes and cross-over of material

Anaphase I

Two diploid cells produced

Anaphase II may be several years delayed

Four haploid gametes form

Fertilisation generates diploid cells

Meiosis procedes normally to anaphase I

Duplication of chromosomes and cross-over of material

Anaphase I

Two diploid cells produced

At anaphase II there is failure of disjunction of two chromatids

Trisomy and monosomy will result if affected gametes are fertilised

Figure 24.3 Meiosis

Figure 24.4 Chromosomal non-disjunction

chromosomes so that one daughter cell will have an extra chromosome (trisomy) while the other is missing a chromosome (monosomy). A pair of chromosomes or sister chromatids may fail to separate, so-called **non-disjunction**, or there may be delayed movement (**anaphase lag**) of chromosomes so that one is left on the wrong side of the dividing wall. The cause is unknown, but the incidence increases with maternal age, as we have discussed when considering Down syndrome. It may also be associated with irradiation, viral infection or familial tendencies.

Polyploidy means that the cell contains at least one complete extra set of chromosomes. Most commonly, this is one extra set, i.e. 69 chromosomes or triploidy. Affected fetuses usually die *in utero* or abort in early pregnancy. The condition can result from fertilisation by two sperm (dispermy) or from fertilisation in which either the sperm or ovum is diploid because of an abnormality in its maturation divisions.

ABNORMAL CHROMOSOME STRUCTURE

Abnormalities in chromosome structure occur when chromosomes are inaccurately repaired after breaks have occurred. **Chromosomal breakage** can happen randomly at any gene locus, but there are some areas that are particularly liable to breakage. The rate of breakage is markedly increased by ionising radiation, certain chemicals and some rare inherited conditions. Structural abnormalities, such as translocations, deletions, duplications and inversions (see figure 23.2, page 294), occur when two break points allow the transfer, loss or rearrangement of chromosomal material.

SINGLE GENE DISORDERS

Single gene disorders can also result from structural abnormalities involving minute areas of the chromosome. These are produced by the same mechanism, i.e. breakage resulting in deletions, etc.

Alternatively, single gene disorders can arise from a **point mutation** at the gene site. Point mutations are usually spontaneous and of unknown cause, but are probably mostly due to copying errors. Substitution of one base within a codon may lead to a different amino acid being inserted into the protein and major pathological effects, e.g. sickle cell disease. This is not, however, inevitable because there are only 20 amino acids but 64 possible codons ($4 \times 4 \times 4$), which is the basis of '**degeneracy of the genetic code**'. For example, an mRNA sequence of GAA or GAG will code for alanine, so some point mutations can alter the codon but have no effect on the amino acid sequence. Approximately 25 per cent of point mutations have no effect.

As well as coding for amino acids, codons also act as start and stop instructions. Messenger RNA employs UAA, UAG or UGA as stop codons. If a point mutation produces a **stop codon**, the amino acid chain will terminate too early, which is the effect of about 5 per cent of point mutations. The ultimate problem is a **frameshift** mutation in which the gain or loss of one or two bases produces a nonsense message because it alters every codon.

Let us look back at the 'cat and rat' sentences that started this part. Hopefully, their significance is now clear.

SHE HAD ONE MAD CAT AND ONE SAD RAT
SHE HAD ONE BAD CAT AND ONE SAD RAT
THE MAD BAD CAT ATE THE ONE SAD RAT
THE MAD SHE CAT ATE THE ONE SAD RAT
THE MAD HEC ATA TET HEO NES ADR AT

- The first sentence is the normal code.
- The second has a point mutation without a frameshift, so there is a 25 per cent probability that it will not have any effect.
- The third sentence has a length mutation, possibly a translocation.
- The fourth sentence is a mutation of the third, in which SHE represents a premature stop codon.
- The fifth sentence changes the sex of the cat and makes nonsense.

MULTIFACTORIAL DISORDERS

All new patients are asked about their 'family history', the idea being that if their parents and siblings suffer from a particular disease, they are at increased risk. Unfortunately, for most diseases, it is not known how great that increased risk may be because the inheritance does not follow simple Mendelian principles but is multifactorial. It is likely that there will be a variety of genes involved, which interact with a number of environmental factors.

Research into multifactorial disorders adopts a similar approach to that into single gene problems. First, it is necessary to identify the diseases with a significant genetic component by comparing the incidence in family groups with the general population. This genetic contribution is termed **heritability**; some examples are given in the small print box.

Heritability: genetic contribution to the aetiology of the disorder	
Disease	**Estimate of heritability (%)**
Schizophrenia	85
Asthma	80
Cleft lip and palate	76
Coronary artery disease	65
Hypertension	62
Neural tube defect	60
Peptic ulcer	35

The next step is to look for genetic, biochemical and immunological features that affected individuals have in common. It is well established that certain HLA types are associated with particular diseases, and this may be helpful in counselling affected families. For example, in a family with ankylosing spondylitis, a first-degree relative has a 9 per cent risk of developing the disease if HLA-B27 positive but less than a 1 per cent risk if HLA-B27 negative.

The ultimate goal is to identify the gene or genes and environmental factor(s) so that those at particularly high genetic risk could attempt to avoid the relevant environmental hazard. At a simple level, this would mean giving vitamin supplements to pregnant women at risk of producing babies with neural tube defects, or advising potential 'arteriopaths' to modify their diet and not smoke.

Diabetes is a disease in which a genetic predisposition is beginning to be better understood. The insulin-dependent (type 1) form was known to be associated with certain HLA types and thought to involve a viral infection in susceptible individuals. Although HLA association need not mean that the HLA genes are involved, study in this case of the histocompatibility areas of chromosome 6 revealed that amino acid 57 in the DQ gene cluster was altered in susceptible individuals. Individuals with aspartate at position 57 had resistance to the disease, whereas mutations substituting alanine, valine or serine increased susceptibility.

CHAPTER 25

CAN GENES CHANGE AFTER BIRTH?

• DNA repair

Genes can change after birth, both by accident and by design. We have already discussed the accidents that can occur in the production of gametes or in the early divisions of the fertilised egg, and these will affect all of the daughter cells, i.e. the whole individual. Now we shall consider the accidents that affect somatic cells after birth and are important in the aetiology of cancer, and the deliberate changes that occur in the genetic code of immune cells to allow them sufficient diversity to tackle the enormous range of potential antigens.

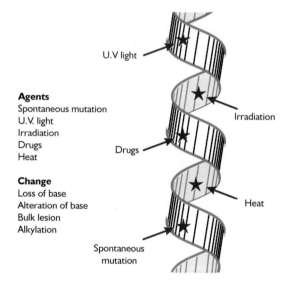

DNA REPAIR

DNA is usually copied accurately, so a genome of 3×10^9 base pairs will change by only 10–20 base pairs per year. This remarkable feat is achieved because there is a variety of DNA repair enzymes that continuously scan the DNA and repair any inaccuracies caused by replication or damage by environmental agents. The double-stranded nature of DNA is essential because the complementary information on the two strands allows the damaged piece to be rebuilt as Figure 25.2 shows.

Any fault in this process will result in an increased number of mutations. This occurs in a number of rare human diseases where there is a

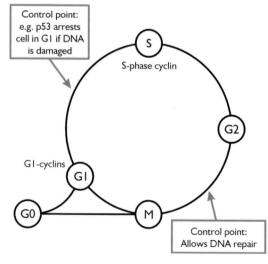

Figure 25.1 Causes of DNA damage and repair points in the growth cycle

DNA damage

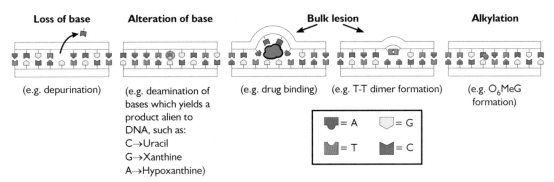

| Loss of base | Alteration of base | Bulk lesion | | Alkylation |

(e.g. depurination)

(e.g. deamination of
bases which yields a
product alien to
DNA, such as:
C→Uracil
G→Xanthine
A→Hypoxanthine)

(e.g. drug binding)   (e.g. T-T dimer formation)

(e.g. O_6MeG
formation)

| = A | = G |
| = T | = C |

Mechanisms of DNA repair

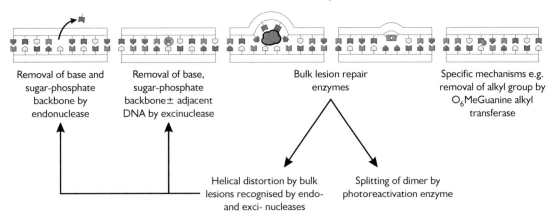

Removal of base and
sugar-phosphate
backbone by
endonuclease

Removal of base,
sugar-phosphate
backbone± adjacent
DNA by excinuclease

Bulk lesion repair
enzymes

Specific mechanisms e.g.
removal of alkyl group by
O_6MeGuanine alkyl
transferase

Helical distortion by bulk
lesions recognised by endo-
and exci- nucleases

Splitting of dimer by
photoreactivation enzyme

DNA reconstitution

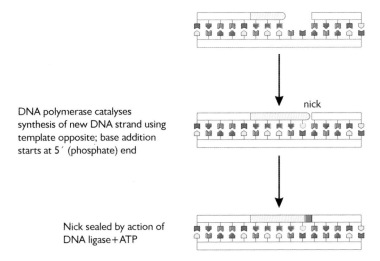

DNA polymerase catalyses
synthesis of new DNA strand using
template opposite; base addition
starts at 5′ (phosphate) end

nick

Nick sealed by action of
DNA ligase+ATP

Figure 25.2 Types of DNA damage and examples of repair mechanisms

failure of the repair systems. In xeroderma pigmentosa, there is a defect in the excision stage of repair. These patients are particularly susceptible to damage induced by ultraviolet radiation and have an increased risk of developing skin cancer. In Bloom's syndrome, there is a defect in one of the repair enzymes, DNA ligase I, and patients with this disorder have an increased risk of all forms of cancer. Ataxia-telangectasia and Fanconi's anaemia are other examples with similar enzyme defects.

There is a saying, 'Where God puts disease, he also puts a cure.' Viruses undoubtedly cause infectious disease and can be one step on the road to cancer. However, they may also provide a possible cure for disease as they may be ideal vehicles for altering the genetic code within human cells. Ultimately, it would be best if patients with single gene disorders could have their defective gene replaced by the correct gene. In theory, this is possible by using a retrovirus to introduce the gene into the affected cells, although, in practice, there are many problems to conquer. The most useful practical application of our rapidly expanding knowledge of the genes is in the manufacture of specific proteins, e.g. insulin and growth hormone.

CHAPTER 26

RECOMBINANT DNA TECHNOLOGY AND THERAPEUTICS

Recombinant DNA involves inserting the relevant gene into a rapidly replicating organism, such as the bacterium *E. coli* or a yeast. These organisms can be cultured continuously, and large amounts of the protein can be produced. First, the gene must be identified, and, once a double-stranded complementary DNA (cDNA) has been prepared, it can be inserted via a plasmid.

How has production of these proteins been of use in therapeutics? The best established examples are hormones. Most people are aware that, until relatively recently, insulin was prepared from pig pancreas and that this method had problems related to its limited supply and to hypersensitivity reactions in the recipients. Recombinant DNA technology has given us a method of producing human insulin synthetically and in unlimited quantities. The advantages of producing proteins in this way are tremendous. We can produce vast quantities of the proteins, and the risk of contamination with infectious agents is eliminated. This particular problem has been highlighted recently because of the contamination of factor VIII by HIV. Factor VIII can now be produced by recombinant technology rather than through the purification of human blood.

Does this new technology have a role in the treatment or prevention of neoplasia? The answer is yes, although this is at present rather limited. Recombinant TNF and IFN-α are being tried in cancer chemotherapy (page 277), and growth stimulators, such as GM-CSF, may help to maintain the body's normal cells during chemotherapy and thus minimise problems such as neutropenia. An interesting example relating to cancer prevention is immunisation against hepatitis B. Now that a synthetically engineered vaccine is available, it is possible to immunise people at high risk and hence reduce the burden of chronic hepatitis and hence hepatocellular carcinoma. Recent evidence suggests that this has been effective in south-east Asia, where the incidence of hepatitis B is high. With increasing understanding of the genes directly involved in cancer, maybe, in time, we will be able to direct treatment at the level of the abnormal gene. Alternatively, chemical mediators might be able to modify the expression of the mutant genes and hence the biological course of the disease.

Is there any more to know, or have we come to the end of the road? Far from it! We are only just beginning to understand the intricate patterns that constitute life, and we have only just embarked on the battle to conquer the genetic code. Our knowledge of the genes involved in disease forms a minuscule part of the whole genetic code. It is a bit like Columbus arriving in America and making a map of the port in which he had landed. The discovery of that piece of land may indeed have been a great achievement, but it was only a small part of the continent, and that continent only a small part of the world. Just as it has been necessary to map out the whole of the world in order to gain an understanding of it, so it will be necessary to map out the whole of the genetic code before we can understand the complex interplay between all the different genes. This task is both necessary and immense, and it is a boring one! The paragraph below is an example of how a tiny part of it might read:

GGATTACCGTACCATAATTCCATGGGATTTACGTTAGCAGTAGTTGATTACGTGCT
GACGTACGTAGCTGACTGTTGCAGTAAGGAGGATTACCGTACCATAATTCCATGGGATT
TACGTTAGCAGTGCGGATTACCGTACCATAATTCCATGGGATTTACGTTAGCAGTAGTTGAT
TACGTGCTGACGTACGTAGCTGACTGTTGCAGTAAGGAGGATTACCGTACCATAATTC
CATGGGATTTACGTTAGCAGTGCGGATTACCGTACCATAATTCCATGGGATTTACGT
TAGCAGTAGTTGATTACGTGCTGACGTACGTAGCTGATGTTGCAGTAAGGAGGATTACCGTAC
CATAATTCCATGGGATTTACGTTAGCAGTGCGGATTACCGTACCATAATTCCATGGGATT
TACGTTAGCAGTAGTTGATTACGTGCTGACGTACGTAGCTGACTGTTGCAGTAAGGAGGAT
TACCGTACCATAATTCCATGGGATTTACGTTAGCAGTGCGGATTACCGTACCATAATTC
CATGGGATTTACGTTAGCAGTAGTTGATTACGTGCTGACGTACGTAGCTGACTGTTGCAGTAA
GAGGATTACCGTACCATAATTCCATGGGATTTACGTTAGCAGTGCGGATTACCGTAC
CATAATTCCATGGGATTTACGTTAGCAGTAGTTGATTACGTGCTGACGTACGTAGCTGACT
GTTGCAGTAAGAGGATTACCGTACCATAATTCCATGGGATTTACGTTAGCAGTGCGGATTAC
CGTACCATAATTCCATGGGATTTACGTTAGCAGTAGTTGATTACGTGCTGACGTACGTAGCT
GACTGTTGCAGTAAGGAGGATTACCGTACCATAATTCCATGGGATTTACGTTAGCAGTG

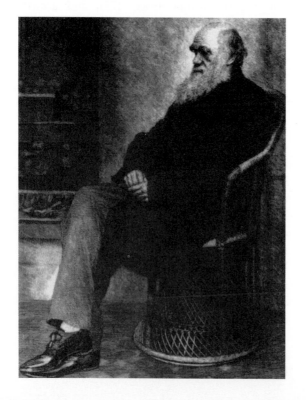

Figure 26.1 Charles Darwin was born at Shrewsbury on 12 February 1809. In 1825 he was sent to Edinburgh to study medicine. However, this was his father's choice, and Darwin later chose to study classics at Cambridge. He joined the *HMS Beagle*, which surveyed the coast of South America for 5 years. On this trip, Darwin pondered on the amazing diversity in nature. He was very religious and believed in the literal truth of the Bible. Thus he was reluctant to publish his heretical theory on evolution, preferring to direct his wife to publish it after his death. However, Alfred Russel Wallace had reached similar conclusions, which he sent to Darwin in 1858. This resulted in both Darwin's and Wallace's ideas being presented to the Linnean Society in London that year, followed in the next year by the publication of the *On the origin of species by means of natural selection*, or the *Preservation of favoured races in the struggle for life*. He died on 19 April 1882 and was buried in Westminster Abbey. (Courtesy of the Wellcome Institute for the History of Medicine)

Can you imagine a book in which every page looked like that, going on and on for 3 000 000 000 letters? It would be one of the most tedious, but useful, books that any one could imagine. Still, we are in favour of the publication of such a book as it would provide a tremendous survival advantage for all pathology textbooks!

FURTHER READING

Connor, J.M. 1992: Genetics and disease. In MacSween, R.N.M., Whaley, K.W. (eds) *Muir's Textbook of Pathology*, 13th edn. London: Edward Arnold, Ch. 2.

Cotran, R.S., Kumar, V., Robbins, S.L. 1989: Genetic Disorders. In *Robbins' Pathologic Basis of Disease*, 4th edn. Philadelphia: W.B. Saunders, Ch. 4.

Dawkins, R. 1989: *The Selfish Gene*, 2nd edn. Oxford: Oxford University Press.

Emery, A.E.H., Rimoin, D.L. 1990: *The Principles and Practice of Medical Genetics*, 2nd edn. Edinburgh: Churchill Livingstone.

Ponder, B.A.J. 1990: Inherited cancer syndromes. In Carney, D., Sikora, K. (eds) *Genes and Cancer*. Chichester: John Wiley.

Talmud, P.J., Humphries, S.E. 1992: Molecular genetic analysis of coronary artery disease: an example of a multifactorial disease. In McGee, J., Isaacson, P.G., Wright, N.A. (eds) *Oxford Textbook of Pathology*, Oxford: Oxford University Press, Ch. 2.7.

APPENDIX 1

BACON, FRANCIS (1561–1626)

Francis Bacon was born on 22 July 1561 at York House, off The Strand, in London. He was the second son of Sir Nicholas Bacon, Lord Keeper, and his second wife, Ann Cooke.

Francis Bacon, although recognised as an important figure in the history of thought, has not really been taken as a serious figure by philosophers. He is, of course, well known to students of literature for his sharp wisdom and clever writing. Besides literature, Francis Bacon also wrote about law, which was his profession, and about the history of the reign of Henry VII. His main works, *The Advancement of Learning* and *Novum Organum* (a presentation of a new method of logic), are, however, philosophical, and it is from his discourse on inductive reasoning that the quote on page 3 comes.

THE ADVANCEMENT OF LEARNING

This consisted of two books, published in 1605. The first is essentially about the value of knowledge, which may seem a bit strange if you are unaware of the opposition to the acquisition of knowledge that existed at the time. The opposition was both religious and social, and many believed that knowledge weakened action. It is not surprising, therefore, that Bacon felt inclined to provide a defence for knowledge.

The second book is about the classification of knowledge and is a reflection of his ordered mind. In Bacon's classification, all knowledge is divided according to the faculties of Memory ('history'), Imagination ('poesy') and Reason ('philosophy'). Although he divided it into separate groups, he believed in the wholeness of knowledge. He did, however, have his own bias, as he put it, in the 'domain of philosophy and the sciences'.

It is true that Bacon has often been rejected and has been criticised for his lack of understanding of mathematics and the scientific advances that were being made at the time. In this, there is an element of truth. What Bacon did, however, was to propagate the idea that it was possible to have a continuous growth of knowledge and to find more knowledge. Until then, there was a preoccupation with hanging on to the old knowledge for fear that it might disappear!

NOVUM ORGANUM

In this book, the teaching was in the form of aphorisms. There is a group of three ideas: the need for a new logic, the attempt to discover the 'forms' of the simple natures, e.g. heat, and the collection of a comprehensive natural history. Bacon believed that these three were tied in with natural history at the base, the laws of physics in the middle and logic as the crown.

A great deal has been written about the philosophical and scientific works of Francis Bacon, and there is considerable literature about his personal and political life. He had a strong association with the royalty and served in Parliament as a member for Melcombe Regis in Dorset and later for Taunton and Liverpool. He fell out of favour in 1621 after admitting charges of bribery.

For those who are interested in reading more about the life of Francis Bacon, the *Encyclopedia Brittanica* is a good starting point. Oxford University Press also produce a series of 'Past Masters', the one on Bacon having been written by Anthony Quinton.

GITANJALI (1961–77)

Gitanjali was born in Meerut, India on 12 June 1961. She died soon after her 16th birthday, on 11 August 1977. That she died of cancer is not particularly remarkable in itself – many children and adults do. What is remarkable is that, born from a realisation of her own mortality, she left us with a record of her fears and worries, her faith and courage. Rabindranath Tagore, who is probably India's greatest poet, is best remembered for his poem entitled 'Gitanjali', which means 'song-offering'. The first verse of Tagore's poem is as follows:

> 'Thou hast made me endless, such is thy pleasure. This frail vessel thou emptiest again and again, and fillest it ever with fresh life.
>
> This little flute of a reed thou hast carried over the hills and dales, and hast breathed through it melodies eternally new.
>
> At the immortal touch of thy hands my little heart loses its limits in joy and gives birth to utterance ineffable.
>
> Thy infinite gifts come to me only on these very small hands of mine. Ages pass, and still thou pourest, and still there is room to fill.'

Gitanjali's wish was that she might live up to her name, and she did. The publication of the poems in the form of a book is remarkable in itself. Gitanjali's mother had discovered the poems hidden around the house among her books and clothes. She tried in vain to get them published until, having almost given up hope, she sent one to *The Illustrated Weekly* of India. They were so moved by it that they decided to publish it.

The book *Poems of Gitanjali* was first published by Oriel Press in 1982.

HARVEY, WILLIAM (1578–1657)

William Harvey was born in Folkestone on 1 April 1578. It may have been April Fools day, but this man provided medicine with the boost it needed to push it out of stagnation. The value of his work is put into perspective when you realise that to be honoured as a Harveian Orator by the Royal College of Physicians is the greatest distinction that one can aspire to.

Harvey undertook his medical training at Caius College, Cambridge, and later in Padua, Italy. In Padua, Harvey studied with Fabricius, who had succeeded Fallopio (of fallopian tube fame). Galileo was the Professor of Mathematics at Padua at the time but does not appear to have been influential in Harvey's development.

Harvey was elected a full fellow of the College of Physicians in 1607 and soon afterwards became Assistant Physician to St Bartholomew's Hospital. This helped to establish his private practice, and, interestingly, his famous patients included James I, Charles I and the Lord Chancellor, Sir Francis Bacon. Although Bacon is given the credit for inductive thinking, it was Harvey who applied it to his investigations of the heart. Harvey, in fact, had very little respect for Bacon and had stated that Bacon 'writes philosophy (science) like a Lord Chancellor; I have cured him of it'.

The quote at the beginning of Chapter 2 is the first paragraph of Chapter 1 of his famous book *De Motu Cordis*. The movements of the heart were so fast and complicated that he often despaired at ever being able to work out the sequence of each of the movements. *De Motu Cordis* evolved in two stages: initially, it was an investigation into the heart beat and the arterial pulse, and only later did Harvey include the investigation of the circulation. Together, it forms one of the most important pieces of scientific work. The book is quite small, 72 pages, and would probably fit into a white coat pocket, but the few remaining copies of the original 1628 edition would set you back a cool £200 000, assuming anybody were willing to sell it!

William Harvey died of a stroke on 30 June 1657.

Much has been written about Harvey, and the Keynes translation of 1928 is believed to be the most accurate. Keynes has written a couple of books on Harvey: *The Personality of William Harvey*, published by Cambridge University Press in 1949, and *The Life of William Harvey*, Oxford University Press, 1966.

HEISENBERG, WERNER KARL (1901–76)

Heisenberg, who is well known for his contribution to quantum mechanics, was born on 5 December 1901, in Würzburg, Germany. He studied physics at the University of Munich, his doctoral thesis, which he presented in 1923, being on turbulence in fluid streams.

In 1927 Heisenberg published his 'uncertainty principle', which says that, in the subatomic world, it is not possible to know both the position and the momentum of a particle accurately. The better we know one variable, the less sure we can be of the other. The important point is that it is not the limitation of the technique of measurement that imposes this law, but simply the limitation of the principle. What this means is that the uncertainty principle is a mathematical way of expressing the limitation of our classical models of looking at the world.

Our classical way of looking at the world is derived from gross appearances, and we have a tendency to divide things into discrete units or, to put it another way, to perceive the world as being particulate. At the subatomic level, this particulate view is an idealisation without any meaning, and it is not possible to describe anything without a reference to the whole. Hence 'entities' such as position and momentum are interrelated and cannot be defined precisely at the same time, since changes in one are tied in with changes in the other. These connections are of a statistical nature, i.e. are probabilities rather than certainties.

This idea of interactions led to the proposal of the concept of the 'S matrix', which is a mathematical model for these interactions. It was this belief in the fundamental principles of a shift from objects to events that lead to the quotation at the end of Chapter 1, just as, in the subatomic world, the various events in the body are a manifestation of the many interactions between the various processes. They are not isolated events but interact and combine in intricate ways in any given situation.

Heisenberg is mainly known for his achievements in physics, but he is also a philosopher trying to understand the relationships that are fundamental in nature. He was awarded the Nobel Prize in 1932.

OSLER, WILLIAM (1849–1919)

Many people believe that Sir William Osler was the most loved and greatest physician of recent times. This was not for his scientific contribution but for his ability to fascinate the young students and for completely transforming medical education and clinical medical training.

Osler was born at Bond Head, Ontario, Canada. His parents were English missionaries who had migrated to Canada, and he was the youngest of nine children. His initial intention was to follow his father into the Church, and he began his studies at Trinity College, Toronto. He changed his mind, however, and enrolled at the Toronto

Medical School in 1868, finishing his medical education at McGill University. Having qualified, he spent the next 2 years travelling around Europe, the longest period being spent with Sir John Burdon-Sanderson at University College, London.

Osler returned to Canada with the intention of entering general practice but within a few months was appointed lecturer in medicine at McGill teaching physiology and pathology to the medical students. The following year, he was appointed Professor. After a decade in Montreal, he went as Professor of Medicine to Pennsylvania and, in 1888, he accepted a post at the new Johns Hopkins Hospital in Baltimore. He was the second of the famous 'Hopkins four', the others being William Welch, chief of pathology, Howard Kelley, chief of obstetrics and gynaecology, and William Halstead, chief of surgery. It was with these three colleagues that Osler revolutionised the medical curriculum.

For the first 4 years at the Johns Hopkins, there were no medical students, and Osler used these years to write *The Principles and Practice of Medicine*, first published in 1892.

In 1904, while visiting the UK, he was offered the Regius Chair of Medicine at Oxford, succeeding Burdon-Sanderson. Osler accepted and started his post in 1905.

Osler's name is associated with three medical conditions: Osler's nodes (tender, red swellings on the palms and fingers in bacterial endocarditis) Osler–Vaquez disease (polycythaemia rubra vera) and the Rendu–Osler–Weber disease (recurrent haemorrhages from multiple telangectasias in skin and mucous membranes).

Osler wrote much about almost everything, especially about the relationship between teacher and student, teacher and teacher, and teacher and patient. The quotation at the end of Chapter 2 is from his book *Counsels and Ideals from the Writings of Sir William Osler*, 1905.

THOMAS, LEWIS

Lewis Thomas is University Professor at the State University of New York at Stony Brook, and President Emeritus of the Memorial Sloan-Kettering Cancer Center in New York. The quotes come from essays that were first published in the *New England Journal of Medicine*, at the invitation of the editor Dr F.J. Ingelfinger. The column was titled 'Notes of a biology-watcher'. These essays were first published in book form in two separate volumes, *The Lives of a Cell* (1974) and *The Medusa and the Snail* (1979), by the Viking Press. These have been combined into one volume, *The Wonderful Mistake*, and published by Oxford University Press (1988). His other books include *The Youngest Science* and *Late Night Thoughts*, produced by Oxford Paperbacks.

FURTHER READING

Bamforth, J., Osborn, G.R. 1958: Diagnosis from cells. *Journal of Clinical Pathology* ii, 473–82.

Capra, F. 1983: *The Tao of Physics*, 2nd edn. Glasgow: Fontana.

Nuland, S.B. 1988: *Doctors. The Biography of Medicine*. Birmingham, Alabama: Gryphon Editions.

Paget, S. 1897: *John Hunter. Man of Science and Surgeon*. London: T. Fisher Unwin.

Pickering, G. 1964: William Harvey, physician and scientist. *British Medical Journal* 2, 1615–19.

Rains, A.J. Harding 1974: *Edward Jenner and Vaccination*. London: Priory Press.

Rather, L.J. 1957: Rudolf Virchow and scientific medicine. *Archives of Internal Medicine* 100, 1007–14.

Sergerist, H.E. 1935: *Great Doctors. A Biographical History of Medicine*. London: George Allen & Unwin.

Weimerskirch, P.J., Richter, G.W. 1979: Hunter and venereal disease. *Lancet* 1, 503–4.

APPENDIX 2

ABBREVIATION	EXPANSION
5HT	5 Hydroxytryptamine (serotonin)
ACTH	Adrenocorticotrophic hormone
ADP	Adenosine diphosphate
AMP	Adenosine monophosphate
APC gene	Adenomatous polyposis coli gene
Apo eg Apo E	Apoprotein
ARDS	Adult respiratory distress syndrome
ATP	Adenosine triphosphate
C eg C3	Complement components
Ca	Cancer or carcinoma in neoplasia diagrams
Ca++	Calcium
CAM	Calmodulin
cAMP	cyclic AMP
CD	Cluster designation
CIN	Cervical intraepithelial neoplasia
DAG	Diacyl glycerol, an intermediate messenger
DCC gene	Deleted in colorectal cancer gene
DIC	Disseminated intravascular coagulation
dsDNA	Double-stranded DNA
DVT	Deep vein thrombosis
ECF	Eosinophil chemotactic factor (a chemotaxin released by the mast cell)
ECG	Electrocardiogram
EDRF	Endothelium-derived relaxing factor
ELAM	Endothelial leucocyte adhesion molecule
Fab	Antibody-interacting end of immunoglobulin molecule
Fc	Complement-interacting end of immunoglobulin molecule
FDP	Fibrin degradation product
G0 phase of cell cycle	Resting phase; cells may re-enter the cell cycle if appropriately stimulated
G1 phase of cell cycle	Pre-synthetic phase
GDP	Guanosine diphosphate
GTP	Guanosine triphosphate

Hb	Haemoglobin
hCG	Human chorionic gonadotrophin
HIV	Human immunodeficiency virus
HTLV	Human T-lymphocyte virus
ICAM	Intercellular adhesion molecule
ICE	Interleukin-1β converting enzyme
IL eg IL2	Interleukin
K+	Potassium
LDL	Low density lipoprotein
LT eg LTC4	Leukotrienes
LTR	Long terminal repeat sequence, containing promotors and enhancers of transcription
LV	Left ventricle
M phase of cell cycle	Mitotic phase
Mac	Macrophage
MCHC	Mean corpuscular haemoglobin concentration
MCV	Mean corpuscular volume
MEN I, IIa, IIb	Multiple endocrine neoplasia syndromes
MHC	Major histocompatibility complex
N	Normal
Na+	Sodium
NBTZ	Nitroblue tetrazolium
NCF	Neutrophil chemotactic factor (a chemotaxin released by the mast cell)
PAF	Platelet activating factor
PCV	Packed cell volume
PDGF	Platelet derived growth factor
PF eg PF4	Platelet factor
PG eg PGD2	Prostaglandin
PMN	Polymorphonuclear cells (ie acute inflammatory cells)
RBC	Red blood cell
RV	Right ventricle
S-phase of cell cycle	DNA synthesis occurs during the S-phase
Th	T helper cell
Tm	T memory cell
Tsc	T suppressor/cytotoxic cells
VCAM	Vascular cell adhesion molecule

INDEX

Note: page numbers in *italics* refer to figures and tables

influenza virus 59
injury 78
insulin manufacture 310
insulin-like growth factors 258
integrase 54
integrins 15
interferon, apoptosis 197
interferon-alpha (IFN-a) 277
  recombinant 311
interferon-beta (IFN-ß) 277
interleukin 258
interleukin-1 (IL-1) 15, 19, 23, 70
interleukin-2 (IL-2) 70, 277
interleukin-5 (IL-5) 70
interleukin-6 (IL-6) 23, 70
intermittent claudication 90
intimal cushion lesions 140
intrauterine death 290
intrauterine infection 290–1
intrinsic factor 130–1
involution 221
iron 208
  deficiency 126–7
  deposition 208–9
  haem/non-haem 211
  normal metabolism *210*
  Prussian blue staining 212
  see also anaemia, iron deficiency
ischaemia 92, 119
islet cell tumours 206

J gene segment 31, 32
jaundice *213*
Jenner, Edward *46, 47*
jugular venous pressure 199

kallikrein 22
Kaposi's sarcoma 250, 252
Kaposi's sarcoma-associated herpes
  virus (KSHV) 251
karyolysis 181
karyorrhexis 181
karyotypes *293, 295*
keratinocyte growth factor 82
kidney
  amyloid 199–200
  ischaemia *166, 167*
killer cells 27, 29
kinin cascade 22
Klinefelter's syndrome 302, *303*
Knudson 260, 261
Koch, Robert 71
Kupffer cells 6

lactate dehydrogenase 178
lactoferrin 18
Langhan giant cell 75, *76*
Langhan-type cells 72
left ventricular failure *166*
leiomyoma, benign *225*
Leishmania 55

Leonardo da Vinci 91
leucocytes 11, 24, 27
  atheromatous plaque 144
leukaemia 247
leukotrienes 15, 16, 18, 115, 117
Lewis, Thomas 5, 18, 317
LFA-1 15
lines of Zahn *102*, 103
lipid A 61
lipids 148–51
lipofuscin 212, 214
lipopolysaccharide 50
  bacterial cell wall 61, 62
lipoprotein 145, *150*, 180
liver
  carcinoma 209, 249, 250
  cirrhosis 21, 22, 84, 181, 187–8
  disease stigmata *187*
  failure in haemochromatosis 208
  fatty change 180–1
  iron deposition 209, *210*
  regeneration 220
  tumours 243, 268
  see also hepatocellular carcinoma
low-density lipoprotein (LDL) 142,
  150, 151
  atheromatous plaque 142, *144*
  cholesterol 148, 153
  familial hypercholesterolaemia 303
  macrophages 77
lung
  Arthus reaction 40
  fibrosis 188
  lobar pneumonia 8–10
  shock 117
lung cancer 135, *224, 226*, 247
  metastatic *273*
  paraneoplastic syndromes 275
  small cell carcinoma 226, 259, 275
  smoking 243
  tumour spread 268
lymph 25
lymph node architecture *26*
lymphatic system
  inflammation 25–7, *28, 29, 30*, 31
  tumour spread 267, *268*
lymphocytes 5, 6, 24, 25
  homing 15, 25
lymphokine-activated killer (LAK)
  cells 277
lymphokines 19, 27, 72
lysogenic conversion 65
lysosomal contents 21
lysosome 17
lysozymes 18, 45

McBurney's point 10
macrophage-derived growth factor 77
macrophages 5, 6, 14, 26, 75–7
  alveoli 45
  chronic inflammation 76

LDL 77
lipid-laden 140
lobar pneumonia 9
multinucleate giant 75
nitric oxide production 22
opsonin recognisation 17
tumour spread 271
MAGE protein family 271
major basic protein (MBP) 18
major histocompatibility complex *see*
  MHC molecules
malaria 44, 288–9
malnutrition, fatty change 180
Malpighi, Marcello 91
Mantoux test reaction *40*, 41
Marfan's syndrome 162
margination 11, 14–15, *16, 17*
Masson-Fontana technique 212
mast cells 6
maternal age 289–90
medullary thyroid carcinoma 206, 275
megakaryocytes 6
melanin 209, 212
melanocytic skin tumours, benign 227
melanoma 247, 271
  risk 242, *243*
membrane bound vesicles 21
membrane pump failure 175
Mendel, Gregor 284
Mendelian inheritance 284, *285, 286,*
  287
menopause 192
menstrual shedding 191, 211
mesothelioma 243
metamorphosis 191
metaplasia 222–3
metastases 230, 267, 268, 273, 274–5
  production 269, *270*
metastatic disease 267, 268
Metchnikoff, Elias 5
methicillin-resistant *Staphylococcus*
  aureus (MRSA) 68
MHC molecules 28, 29, 31
microaneurysm 161, *162, 166*, 167
microsatellites 263
microvasculature, inflammation 4
mismatch repair genes 262–3
mitotic figures 266
mobility, healing 83
molecular recognition *30*
Monckeberg's medial calcific stenosis
  141
monocytes 6
monokines 19
monosomy 306
mosaicism 293, 295
mouth, defences 45
mRNA 297
mucociliary clearance 45
mucociliary defence, respiratory tract
  59